HORMONES

AND

THE FETUS

Volume II

Book Title of Related Interest

PASQUALINI and KINCL

Hormones and the Fetus Volume I
Production, concentration and metabolism during
pregnancy

Journal Titles of Related Interest

Cellular Signalling

Current Advances in Physiology

Journal of Steroid Biochemistry and Molecular Biology

Progress in Growth Factor Research

Reproductive Toxicology

HORMONES

AND

THE FETUS

Volume II

by

JORGE R. PASQUALINI

CNRS Steroid Hormone Research Unit,
Foundation for Hormone Research,
26 Boulevard Brune, 75014 Paris, France

FRED A. KINCL✝

The City University of New York,
Staten Island, New York, USA

and

CHARLOTTE SUMIDA

CNRS Steroid Hormone Research Unit,
Foundation for Hormone Research,
26 Boulevard Brune, 75014 Paris, France

PERGAMON PRESS

A Member of the Maxwell Macmillan Pergamon Publishing Corporation

OXFORD · NEW YORK · BEIJING · FRANKFURT
SÃO PAULO · SYDNEY · TOKYO · TORONTO

U.K.	Pergamon Press plc, Headington Hill Hall, Oxford OX3 0BW, England
U.S.A.	Pergamon Press, Inc., Maxwell House, Fairview Park, Elmsford, New York 10523, U.S.A.
PEOPLE'S REPUBLIC OF CHINA	Pergamon Press, Room 4037, Qianmen Hotel, Beijing, People's Republic of China
FEDERAL REPUBLIC OF GERMANY	Pergamon Press GmbH, Hammerweg 6, D-6242 Kronberg, Federal Republic of Germany
BRAZIL	Pergamon Editora Ltda, Rua Eça de Queiros, 346, CEP 04011, Paraiso, São Paulo, Brazil
AUSTRALIA	Pergamon Press Australia Pty Ltd., P.O. Box 544, Potts Point, N.S.W. 2011, Australia
JAPAN	Pergamon Press, 5th Floor, Matsuoka Central Building, 1-7-1 Nishishinjuku, Shinjuku-ku, Tokyo 160, Japan
CANADA	Pergamon Press Canada Ltd., Suite No. 271, 253 College Street, Toronto, Ontario, Canada M5T 1R5

First edition 1991

Library of Congress Cataloging-in-Publication Data
Pasqualini, Jorge R.
Hormones and the fetus.
Includes bibliographies and index.
Vol. II by: Jorge R. Pasqualini, Fred A. Kincl, Charlotte Sumida.
Contents: v. I. Production, concentration and metabolism during pregnancy.—v. II. [without special title]
1. Obstetrical endocrinology. 2. Placental hormones. I. Kincl, Fred A. II. Sumida, Charlotte. III. Title. [DNLM: 1. Hormones—Physiology. 2. Hormones—Biosynthesis. 3. Maternal-fetal exchange. 4. Reproduction. 5. Fetus. W 210.5 P284h]
RG558.5.P37   1985   612'.647   84-344

British Library Cataloguing in Publication Data
Pasqualini, Jorge R.
Hormones and the fetus.
Vol. II
1. Man. Foetuses. Development. Role of hormones
I. Title II. Kincl, Fred A. III. Sumida, Charlotte
612.647

ISBN 0-08-035720-2

Printed in Great Britain by BPCC Wheatons Ltd., Exeter

Contents

Preface

Volume I of *Hormones and the Fetus* covered the quantitative and qualitative aspects of different hormones in the three compartments (fetal, placental and maternal) of the human and other mammalian species, the transfer between the compartments and the qualitative and quantitative hormonal changes involved before and during parturition.

This second volume of *Hormones and the Fetus* gives a general idea of the mechanism of action of the different hormones during fetal development.

The first chapter of Volume II includes the interaction of different hormones with fetal plasma and other biological fluids of the fetal and placental compartments. Despite the fact that at present the role of this interaction is not very clear, one can accept that the binding of the hormone to these proteins could be a control of the biological activity or to serve as a reserve source for the active hormone. Some proteins bind specifically and with high affinity to limited species: progesterone binding globulin in the guinea-pig and other hystricomorphs; α-fetoprotein, which is present in most species, binds specifically and with high affinity estradiol in only two species, the rat and the mouse; uteroglobin in the uterine fluid of the rabbit.

The second chapter of this volume covers the presence of receptors of the various hormones and the biological hormonal responses in different fetal tissues and in the placenta. The discovery in the early seventies of estrogen receptors and mineralo-corticoid receptors in the fetal compartment (J.R. PASQUALINI's Laboratory) has opened new possibilities for the investigation of the mechanism of action of hormones during embryonic and fetal life. The presence of receptors in the fetal compartment was extended to other steroid hormones and polypeptide hormones and interesting correlations were found between the presence of these receptors and the biological responses, indicating that many biological activities of the hormone are initiated during fetal life and their receptors could be an obligatory step in the mechanism of the hormone action.

The third chapter deals with sex differentiation and fetal endocrinology, including gonadal sex and the hormonal control of sexual development. In this chapter, the work on the origin of germ cells and the development of the gonads was carried out by Dr J.E. JIRASEK from Czechoslovakia to whom we would like to express our deepest thanks. This chapter also includes a general idea of the teratological effect of steroid hormones during fetal life.

We would like to thank the staff of Pergamon Press, in particular Mr Richard Marley, and Ms S.Y. MacDonald (CNRS Steroid Hormone Research Unit, Foundation for Hormone Research) for their efficient collaboration in the preparation of this book.

J.R. PASQUALINI

1

The Binding of Hormones in Maternal and Fetal Biological Fluids

Contents

Introduction

Many hormones secreted from specific organs are bound to carrier proteins in blood. The interaction is reversible and depends on the type of hormone, the animal species and physiological conditions. During pregnancy the binding of hormones to plasma proteins usually increases. For example, the plasma concentration of corticosteroid binding globulin (CBG) is many times higher during gestation in many species.

Some plasma binding proteins may be found only in specific animal species, e.g. progesterone binding globulin (PBG) appears in guinea-pigs and other hystricomorphs but not in other species (see Section 1.2.1). Another interesting example is α-feto-protein, probably present in most mammals, which binds specifically and with high affinity estradiol in only two species: the rat and the mouse.

These interactions between a hormone and a binding protein may have several functions: 1. *to control the biological activity* of the hormones since only the unbound, unmetabolized hormone exerts biological activity. This aspect is of importance because the production rates of many hormones (progesterone, estrogens, corticosteroids) increase very significantly during pregnancy (see Volume I, Chapter 3); 2. *to serve as a reserve* of the potentially active hormones, since the enzymatic systems which transform a hormone into an inactive metabolite either do not operate, or do so to a very limited extent, on the hormone–protein complex; 3. to facilitate the *transport of hormones*, an aspect of probably limited importance since the binding of the same hormone differs from species to species, and the hormones can reach their target organs by simple diffusion from the blood.

TABLE 1.1. *Concentrations and Molecular Weights of Some Steroid Hormone Binding Proteins in Human Plasma*

Protein	Concentration		Molecular weight
	μM	mg/l	Da
Albumin	550.0	37 950	69 000
α_1-Acid glycoprotein (AAG)	18.0	738	41 000
Corticosteroid binding globulin (CBG)	0.7	36	52 000

The interaction of various hormones with plasma proteins presents significant differences in the physicochemical characteristics of the binding, particularly in their affinity and specificity. In addition, the interaction of hormones with plasma proteins is influenced by the relative concentration of the other blood proteins. For instance the concentration of albumin, which binds most steroids with low affinity, is 1000 times greater than that of corticosteroid binding globulin (CBG) and thirty times greater than that of α_1-acid glycoprotein (AAG) (Table 1.1). Finally, the presence of the other hormones may influence the hormone–plasma protein binding.

In this chapter we give a general outline of the main characteristics of the proteins which interact with hormones present in the plasma of the fetal or maternal compartments and in amniotic fluid during the course of gestation in humans and other mammals. (For a recent and exhaustive review of steroid–protein interaction, except the binding to receptor, see Westphal, 1986.)

1. The Binding of Progesterone and of Progesterone Derivatives in Plasma During Gestation

Progesterone is associated mainly with three plasma proteins: corticosteroid binding globulin (CBG), human serum albumin (HSA), and α_1-acid glycoprotein (AAG). The distribution of progesterone binding to various proteins is shown in Table 1.2. Half of

TABLE 1.2. *Distribution of Progesterone Bound to Different Proteins During Human Pregnancy*

	%
Albumin (HSA)	50–52
Transcortin (CBG)	42–47
α_1-Acid glycoprotein (AAG)	1
Unbound	5–7

Quoted from Westphal (1966); Rosenthal *et al.* (1969).

TABLE 1.3. *Affinity Constants of Progesterone Binding Proteins in Human Serum*

Protein	Association constant $(K_a)(10^6\ M^{-1})$	
	4°C	37°C
CBG	700	90
AAG	1.5	0.6
HSA	0.36	0.18

Quoted from Westphal *et al.* (1977a,b).

the progesterone present is associated with serum albumin which, in spite of its low affinity for progesterone (see Table 1.3) binds large amounts because it is present in very high concentrations (see Table 1.1).

1.1. In Humans

The production rate and plasma concentration of progesterone increase very significantly during pregnancy (see Volume I, Chapter 3) but only a small fraction of the native hormone, 5–7% of the total circulating progesterone, is present in an unbound form. The percentages of unbound progesterone, the absolute values during the luteal phase, during the first trimester and at term, and in the umbilical vein are shown in Table 1.4. Batra *et al.* (1976) found that unbound progesterone increased with the advance of pregnancy and reported values of 6% of the total progesterone at week 24 of gestation and 13% at term (Fig. 1.1). Rosenthal *et al.* (1969) give values of only 1.8%, while Yannone *et al.* (1969) report a range between 1.3 and 11%. The

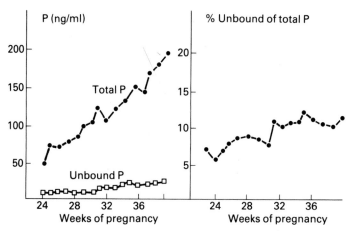

FIG 1.1. Mean Concentrations of Total and Unbound Progesterone (P) in the Last Trimester of Human Pregnancy.
Quoted from Batra *et al.* (1976).

TABLE 1.4. *Concentrations of Bound and Unbound Progesterone in Plasma During the Human Menstrual Cycle and in Pregnancy*

Plasma	Bound		Unbound		Total
	%	ng/ml	%	ng/ml	ng/ml
Luteal phase	95.2	16	4.8	0.8	17
Pregnancy:					
First trimester	95.1	39	4.9	2.0	41
Term	95.0	152	5.0	8.0	160
Umbilical vein (Term)	93.0	733	7.0	55.0	788

Quoted from Tulchinsky and Okada (1975).

discrepancies may be due to the different methods used for the measurement. A significant increase in absolute values of unbound progesterone would influence its biological activity during gestation.

Immediately after birth (1–3 h), the plasma concentration of progesterone abruptly decreases, while the percentage of the unbound fraction increases. In the newborn the rise in the concentration of unbound progesterone increases, possibly the result of a significant increase in corticosteroids during labor, which compete with progesterone for binding, or the decrease in the concentration of CBG due to the decreased production of estrogens.

1.2. In Other Mammals

1.2.1. EFFECTS OF PROGESTERONE BINDING GLOBULIN (PBG)

In 1967, Heap and Deanesly observed drastic changes in progesterone metabolism during gestation in the guinea-pig, and in 1969 two groups, Diamond *et al.* and Heap found in the serum of pregnant animals of the same species, a protein which specifically bound progesterone with high affinity. This unique plasma protein has so far been found also in related species (chinchillas, cuis, degu, coypus, viscachas, casiraguas and tuco-tucos) (Heap and Illingworth, 1974; Ackland *et al.*, 1979) during gestation.

1.2.1.1. Purification of PBG

The concentration of PBG can reach a value of 1 g/l (see Table 1.12) in the maternal serum of pregnant guinea-pigs. The protein has been purified by ammonium sulfate precipitation, gel filtration, ion-exchange chromatography and electrophoresis (Lea, 1973; Milgrom *et al.*, 1973; Burton *et al.*, 1974). A practical procedure was described by Stroupe and Westphal (1975a) who used an acid chromatography column of sulfopropyl Sephadex (pH 4.5) which allows the adsorption of most of the other serum proteins. As PBG has a low isoelectric point (pI 2.8), it is eluted from this column in the void volume. The partially purified PBG was then subjected to affinity

Hormones and the Fetus

chromatography using activated Sepharose 4B condensed with the 17-hemisuccinate of 19-nor-testosterone or the hemisuccinate of deoxycorticosterone (Cheng *et al.*, 1976). Purified PBG was obtained after elution from the affinity chromatography column using 10 μM of progesterone or of 5α-pregnane-3,20-dione solutions.

1.2.1.2. Structure and Physicochemical Properties of PBG

Progesterone binding globulin is rich in carbohydrates (71%) (Table 1.5). Using Sephadex G-200 columns, Burton *et al.* (1974) reported that PBG is composed of two forms: *PBG-I*, with a molecular weight of 117 300 Da and *PBG-II* of 78 400 Da. The presence of various carbohydrates in the two forms of PBG are shown in Table 1.6 and the details of amino acid composition (in %) in Table 1.7. The physicochemical properties of PBG and of the two forms PBG-I and PBG-II are summarized in Table 1.8. The low values of pI agree with the predominance of acid components.

TABLE 1.5. *Composition of Progesterone Binding Globulin (PBG)*

Composition		Percent
Carbohydrates (Total 71%)	Fucose	1.5
	Hexosamine	23.5
	Hexose	29.0
	Sialic acid	17.0
Polypeptides		28.0

Quoted from Harding *et al.* (1974); Stroupe and Westphal (1975a); Westphal *et al.* (1977a,b); Evans *et al.* (1982).

TABLE 1.6. *Composition of Progesterone Binding Globulin: PBG-I and PBG-II*

	PBG-I		PBG-II	
	Mol. wt: %	117 300 g/mol	Mol. wt: %	78 400 g/mol
Carbohydrate total	72.5	85 000	62.4	48 000
Hexose	27.7	32 500	24.5	19 200
N-Acetylhexosamine	31.3	36 700	25.0	19 600
Fucose	0.8	900	0.7	500
Sialic acid	12.7	14 900	12.3	9 600
Polypeptide total	23.6	27 700	32.8	25 700
Ash	1.8	2 100	2.3	1 800
Total	97.9	114 800	97.5	76 400

Quoted from Burton *et al.* (1974).

TABLE 1.7. *Amino Acid Composition of PBG-I and PBG-II*

	PBG-I %	PBG-II %
Ala	4.3	4.7
Arg	4.8	4.6
Asp	10.4	9.7
Glu	13.2	14.5
Gly	4.3	5.2
His	1.8	1.7
Ile	3.7	3.4
Leu	10.1	9.8
Lys	5.0	5.3
Phe	8.3	7.2
Pro	4.6	4.8
Ser	8.3	8.9
Thr	5.8	5.7
Tyr	2.4	2.2
Val	5.3	5.2

Quoted from Burton *et al.* (1974).

TABLE 1.8. *Physicochemical Properties of Progesterone Binding Globulin (PBG)*

	PBG	PBG-I	PBG-II
Molecular weight ($\times 10^{-3}$)	77–88	117	78
Sedimentation coefficient (S)	4.5	6.1	5.2
Isoelectric point (pI)	2.8–3.6	–	–
Absorbance ($E^{1\%}_{1\,cm,\,280\,nm}$)	4.9–7.3	4.4	5.0
Diffusion coefficient $[D^0_{20,w}(cm^2/s) \times 10^7]$	5.1	–	–
Partial specific volume ($\bar{v}$, ml/g)	0.68	0.66	0.66
Half-life ($t_{\frac{1}{2}}$)	2 days		

Quoted from Lea (1973); Milgrom *et al.* (1973); Burton *et al.* (1974); Stroupe and Westphal (1975b); Cheng *et al.* (1976).

1.2.1.3. Physicochemical Characteristics of the PBG–Progesterone Complex

The association constant Ka of the binding of progesterone to PBG is 2.2×10^9 M^{-1} at 4°C and 0.35×10^9 M^{-1} at 37°C (Stroupe and Westphal, 1975b). The affinity constants of PBG for different steroids (Table 1.9) indicate that the PBG–steroid interaction decreases with increasing steroid polarity. The data suggest that this interaction is hydrophobic in nature. The affinity for a synthetic progestagen, medrogestone, is two times that of progesterone and the Ka for cortisol is 1/1000 that of progesterone.

Hormones and the Fetus

TABLE 1.9. *Affinity Constants of the Binding of Various Steroids to Progesterone Binding Globulin*

Steroid	K_a (10^8 M^{-1})
Progesterone	20
Deoxycorticosterone	10
Testosterone	2.9
Testosterone acetate	9.2
Corticosterone	0.2
Cortisol	0.02
Medrogestone (6,17α-Dimethyl-4,6-pregnadiene-3,20-dione)	45.5

Quoted from Stroupe and Westphal (1975b).

PBG–progesterone complex is relatively resistant to temperature and pH changes. After 30 min of heating at 50°C, 70–80% of progesterone is still bound with high affinity (MacLaughlin and Westphal, 1974) (Table 1.10). The isolation of PBG in pure form allows the measurement of the binding equilibrium between the hormone and the macromolecule. Quenching of the strong fluorescence signal of the interaction of PBG and 3-oxo-4-ene steroids provides a sensitive indicator to study the association and dissociation rate constants. Stroupe and Westphal (1975b) used the stopped-flow fluorometry method and evaluated the association rate constants (k_{+1}) between progesterone and PBG to be 8.6×10^7 M^{-1} s^{-1} at 20°C, with a half-life of 22.5 min. The dissociation rate constant (k_{-1}) at the same temperature was 0.053 s^{-1} with a half-life of 13.1 s. In PBG, as well as in the two forms of PBG (I and II) there is one steroid binding site per molecule (Stroupe and Westphal, 1975b; Westphal *et al.*, 1977a,b).

The kinetic parameters of the steroid hormone–protein complex are of physiological and biological importance. A faster binding of the hormone to plasma proteins facilitates the protective mechanism against an enzymatic attack of the hormone and avoids an excess of the circulating unbound progesterone. A rapid dissociation provides a ready source of the biologically active hormone.

TABLE 1.10. *Physicochemical Properties of the PBG–Progesterone Complex*

Association constant (K_a)	4°C	2.2×10^9 M^{-1}
	22°C	1.1×10^9 M^{-1}
	37°C	0.35×10^9 M^{-1}
Association rate constant	4°C	2.2
k_{+1} (M^{-1} sec^{-1} × 10^{-1})	37°C	16.2
Dissociation rate constant	4°C	0.0095
k_{-1} (sec^{-1})	37°C	0.39
Thermostability between 4–40°C	100–80%	unchanged
Effect of pH between 7 and 10	95–100%	unchanged

Quoted from Stroupe and Westphal (1975b).

In contrast to plasma protein binding, the dissociation rate of the hormone–receptor complex in the target tissue is about 500 times lower: the half-time of dissociation of rat liver glucocorticoid receptor at 37°C is 13 min (Koblinsky *et al.*, 1972) while that of the PBG–progesterone complex (same temperature) is only 1.8 s. The longer binding of a hormone to a receptor molecule is necessary for the different steps of the hormone action and genome expression.

1.2.1.4. Steroid Conformation, Crystal Structure and Binding

The binding of a steroid to a macromolecule is a function of different parameters: polarity, chemical structure, optimal contact and spatial relationship. In the last factor, the steric hindrance of a substituent in the steroid moiety can significantly alter the affinity of the complex (see for review Westphal, 1986).

In recent years a comparison of the crystallographic steroid conformation and dimensional data has been extensively used to correlate a structure with biological activities (for a review see Duax and Norton, 1975; Duax *et al.*, 1988; Griffin *et al.*, 1984). An important condition required to validate the application of crystallographic steroid conformation to biological function is that the conformational structure revealed by X-ray crystallographic data must be similar to that of the steroid-protein binding in aqueous solution. In the case of PBG–progesterone complex there is a good correlation between the binding affinity and the planar structure, e.g. progesterone and 5α-dihydroprogesterone have a significantly higher affinity for PBG than 5β-dihydroprogesterone (angular structure).

The volume of space of one molecule of progesterone is 448 Å³ (5.2 × 6.3 × 13.8 Å) (Westphal, 1958). At 40 days of gestation, maternal plasma contains around 50 μg/100 ml of progesterone, indicating that each unbound progesterone molecule is surrounded by a solvent volume of more than 100 million times its own.

1.2.1.5. Concentration in Maternal and Fetal Plasma of Guinea-pig

Westphal (1971) measured progesterone binding activity in the serum of pregnant and lactating guinea-pigs using the combining affinity *C*, a concept introduced by Daughaday in 1958a,b. The combining affinity is defined as:

$$C = \frac{[Sbd]}{[S][Pt]} \text{ g/l}$$

where *Sbd* is the concentration of the bound fraction of the steroid, *S* the unbound, and *Pt* the total protein.

The equilibrium dialysis method using tritiated progesterone reveals that at 40–50 days of gestation the levels of PBG reach a maximal concentration in the maternal plasma of more than 1 g/l (1.2×10^{-5} mol) (Fig. 1.2(a)). Significant amounts are found from 20 days post-coitum, and there is a sharp decrease after 50–55 days of gestation, and particularly after birth (Lea *et al.*, 1976; Evans *et al.*, 1981, 1982). Figure 1.2(b) shows that there is a parallel increase in progesterone levels and PBG concentration. Quantitatively, there is a large molar excess of PBG over progesterone; in early gestation the PBG ratio to progesterone is about ten and increases many times at 40–50

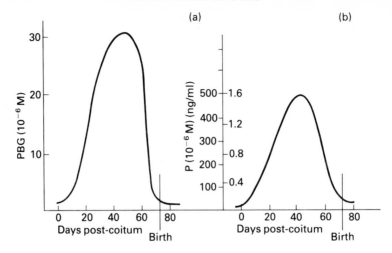

FIG 1.2. Progesterone Binding Globulin (PBG) and Progesterone (P) Plasma Concentrations in Guinea-pig during Gestation.
Quoted from Lea *et al.* (1976).

TABLE 1.11 *Concentration of Progesterone Binding Globulin
(PBG) in Pregnant and Nonpregnant Guinea-pigs and in the
Amniotic Fluid*

	PBG	
	μg/ml	10^{-6} M*
Maternal plasma (days of gestation)		
11–13	ND	ND
14–19	40–200	0.5–2.2
20–27	280–760	3.5–9.5
28–36	740–1180	9.2–14.8
37–45	960–2000	12–25
45–65	640–1200	8–19
Fetal plasma	2.77 ± 0.32	–
Umbilical artery	1.79 ± 0.40	–
Umbilical vein	2.90 ± 0.88	–
Amniotic fluid	0.47 ± 0.03	–
Nonpregnant females	2.10 ± 0.13 (SE)	
Males	1.54 ± 0.24 (SE)	

ND: Not detectable; *1 g PBG ~ 1.2×10^{-5} mol.
Quoted from Diamond *et al.* (1969); Heap and Illingworth (1974); Perrot and Milgrom (1978); Evans *et al.*
(1981).

TABLE 1.12. *The Concentrations of Progesterone Binding Globulin in Plasma of Different Hystricomorph Rodents During Gestation and its Physicochemical Properties*

	g/l	μM	Binding capacity ($\times 10^{-6}$ M)	Association constant $K_a \times 10^9$ M^{-1}
Chinchilla (*Chinchilla laniger*)	1.3	16	–	–
Coypu (*Myocastor coypus*)	1.2	15	4.8	1.2
Cuis (*Galea musteloides*)	0.8	10	2.0	0.3
Casiragua (*Proechimys guairae*)	0.6	7	7.9	3.3
Plain viscacha (*Lagostomus maximus*)	0.3	4	0.5	2.3
Tuco-tuco (*Ctenomys talarum*)	0.2	3	–	3.5
Degu (*Octogon degus*)	0.2	3	5.0	1.1
Guinea-pig	0.8	10	7.7	1.6

Quoted from Illingworth *et al.* (1973); Heap and Illingworth (1974); Ackland *et al.* (1979); Heap *et al.* (1981).

days of gestation. As a result, the percentage of circulating unbound progesterone, the physiologically active hormone, is very low.

PBG is also found in the fetal plasma of guinea-pig (40–60-day-old fetus) (Castellet and Pasqualini, 1973; Millet and Pasqualini, 1978; Perrot and Milgrom, 1978). The progesterone receptor is present in this compartment mainly in the uterus and ovaries (Pasqualini and Nguyen, 1980). Comparison of the physicochemical properties of the interaction of progesterone with the receptor and with PBG shows differences in the characteristics of these two complexes (see Table 2.18, Chapter 2, Section 1.1.1.1). PBG is mainly found in the plasma; it does not penetrate and is not synthesized in the progesterone target organs, such as the uterus.

The PBG concentrations in maternal and fetal plasma, in the umbilical artery and vein and amniotic fluid are indicated in Table 1.11. Using an immunoenzymatic assay, only very low levels of PBG were found in nonpregnant females and in males (Perrot and Milgrom, 1978). It is interesting to note that PBG is present in the milk of lactating guinea-pigs with a concentration of 26.5 ± 12 nM on day 1 post-partum (Raymoure and Kuhn, 1980). The plasma concentrations of PBG in other hystricomorph rodents are indicated in Table 1.12. The table also shows the binding capacities and the association constants of PBG in these species.

As a result of the high concentrations of PBG, the metabolic clearance rate of progesterone decreases drastically in pregnant guinea-pigs, from a value of 1128 ± 7.0 to 8.3 ± 0.8 l plasma/day/kg (Heap, 1970; Illingworth *et al.*, 1970). The high affinity binding influences progesterone extractibility from plasma; in nonpregnant animals most of the hormone (95%) is extracted with ether, but in pregnant guinea-pig only 16–18% is obtained with that procedure and for a complete extraction, plasma proteins must be denatured with NaOH.

1.2.1.6. The Origin of PBG

PBG is synthesized most likely by the placenta. Metz *et al.* (1977) used immunohistochemical techniques to localize PBG in the synctiotrophoblast of the guinea-pig placenta and Perrot-Applanat and David-Ferreira (1982) located the protein in different organelles: the rough endoplasmic reticulum, Golgi apparatus and perinuclear space of the same organ. The latter authors were unable to localize PBG in the liver, muscles, heart, lungs, kidneys, ovaries or uterus. The origin of the PBG present in fetal plasma remains to be elucidated.

In the guinea-pig the concentrations of PBG rise sharply by the period of 15–20 days of gestation, which coincides with the time when the definitive placenta is established and the developing allantois establishes close contact with the chorion. However, in the viscacha PBG rises 1–2 weeks before the time of formation of the definitive placenta and in the casiragua the increase in PBG is 10 days after the formation of the allantochorionic placenta. These data also indicate that the origin and the mechanism of control of PBG remain to be elucidated.

What is the physiological role of PBG which is present in a limited number of species and only during gestation? Despite the fact that this protein can control progesterone activity, the reason for the very high concentrations present in both maternal and fetal compartments is an important aspect to be elucidated.

2. Estrogen Binding During Gestation

2.1. Alpha-Fetoprotein (AFP)

In 1956, Bergstrand and Czar discovered in the human fetal plasma a protein called α-fetoprotein (AFP), which was not detected in the plasma of children or adults. This protein accounted for 10% of the total fetal serum proteins (Bergstrand and Czar, 1957). It was demonstrated that the physicochemical properties of this protein differed from those of another fetal protein 'the fetuin' found previously by Pedersen in 1944 in the fetal sera of bovine and other animal species (Pedersen, 1947; Putnam, 1965). It can be remarked that fetuin throughout the gestational period of different species (e.g. sheep, cattle, pigs, goats) is quantitatively one of the most important proteins. It constitutes up to 5 g/l of fetal plasma (Dziegielewska *et al.*, 1980).

AFP gained considerable importance in the studies on the mechanism of action of steroid hormones when it was observed that AFP bound estradiol with high affinity in two species: rat and mouse, like the binding of estrogens to the receptor molecule (Soloff *et al.*, 1971; Nunez *et al*, 1971a; Uriel *et al.*, 1972; Savu *et al.*, 1972).

Another attractive aspect of this protein is its presence in the serum of mice bearing primary hepatomas (Abelev, 1963, 1968) and in the serum of humans with primary hepatocellular carcinoma (Tatarinov, 1965). Elevated serum concentrations of AFP are not only found in tumors of gonadal or extragonadal origin (Abelev *et al.*, 1967; Masopust *et al.*, 1968; Nørgaard-Pedersen and Axelsen, 1978), but also in some major abnormalities of intrauterine life, including neural tube defects, intrauterine fetal distress and following fetal death (Aliau *et al.*, 1973; Brock and Sutcliffe, 1972; Brock and Scrimgeour, 1972; Nørgaard-Pedersen *et al.*, 1975; Weiss *et al.*, 1978; Milunsky *et al.*, 1980).

2.1.1. PURIFICATION AND PHYSICOCHEMICAL PROPERTIES OF AFP

Purification of AFP was achieved by different methods including column chromatography on Sephadex C-50, hydroxyapatite, DEAE-Sephadex A-25, electrophoresis on polyacrylamide gels and affinity chromatography on immunoadsorbent columns of Sepharose coupled with rabbit antibodies against rat adult serum proteins.

The examination on analytical polyacrylamide-gel electrophoresis of AFP from rat amniotic fluid revealed a microheterogeneity of this protein composed of two bands: α_1-fetoprotein, moving slowly and corresponding to about two-thirds of the total protein, and α_2-fetoprotein moving fast (Versee and Barel, 1978a,b). This property of AFP was already reported in fetal serum of human (Alpert *et al.*, 1972) and rat (Aussel *et al.*, 1973).

The molecular weight of AFP is around 70 000 Da and is similar for the two forms. A molecular weight of 65 000 Da was found in human fetal plasma and of 70 000 Da in the plasma of hepatoma patients and fetal mice (Nishi, 1970; Watabe, 1974).

Further studies using *Ricinus communis* agglutinin fractionation (Kerckaert *et al.*, 1977) and concanavalin-A-Sepharose (Soloff *et al.*, 1976) revealed the presence of at least nine molecular variants of AFP.

Guinea-pig AFP can be separated into three electrophoretic variants in nondenaturing polyacrylamide gel with respective isoelectric points of 5.0, 5.12 and 5.54 (Gourdeau and Belanger, 1983).

AFP has a tendency to aggregate in a dimer form with a molecular weight of 140 000 Da or in trimeric polymer. All of these oligomeric forms are a consequence of the experimental conditions (Ruoslahti and Seppala, 1971; Yachnin *et al.*, 1977).

AFP has a sedimentation coefficient of $4.5-4.8$ S, an isoelectric point (pI) of $4.7-5.0$, a diffusion constant $(D_{20,w})$ of $5.7-6.6$ $(10^{-7}$ cm^2/s) and an absorbance $E_{1\,cm}^{1\%}$ of $4.15-5.30$ (at 278 nm).

2.1.2. CHEMICAL COMPOSITION OF AFP

About 93% of the molecule 65 000 Da, corresponds to the peptide portion and 5300 Da to carbohydrates. Studies on the amino acid composition revealed a similarity (qualitatively and quantitatively) among different species: in the human, rat and mouse, as well as in the chicken (Table 1.13). The carbohydrate fraction contains mainly hexose, hexosamine and sialic acid (Table 1.14).

2.1.3. BINDING OF AFP TO ESTROGENS

Although the presence of AFP has been described in the fetal serum of most mammalian species, the protein binds estrogens specifically and with high affinity only in the rat and mouse (Soloff *et al.*, 1971; Nunez *et al.*, 1971b; Raynaud *et al.*, 1971; Savu *et al.*, 1974b). No specific binding of AFP to these hormones was found in the fetal plasma of human (Swartz and Soloff, 1974), cow, rabbit, chicken (Attardi and Ruoslahti, 1977) or guinea-pig (Pasqualini *et al.*, 1976; Gourdeau and Belanger, 1983). In the rat, the binding affinity for estrogens is higher at 5 days of age and disappears at 3–4 weeks of age, and in the mouse maximal affinity values are found in the 18-day-old fetus. The [^{3}H]-estrogen-AFP complex has a sedimentation coefficient of 4.5 S. Maximal values are found in the plasma of 20-day-old rat fetuses (Raynaud *et al.*, 1971). There is one molecule of estrogen bound per AFP molecule (Aussel and Masseyeff, 1977; Versee and Barel, 1978b).

TABLE 1.13 *Amino Acid Composition of α-Fetoprotein in Different Animal Species (expressed as mol/1000 moles)*

Amino acid	Human[1]	Rat[2]	Mouse[3]	Chicken[4]
Asp	87	92	78.6	99
Thr	65	50	54.4	50
Ser	66	58	80.2	54
Glu	197	159	154.0	147
Pro	38	49	44.0	44
Gly	47	47	46.5	34
Ala	90	89	77.3	54
Cys	20	46	61.5	28
Val	48	41	40.3	36
Met	8	22	18.9	29
Ile	44	47	51.6	55
Leu	94	102	103.5	99
Tyr	28	24	19.3	28
Phe	48	39	43.6	47
Lys	64	83	68.5	81
His	22	33	21.5	24
Arg	31	36	33.1	62
Trp	3	2	3.0	–

Quoted from: [1]Nishi (1975); [2]Watabe (1974); [3]Hassoux *et al.* (1977); [4]Ido and Matsuno (1982).

TABLE 1.14. *Carbohydrate Composition of α-Fetoprotein in the Fetal Serum of Different Species (in percentage of total composition)*

Carbohydrate	Human[1]	Bovine[2]	Rat[3]	Mouse[4]
Hexose	2.2	2.7	–	1.5
Hexosamine	1.2	2.4	2.0	2.2
Sialic acid	0.9	1.8	2.0	1.0
Total carbohydrate	4.3	6.9	–	4.7

Quoted from [1]Ruoslahti and Seppala (1971); [2]Aliau *et al.* (1978); [3]Versee and Barel (1978a,b); [4]Zimmerman *et al.* (1976).

Affinity constants for the binding of different estrogens to rat AFP are indicated in Table 1.15. The affinity for estrone is higher than that for estradiol and that for diethylstilbestrol is very weak. This difference in binding of AFP to natural and synthetic estrogens is extensively used to differentiate AFP from the estrogen receptor protein, which in general binds most estrogens with high affinity. Another synthetic estrogen, RU-2858, which binds the estrogen receptor with very high affinity shows no specific binding to AFP (Raynaud, 1973). This estrogen was used recently to characterize estrogen receptors in the fetal uterus and ovary of the rat (Nguyen *et al.*, 1988).

TABLE 1.15. *Association Constants (K_a) and Competition of Estrogens and Other Steroids for Estradiol Bound to Rat α-Fetoprotein*

	K_a ($10^8 \times M^{-1}$)	% of inhibition
Estradiol	1.3	100
Estradiol-17α	–	70
Estrone	2.8	108
Estriol	0.04	53
17α-Ethinyl estradiol	0.06	40
2-Hydroxy-estrone	0.04	32
6α-Hydroxy-estrone	–	105
16α-Hydroxy-estrone	–	35
15α-Hydroxy-estriol (Estetrol)	–	0
Testosterone	–	0
Androstanediol (5α-androstane-3β,17β-diol)	–	15
Pregnanolone	–	0
Progesterone	–	20

Quoted from Laurent *et al.* (1975); Aussel and Masseyeff (1978).

The affinity constant does not vary significantly with temperature. For example the estrone–AFP complex has at 5°C a K_a of 3.0×10^8 M^{-1}; at 23°C, 2.4×10^8 M^{-1} and at 37°C, 1.7×10^8 M^{-1} (Aussel and Masseyeff, 1978). The data indicate the thermostability of the AFP–estrogen complex, which is in opposition to that for the estrogen–receptor complex which is very sensitive to temperature. The association rate constants (k_{+1}) for estrone–AFP and estradiol–AFP complexes are respectively: 1.4×10^6 and 1.1×10^6 M/s and the dissociation rate constants (k_{-1}): 3.1×10^{-3} and 4.6×10^{-3} s^{-1} (Keel and Abney, 1984).

An interesting observation was made by Benassayag *et al.* (1977, 1979) that nonesterified unsaturated fatty acids can compete with estradiol for the AFP binding site. These fatty acids include linoleic, oleic and arachidonic acids (Aussel and Masseyeff, 1983a,b). The inhibitory effect of unsaturated fatty acids on the interaction with the estrogen–AFP complex is dose-dependent. It is suggested that these fatty acids, binding in the vicinity of the estrogen binding sites, can release the hormone and induce specific cellular responses.

AFP can also bind tryptophan methylester and related compounds with high affinity which compete with estrogens. The binding is stereoselective and pH-dependent, suggesting that the protease substrate binding site on AFP is spatially close to the estrogen binding site (Baker *et al.*, 1980). The substitution of *p*-nitrophenyl for the methyl group in the acetyltryptophan methyl ester results in a 10^5 increase in affinity for AFP, consequently *N*-benzyloxycarbonyl-tryptophan *p*-nitrophenyl ester is bound to AFP with a K_d of 3.9×10^{-9} M (Baker *et al.*, 1982).

2.1.4. Biosynthesis and control of AFP

AFP is synthesized in the embryonic liver (Gitlin and Boesman, 1967) of different species and in the yolk sac (Gitlin and Perricelli, 1970). Kekomaki et al. (1971) demonstrated that perfusion of isolated liver of 14–20-week-old human fetuses resulted in a release of AFP of 19–26 μg/min. Using the autoradiography method and labeled estrogens, Uriel et al. (1973) demonstrated the intracellular localization of AFP in the liver of fetal and newborn rats. In the fetal liver the synthesis of AFP is localized in a small population of the parenchymal hepatocytes (Tuczeck et al., 1981). This origin of AFP was confirmed by the presence of AFP-mRNA in the yolk sac (Miura et al., 1979) and in the fetal liver of the mouse (Koga et al., 1974).

A variant of AFP with a molecular weight of 65 000 daltons was reported by culture of a mutant-transformed rat fetal liver cell line (the SV 40 tsA). This protein is encoded by a mRNA of 16 S, while the mature AFP is encoded by a mRNA of 20 S (Yang Chou and Savitz, 1986). The data indicated that transcriptional regulation is responsible for the changes in AFP in transformed cells.

Comparison of the primary amino acid sequences of albumin and AFP of several mammalian species revealed the presence of three closely related domains with identical structure (Gorin et al., 1981). The data support the hypothesis that these two proteins arose in evolution as the consequence of a duplication in a common tripartite ancestral gene (Kioussis et al., 1981). All this information leads to the conclusion that there exist different variations of AFP which depend on the animal species and the experimental conditions for their biosynthesis.

Different toxic agents provoke a significant increase in AFP; for instance, administration of carbon tetrachloride to rats during liver regeneration stimulates the production of AFP five-fold (Aussel et al., 1980). Hepatochemical carcinogens also produce an important increase in AFP production, e.g. N-Z-fluorenylacetamide (Sell et al., 1981) and 3′-methyl-4-dimethyl-amino-azo-benzene (Woods, 1983; Yang Chou and Savitz, 1986).

Steroid hormones, particularly estrogens, can play an important role in the control of AFP levels; this was demonstrated after a dose of 10 mg of estriol administered to adult mice increased the plasma concentration from 20 ng/ml (nontreated animals) to 12 500 ng/ml after 5 days of treatment (Kotani et al., 1987). The data could be related to the fact that the administration of large doses of estrogen to adult mice provokes an intense proliferation of hepatocytes (Fujii and Kotani, 1986). On the other hand, glucocorticoids (e.g. dexamethasone) can suppress serum AFP levels (Gourdeau and Belanger, 1983).

2.1.5. AFP and the nervous system

Using immunohistochemical methods, studies by various groups demonstrated the intracellular localization of AFP in the neural crest and neural tube derivatives of mammals (Benno and Williams, 1978; Mollgard et al., 1979; Pineiro et al., 1979; Trojan and Uriel, 1979; Uriel et al., 1981b) and in birds (Moro and Uriel, 1981), during the period of their differentiation. In the rat the localization of AFP in brainstem nuclei and intracranial ganglia precedes that of the cerebral cortex and hippocampus (Trojan and Uriel, 1980).

Studies *in vivo* (Pineiro *et al.*, 1982; Villacampa *et al.*, 1984; Trojan and Uriel, 1986) and *in vitro* (Schachter and Toran-Allerand, 1982) strongly suggest that the intracellular presence of AFP in developing neurons results from exogenous protein uptake rather than *in situ* production. The data of the selective accumulation of AFP in the fetal nervous system after injection of labeled AFP ([125I]-AFP) into the maternal compartment (see Fig. 1.3(a)) gives support to the hypothesis that the presence of AFP in the developing nervous system of mammals and birds is primarily of exogenous origin

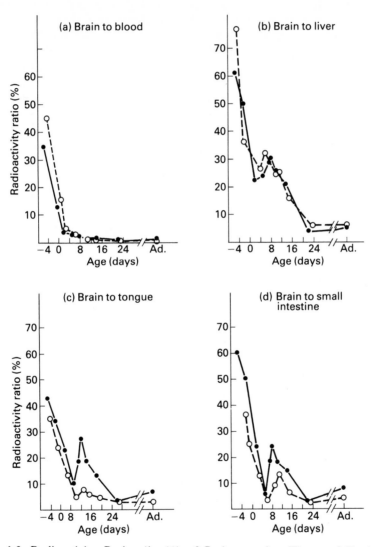

FIG 1.3. Radioactivity Ratios (in %) of Brain to other Tissues of Fetal and Post-natal Rats 4 h (○) and 24 h (●) after Administration of [125I]-α-Fetoprotein Quoted from Villacampa *et al.* (1984) with the permission of *Developmental Brain Research*.

(Villacampa *et al.*, 1984). These authors observed that the maximum uptake of radioactivity in the rat is found in the fetal brain before day 16 of fetal development and rapidly declines with the progress of gestation, and they suggest that maternal blood AFP, after crossing the placental barrier, enters into the fetal circulation and accumulates in the cerebrospinal fluid due to the high permeability for AFP (and other serum proteins) of the immature choroid plexus (Mollgard *et al.*, 1979).

Villacampa *et al.* (1984) observed a bimodal pattern when plotting the radioactivity ratios of brain to other tissues after administration of [^{125}I]-AFP (see Fig. 1.3(b–d)). They suggest that this corresponds to two different periods of neural growth and differentiation (day 16 of fetal development and day 8 post-natal) which can be associated with regional areas of brain development, and they concluded that the preferential localization of AFP in a given area is dependent on the maturity of the area at the time of the observation. Kovaru *et al.* (1985) found that the maximal intracellular localization of AFP in the brain of the fetal pig is found in the middle of gestation, whereas in the fetal thymus the highest values are found at the end of gestation. Since AFP is present during the organizing process of neural differentiation, it is concluded that this protein can play an important role during the different steps of this period.

2.1.6. AFP CONCENTRATIONS DURING DEVELOPMENT

In humans and various animal species, AFP appears very early in fetal development, increases significantly to a maximal concentration during this period and decreases rapidly during the perinatal phase. The rat is the only species that conserves high levels of AFP during a relatively long post-natal period.

The concentration of AFP in biological fluids (plasma, amniotic fluid) or in organs is currently evaluated by radio-immunoassay (RIA) using an anti-AFP antibody prepared by immunization of rabbits with purified human AFP. A sensitivity of 0.1–1 ng/ml can be obtained using highly diluted antibodies. AFP can also be measured with a great variety of other methods including immunoelectrophoresis, double diffusion, electroimmunoosmophoresis, immunoautoradiography, latex-agglutination, passive hemagglutination, enzyme-immunoassay; however, RIA is one of the most sensitive and practical techniques (for details see Caballero *et al.*, 1977; Delpre and Gilat, 1978; Wong *et al.*, 1979; Brummund *et al.*, 1980; Gardner *et al.*, 1981; Yamamoto *et al.*, 1986). Very sensitive determinations of AFP were obtained with RIA using monoclonal antibodies (Nomura *et al.*, 1983).

2.1.6.1. In Humans

In fetal serum, AFP achieves a maximum concentration of 2–3 mg/ml at 14 weeks of intrauterine life and declines gradually to 15–100 ng at birth and further to a mean normal adult level of 2–3 ng/ml by two years old (Seppala and Ruoslahti, 1976; Sykes and Dennis, 1977). In amniotic fluid, considerably lower concentrations of AFP parallel those of fetal serum with a significant decrease during the third trimester of pregnancy (Fig. 1.4).

In the maternal serum, AFP increases progressively as pregnancy advances (Fig. 1.4). The evaluation of AFP in maternal plasma, as well as in amniotic fluid, is of

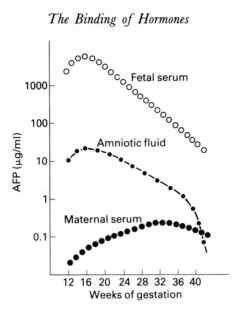

FIG 1.4. α-Fetoprotein (AFP) in Fetal and Maternal Sera and in Amniotic Fluid
during Human Pregnancy.
Quoted from Seppala (1975); Caballero *et al.* (1977) and Ruoslahti *et al.* (1978).

particular importance as high values of AFP in the fetus reflect an open neural tube or certain other birth defects (see the Introduction of this section).

The possible correlation between fetal sex and AFP levels has been studied by different authors with conflicting results: Sowers *et al.* (1983), between 16 and 19 weeks of gestation, and Lardinois *et al.* (1972), during the third trimester, found higher values of AFP in mothers bearing a male than those bearing a female fetus, whereas Milunsky *et al.* (1980) found no differences in maternal serum AFP levels between 12 and 32 weeks of gestation when comparing the two sexes.

Caballero *et al.* (1977) observed that at birth the fetal serum concentration of AFP was twice as high in boys as in girls; however, no differences were found in the maternal sera. Obiekwe *et al.* (1985) confirmed the data that AFP concentrations are higher in male than in female fetuses. They observed no significant difference in AFP levels between umbilical arterial and venous sera. These findings can be explained by the long half-life of AFP (3.5 days) (Gitlin, 1975) and a net clearance during a single circulation time that is undetectable. These authors also observed a higher concentration of AFP in subjects giving birth at less than 40 weeks of gestation (Fig. 1.5).

Studies in a large number of patients have failed to demonstrate any relationship between the concentration of AFP in maternal serum and amniotic fluid (Barford *et al.*, 1985). As the concentration curves of AFP in maternal serum, amniotic fluid and fetal serum differ considerably in relation to gestational age, it is concluded that the evaluation of maternal serum AFP as a test for fetal anomalies must be based upon large population studies and the determination of 'normal values' by reference laboratories at each age of gestation.

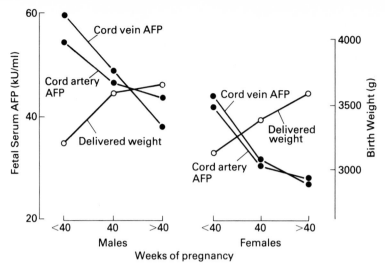

FIG 1.5. Concentration of α-fetoprotein (AFP) in Human Umbilical Artery and
Vein, and Birth Weight in Relation to Gestational Age at Birth.
Quoted from Obiekwe *et al.* (1985) with the permission of *Acta Obstetrica Gynecologia
Scandinava.*

2.1.6.2. In Different Animal Species

In rats and mice maximal values in the levels of AFP are found at the end of
gestation. However, in guinea-pigs, bovines and monkeys, the highest concentrations of
this protein are around the middle of gestation. The concentration of AFP can reach
very high values (e.g. in the fetal serum of the rat at 13 days of gestation AFP is

TABLE 1.16. *Concentration of α-Fetoprotein in Different Species at the Period of
Gestation of Maximal Levels*

Species	Serum		Fluid μg/ml	Maximum values of AFP Days of gestation	Adult serum ng/ml
	Fetal mg/ml	Maternal μg/ml			
Rat	8–10	50–60	1500	8–10	<30
Mouse	5–7				
Guinea-pig	3–5	5–6	100–200	35	400–2000
Rabbit	6	–	–	24	–
Ovine	1.8–2.5	–	17–23	50–70	–
Monkey		0.3–0.6	–	100	–
Human	2–5	0.5–0.8	–	90–100	4–10

Quoted from Gitlin and Boesman (1966); Seppala and Ruoslahti (1972);
Pihko and Ruoslahti (1973): Sell (1974); Bhargava *et al.*, (1979); Linkie
and La Barbera (1979); Smith *et al.* (1979); Aliau *et al.* (1980); Clarke
(1980); Gourdeau and Belanger (1983).

9–10 mg/ml). Table 1.16 gives levels of AFP at the period when they are the highest in different compartments and for various species. Figures 1.6 and 1.7 indicate examples of fetal serum concentrations of AFP during development of different animal species. The rat maintains relatively high plasma concentrations of AFP after birth: 4 mg/ml at 2–3 days, 0.4 mg/ml at 10–18 days, 63 ng/ml at 21 days old, and 200–300 ng/ml at 32 days old. In the adult rat, the values are 10–20 ng/ml.

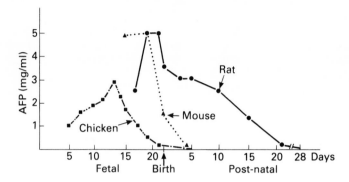

FIG 1.6. Ontogenesis of α-fetoprotein (AFP) in the Sera of Rat, Mouse and Chicken. Quoted from Savu *et al.* (1974b); Nunez *et al.* (1976); Slade and Milne (1978).

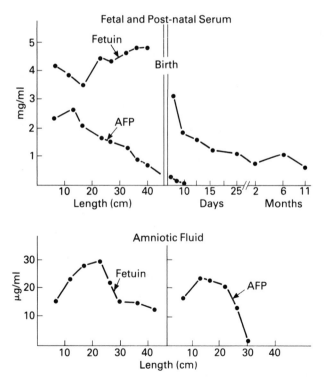

FIG 1.7. α-Fetoprotein (AFP) and Fetuin in the Ovine during Ontogenesis. Quoted from Aliau *et al.* (1980) with the Permission of the *International Journal of Biochemistry.*

TABLE 1.17. *Concentrations of α-Fetoprotein in Different Tissues and Fluids of the Bovine Embryo at Early Gestation*

	AFP (ng/mg protein)			
Days of gestation	14–22	25–27[a]	31–36	40–46
Maternal serum	0.13	0.21	0.18	0.17
Fetal tissues				
Blood	NA	NA	450–74 700	NA
Liver	NA	600	205 000	71 000
Urine	420	NA	35 000	70 000
Conceptus membrane	NA	27 300	8 500	11 200
Whole embryo	5.3	36 000	45 000	80 000
Yolk sac	NA	59 700	40 800	NA
Allantoic fluid	220	39 000	40 800	30 000
Amniotic fluid	NA	233 000	125 000	115 000

NA: not available;
[a]Pre-implantation.
Quoted from Janzen *et al.* (1982).

In the bovine embryo Janzen *et al.* (1982) found that AFP can be first detected by day 14 in trophoblasts and the secretion of AFP into the allantoic fluid occurred by day 16. These authors evaluated AFP in different embryonic tissues and fluids during the pre- and postimplantation period and found levels 560–1 500 000 times higher than those found in maternal serum. Table 1.17 gives an example of the concentration of AFP in different tissues and fluids in the bovine embryo at early gestation. It is to be remarked that the levels of AFP in maternal serum are similar to those found in nonpregnant cows (0.11–0.35 ng/mg protein) (Janzen *et al.*, 1982). These authors also confirmed that the major sites of AFP synthesis are the yolk sac and the fetal liver, and conclude that the synthesis of bovine AFP is not initiated by events associated with implantation.

2.1.7. HALF-LIFE AND FETAL–MATERNAL TRANSFER OF AFP

AFP is one of the few exceptions of macromolecules which can cross the placenta (see Volume I, p. 97). Using [^{125}I]-labeled AFP it was demonstrated that the route of transfer between the fetal and maternal compartments is a function of the animal species and of the period of gestation considered.

Mears *et al.* (1981) showed in the cow that ^{125}I-AFP injected into the fetal circulation readily crosses the placenta in the last third of pregnancy and that the fetal–maternal transfer of AFP via the amniotic sac is of secondary importance. In human and in sheep amniotic fluid levels of AFP decline markedly after the first third of pregnancy (Brock, 1978; Lai *et al.*, 1978) but the maternal serum concentration of AFP continues to rise, indicating that as gestation advances increased placental permeability, rather than transamniotic transfer, is the major route of passage of AFP from the fetus to the mother.

The half-life of AFP shows that it is 3.5 days in the human (Gitlin, 1975), 36 h in the ovine (Mears *et al.*, 1981) and 12–15 h in the pregnant rat (Sell and Alexander, 1974). The half-life of AFP varies in the different compartments, e.g. Mears *et al.* (1981) calculated in the pregnant ovine that the $t_\frac{1}{2}$ is 36 h in maternal plasma, 16.3 h in fetal plasma, and 42.4 h in amniotic fluid. These differences in the half-lives of AFP could be related to the transfer between the different compartments.

2.1.7.1. Biological Importance of AFP

AFP has been extensively characterized as an oncodevelopmental gene product in most animal species and has been found to be of important clinical use in monitoring neoplastic diseases and in obstetric surveillance of feto-placental abnormalities (see Introduction of this Section). With the present knowledge we can establish that the main biological and physiological functions of AFP include:

1. In two rodents, the rat and the mouse, by binding estrogens, AFP impairs the biological activity of estradiol by regulating the concentration of the unbound hormone. This hypothesis is supported by Aussel *et al.* (1981a), who demonstrated that administration of AFP to normal adult rats provoked a decrease in ovarian function. Also, it was observed that the presence of AFP in immature mice suppresses the uterotropic responses to estrogens (Mizejewski *et al.*, 1983). The binding of estrogens to AFP can prevent the formation of biologically inactive metabolites by enzymatic attack. On the other hand, in a number of animal species (including the human) the fetus can be protected from the excess of estrogens either by the formation of estrogen sulfates (a reversible process) since sulfotransferase activity can be very intense in the fetal compartment (see Vol. I, Chapter 2, Section 2), or by the binding of estrogens to other plasma proteins (e.g. sex steroid-binding protein: SBP).

2. The relatively strong binding of AFP to fatty acids may have regulatory effects as free fatty acid levels and distribution can be involved in the control mechanisms during periods of active cellular development (Vallette *et al.*, 1980).

3. Are AFPs involved in the mechanism of the immuno system? Recent information allows to conclude that AFP can play an important role in this concern, but the data suggest that AFP can stimulate or inhibit the immuno response. Vallette (1986) proposed that the immunological control by this protein can be explained by the presence of different forms of AFP (holoforms); each of these forms could have different hydrophobic ligands which can determine the interaction with the target cell (e.g. lymphocytes) and consequently provoke the biological action.

4. The localization of AFP in different areas of the fetal central nervous system (CNS) at an early period of development suggests that this protein could be involved in cell differentiation of the neuronal tissues; however, complementary information is needed to establish a biological role of AFP in the CNS.

5. The fact that estrogens can induce a large and prolonged elevation of serum AFP (Kotani *et al.*, 1987) and that the glucocorticoid dexamethasone reduces the basal plasma levels of AFP (Belanger *et al.*, 1981; Gourdeau and Belanger, 1983) suggests a

direct interaction of hormones in the synthesis of AFP. This information and the control of ovarian function by AFP (Aussel *et al.*, 1981b) suggests that AFP could also be involved in the production of gonadal steroids.

6.   During pregnancy the evaluation of AFP is of particular importance in the detection of fetal disorders including congenital nephrosis, neural tube defects, fetal hydrocephalus, fetal examphalos and intrauterine fetal death. Its assessment is also of value for early detection of primary hepatocellular carcinoma. In addition, new perspectives of the importance of AFP in pathology were opened with the detection of this protein in human breast cancer cells (Sarcione and Hart, 1985) and the findings of a significant increase in AFP in the plasma of post-menopausal women with primary breast carcinoma (Sarcione and Biddle, 1987).

7.   As AFP interacts with steroid hormones in only two species, the generalization of the physiological role of this protein in another species is still a basic problem to be clarified.

3. Androgen Binding Proteins

Androgens can bind specifically and with high affinity various proteins which differ in physicochemical characteristics and biological functions from the typical androgen receptor protein. These proteins include sex steroid-binding protein (SBP), androgen-binding protein (ABP), prostatic steroid-binding protein (PSB), prostatein, estramustine-binding protein, and prostatic α-protein. In this section we will describe only SBP, a protein which increases significantly during pregnancy, and is found in both fetal and maternal plasma; the other proteins are present during extrauterine life. The general properties and functions of these proteins have been described in various reviews (see Heyns, 1977; Bardin *et al.*, 1981; De Phillip *et al.*, 1982; Judge *et al.*, 1983; Westphal, 1986).

3.1. Sex Steroid-binding Protein (SBP)

SBP was discovered in the mid-sixties by two groups: Rosenbaum *et al.* 1966 and Mercier *et al.*, 1966. This protein binds with high affinity not only androgens (e.g. testosterone, 5α-dihydrotestosterone) but also estrogens. Table 1.18 summarizes the physicochemical characteristics of SBP.

SPB can be evaluated using a great variety of methods which include: equilibrium dialysis, ammonium sulfate precipitation, DEAE-cellulose disc, florsil adsorption, gel filtration, PAGE, radioimmunoassay. Using this last method SBP could be measured in a plasma volume of 5 μl. In general, SBP binds 5α-dihydrotestosterone with higher affinity than testosterone, but the affinity and relative binding affinity varies from species to species. It can also bind the synthetic androgen R-1881 and the synthetic estrogen R-2858. It is to be remarked that the characteristic of the high affinity of SBP for synthetic steroids is in contrast to that of α-fetoprotein which only binds the natural estrogens. Table 1.19 indicates the relative binding affinity (RBA) for different steroids in various animal species.

TABLE 1.18. *Physicochemical Characteristics of Sex Steroid-Binding Protein (SBP)*

	Human	Bovine	Rabbit	Dog
Molecular weight	88 000	89 500	74–78 000	76 000
Molecular weight of subunit(s)	16 000	28 400	36 500	40 000
	44 000	52 000	46 000	48 000
	50 000	48 000	43 000	44 000
Sedimentation coefficient (S)	4.1–5.3	5.3	4.4–4.6	5.0
Isoelectric point (pI)	5.5	4.8	5.2	–
Association constant				
$K_a (\times 10^8 \, M^{-1})$	9.3–13	1.1	7.0	5.6
Carbohydrate (%)	11–32	17	30	5.5

Quoted from Bohn (1974); Hansson *et al.* (1975); Suzuki *et al.* (1977; 1979); Mercier-Bodard *et al.* (1979); Petra *et al.* (1983); Strel'chyonok *et al.* (1983); Suzuki and Sinohara (1984).

TABLE 1.19. *Relative Binding Affinity of Sex Binding Protein to Different Steroids in Various Species*

	Human[a]	Chimpanzee[a]	Rhesus[a] monkey	Rabbit[b]	Dog[c]
5α-Dihydrotestosterone	100	100	100	100	100
Testosterone	79	92	87	33	42
R-1881	–	–	–	–	88
5α-Androstane-3β, 17β-diol	101	104	97	18	35
5α-Androstane-3α, 17β-diol	104	101	100	32	13
19-nor-Testosterone	–	–	–	25[d]	7
5-Androstene-3β, 17β-diol	–	–	–	18	–
Estradiol	33	57	55	5	2.5
Estrone	0	0	20	6	21.0
Estriol	0	0	0	2	–
R-2858	–	–	–	–	–
DES	0	0	0	–	–

Quoted from [a]Renoir *et al.* (1980); [b]Mahoudeau and Corvol (1973); [c]Dube *et al.* (1979); [d]Rosner and Darmstadt (1973).

3.1.1. IN HUMAN PREGNANCY

3.1.1.1. Maternal Plasma

In earlier studies, Rivarola *et al.* (1968) demonstrated that SBP increases very significantly during pregnancy, and this was confirmed by others who evaluated this increase at five to ten-fold, as compared with the levels in the nonpregnant state

TABLE 1.20. *Concentration of Sex Binding Protein (SBP) During the Human Life Evolution*

	SBP Concentration	
	nM	μg/ml
Pregnancy (weeks)		
5–9	111 ± 20	7.1
10–14	310 ± 106	19.9
15–19	479 ± 237	30.7
20–24	516 ± 268	33.1
25–29	644 ± 137	41.3
30–34	648 ± 189	41.5
35–40	544 ± 173	34.9
Post-partum (1–5 days)	418 ± 129	26.8
Female 5 years		4–9
10 years		3–8
15 years		2–5
Male 5 years		4–12
10 years		3–8
15 years		2–4
Nonpregnant women	65 ± 27	4.2
Adult men		
Post-menopausal	137–148	

Quoted from Uriel *et al.* (1981a); Helgason *et al.* (1982); Maruyama *et al.* (1987).

(Anderson *et al.*, 1976; Uriel *et al.*, 1981a) (Table 1.20). The maximal values of SBP during pregnancy are found between 25 and 35 weeks of gestation with a plasma concentration of 480–830 nM; on post-partum days (1–5) these values average 400 nM, and in the nonpregnant state 65 ± 27 nM (Uriel *et al.*, 1981a). Figure 1.8 indicates the average concentrations and variations of SBP throughout pregnancy. The levels of circulating testosterone increase very significantly during pregnancy but, as a consequence of the increase in SBP, the free testosterone concentration (the biologically active fraction) remains within the range found in nonpregnant women, at least until the 28th week of gestation (Bammann *et al.*, 1980). The data suggest that the increase in the total testosterone level before week 28 is the consequence of the decreased metabolic clearance rate.

3.1.1.2. Fetal Plasma

The evaluation of SBP in fetal plasma gives levels of 70–75 nM at mid-pregnancy and 100–120 nM at term (Abramovich *et al.*, 1978), values which represent respectively 7 and 5 times less than the levels of SBP in maternal plasma. Chaussain *et al.* (1978) evaluated SBP in cord blood and found a concentration range of 0.80–1.60 μg/100 ml with a mean of 1.27 ± 0.3 (SD) μg/100 ml and observed no significant sex differences.

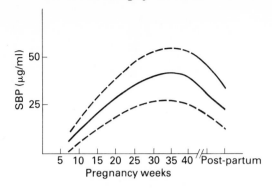

FIG 1.8. Concentration of Sex Steroid Binding Protein (SBP) in Maternal Plasma throughout Human Pregnancy.
Quoted from Uriel *et al.* (1981a).

Binding capacity of SBP is influenced by variations of sex steroid hormones; this capacity is decreased by testosterone and increased by estrogens (Vermeulen *et al.*, 1969). Consequently, increases in estrogen concentrations raise SBP, whereas a rise in androgens decreases it. Forest *et al.* (1973, 1974) demonstrated that plasma testosterone levels are elevated at birth in both sexes and decrease during the first week of life. In male infants SBP binding capacity increases from birth to 3 months and decreases to normal prepubertal levels at 6 months and correlates significantly with plasma testosterone and estradiol levels (Fig. 1.9). In female infants individual values of SBP range between 1.2 and 14.5 μg/100 ml without correlations with age or plasma estradiol levels (Chaussain *et al.*, 1978).

SBP can play an important role in sex steroid action; increases of SBP concentration could be a factor of feminization and decreases of SBP can have a masculinizing effect.

3.1.1.3. Amniotic Fluid

In 1972, Caputo and Hosty characterized the presence of SBP in the amniotic fluid and obtained concentration values of 21–24 nM which are similar to those found in the maternal serum (Caputo and Hosty, 1974). The authors suggest that SBP in the amniotic fluid is of maternal origin.

Wu *et al.* (1979) reported in the amniotic fluid at mid-pregnancy significantly higher binding of estradiol and testosterone to specific proteins than that of estrone or androstenedione and conclude that the possible biologic activity of steroids in this fluid may depend on the dynamic balance between the free, the specific protein-bound, and the nonspecific protein-bound steroids.

3.1.2. IN DIFFERENT ANIMAL SPECIES

In contradiction to the human, in most other mammals SBP is undetectable during fetal development as well as in the maternal plasma. Only in Macaque monkeys and in rabbits was the presence of a protein with the physicochemical characteristics of SBP and which binds testosterone and dihydrotestosterone specifically demonstrated. The

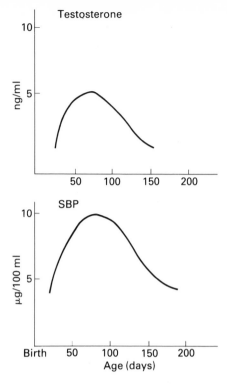

FIG 1.9. Sex Steroid Binding (SBP) Capacity and Testosterone Concentration in Males during the First Year of Life.
Quoted from Chaussain *et al.* (1978) with the Permission of *Acta Paediatrica Scandinavica.*

presence of SBP in other species (rat, little brown bats, bovine, dog, chimpanzee, baboon) is only detected in extra-uterine life. In the fetal rabbit during sexual organogenesis, SBP was found with a similar binding capacity for testosterone and 5α-dihydrotestosterone (73–84%). The binding was also similar for both sexes. However, the binding capacity for these two steroids was higher in the maternal plasma (87–94%) (Veyssiere *et al.*, 1979). As in humans, SBP in rabbits increases after administration of the thyroid hormone (Yosha *et al.*, 1984).

In Macaque monkeys SBP concentration in maternal plasma increases significantly until 28 days of gestation, remains at elevated levels until mid-pregnancy and decreases to low values in the last part of gestation (Schiller *et al.*, 1978).

4. Corticosteroid Binding Globulin (CBG)

The first information that corticosteroid hormones, cortisol, corticosterone, circulate in the plasma largely as a complex formed with an α-globulin was described by Daughaday (1958a,b).

This protein, called corticosteroid binding globulin (CBG), was also named 'transcortin' by other groups (Slaunwhite and Sandberg, 1959). The importance of

CBG during pregnancy is that this protein increases significantly in most animal species, in both the maternal and fetal compartments.

One of the first studies on the control of CBG showed that this protein is strongly stimulated by estrogens (Peterson *et al.*, 1960). As estrogen hormones increase significantly during gestation, it was suggested that the higher quantity of CBG found in maternal and fetal plasma is the consequence of the high production of estrogens. Most of the studies demonstrated that the liver is the principal organ of CBG biosynthesis.

4.1. Plasma Concentration of CBG during Gestation in Different Animal Species

The period of gestation during which CBG concentration is maximal is variable from species to species. In general, the plasma concentration is higher in the maternal plasma than in the fetal plasma, with an abrupt decrease after birth.

Using single radial immunodiffusion, Van Baelen *et al.* (1977a) evaluated the CBG concentration in pregnant rats. Figure 1.10 indicates that maximal values of CBG are found in both maternal and fetal sera at 16–18 days of gestation. The same authors found that dexamethasone provokes a significant decrease in the CBG levels in both compartments. Using radioimmunoassay, Raymoure and Kuhn (1983) also found high values of CBG in the maternal compartment of the same animal species and relatively high values of CBG (0.36 μM) were evaluated in the milk of lactating rat (day 6) (Pearlman *et al.*, 1981).

In the mouse, Lindenbaum and Chatterton (1981) reported a CBG concentration of 23 μM during days 13–18 of gestation and only 0.9 μM during days 11–18 of lactation.

In the guinea-pig, maximal concentrations of CBG are found at the end of gestation in both the maternal and fetal sera. The CBG levels reach 18–22 μM in the maternal

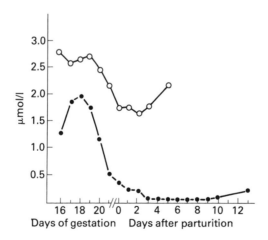

FIG 1.10. Plasma Concentration of Corticosteroid Binding Globulin (CBG) in Fetal and Neonatal Rats (●) and in Pregnant and Lactating Rats (○). Quoted from Van Baelen *et al.* (1977a,b).

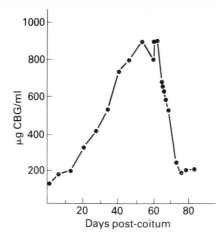

FIG 1.11. Plasma Concentration of Corticosteroid Binding Globulin (CBG) in
Pregnant Guinea-pig.
Quoted from Goodman *et al.* (1981).

sera at 50–68 days of gestation (Fig. 1.11) (Goodman *et al.*, 1981). The values are
2.0–2.2 μM in the fetal serum and no significant differences are found between male
and female fetuses (Dalle *et al.*, 1980).

In bovine the capacity binding for cortisol in the pregnant cow is about 3 μg/100 ml
and reaches values of 5 μg/100 ml in the lactating cow (Krulik and Svobodova, 1969).
This is an exception in relation to most mammals in which it was observed that CBG
decreased after birth. It is also to be remarked that in this species CBG is not stimulated
by estrogen administration.

In the fetal lamb the binding capacity of CBG increases from 1–2 μg/100 ml at
80–100 days of gestation to 6–8 μg/100 ml at term (Fig. 1.12) (Ballard *et al.*, 1982).
The concentration of CBG decreases drastically after birth and at 14 days of life CBG
values are only 0.5–1.0 μg/100 ml.

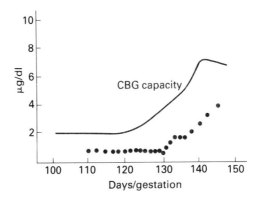

FIG 1.12. Corticosteroid Binding Globulin (CBG) Capacity and Total Plasma
Corticosteroid Concentrations in Fetal Sheep.
Quoted from Ballard *et al.* (1982).

In the pregnant baboon, Oakey (1975) evaluated the cortisol binding capacity in the maternal serum (60–120 days of gestation) to be $59 \pm 6.4\,\mu g/100$ ml, and at term $43.3 \pm 4.9\,\mu g/100$ ml. In the fetal serum collected between 100 and 132 days of gestation the values were similar to those of the corresponding maternal serum, but at term were only 50% of the maternal levels. The cortisol binding capacity from nonpregnant baboons was $34.4 \pm 5.5\,\mu g/100$ ml.

In the Rhesus monkey (*Macaca mulatta*), the fetal CBG capacity at term was found to be $20.6 \pm 2.1\,\mu g/100$ ml, not significantly different from the $18.1 \pm 1.4\,\mu g/100$ ml found in the corresponding maternal sera (Beamer *et al.*, 1972). After birth, the CBG binding capacity decreases to $5-10\,\mu g/100$ ml and increases to $20-25\,\mu g/100$ ml in the adult. In this species, and in opposition to most mammals, CBG concentrations are similar in both pregnant and nonpregnant animals.

In humans, in the maternal compartment the CBG concentrations reach maximal values at term ($1.24 \pm 0.9\,\mu M$) which are considerably higher than those in the fetal compartment ($0.25 \pm 0.03\,\mu M$). In the newborn, the CBG capacity remains at the low levels and increases at 1 year of life to $0.48 \pm 0.1\,\mu M$, a value close to that found in adults (Hadjian *et al.*, 1975).

4.2. Biosynthesis of CBG

Data obtained from different animal species confirm that the liver is the main organ where CBG is synthesized. Perrot-Applanat *et al.* (1981) using immunoperoxidase–cytochemical methods localized the presence of CBG in the hepatocytes from pregnant and nonpregnant guinea-pigs; the CBG-stained hepatocytes were accumulated mainly in the peripheral regions of the lobules and around the portal space. The CBG-mRNA (16 S) were isolated in the liver of pregnant guinea-pig and the concentration of translatable CBG-mRNA in the liver of pregnant guinea-pigs (40–60 days of gestation) was three to four times that in the liver of nonpregnant animals ($\sim 2-3\%$ vs $0.5-1\%$ of total mRNA activity) (Perrot-Applanat and Milgrom, 1979).

In the rat, Feldman *et al.* (1979) calculated that in the perfused liver approximately 18 pmol g/h of CBG binding sites were secreted, a value which represents $\sim 20\%$ of the total CBG content of a rat per day. Confirmatory evidence that the liver is the main organ of the biosynthesis of CBG was also obtained in this species by Wolf *et al.* (1981) who demonstrated the isolation of CBG mRNA from rat liver *in vitro*.

4.3. Control of CBG

It is well established that corticosteroid (natural or synthetic) provokes a significant decrease in CBG capacity, as was observed in different species. In rats, the administration of cortisol, prednisolone, dexamethasone, reduces plasma CBG to low levels (Komissarenko *et al.*, 1969; Yamamoto and Ohsawa, 1976) (for details see Westphal, 1971 and 1986). A similar effect is provoked by ACTH (Acs and Stark, 1973). On the other hand, adrenalectomy provokes an increase in CBG (Perrin and Forest, 1975).

Similar to corticosteroids, different androgens, testosterone, 5α-dihydrotestosterone and 5α-androstane-3α, 17β-diol decrease the blood concentration of CBG. The data can explain that the plasma concentration of CBG in female rats is about twice that in males (Van Baelen *et al.*, 1977b). The inhibitory effect of androgens is confirmed by the demonstration that gonadectomy can abolish the difference in plasma CBG concentration between male and female rats (Van Baelen *et al.*, 1977b).

4.4. Physicochemical Properties of CBG

Affinity-chromatographic methods provide one of the best techniques for the purification and isolation of CBG. Using these procedures, Bernutz *et al.* (1979) obtained a molecular weight of 50 700 for human CBG. The CBG isolated from rat gives two variants with apparent weights of 56 000 and 62 500 respectively (Chader and Westphal, 1968). Using serum of adrenalectomized rats, Favre *et al.* (1984) obtained also the presence of two electrophoretic variants of CBG with mol. wt of 65 900 and 75 800 respectively. In a cell-free translation system Wolf *et al.* (1981) isolated a CBG which migrated in SDS-gel electrophoresis with an apparent mol. wt of 41 000. This difference

TABLE 1.21. *Amino Acid and Carbohydrate Composition of CBG in Different Animal Species*

	Human[1]	Guinea-pig[2]	Rat[3]
Lysine	15	10.4	14
Histidine	9	9.2	6
Arginine	9	11.6	7
Aspartic acid	35	31.6	46
Threonine	22	20.1	19
Serine	30	23.7	33
Glutamic acid	31	25.1	30
Proline	11	14.0	12
Glycine	21	13.9	14
Alanine	23	21.4	13
Cystine $\frac{1}{2}$	2	2.9	2
Valine	24	10.8	16
Methionine	11	7.5	13
Isoleucine	15	14.6	13
Leucine	37	39.3	34
Tyrosine	10	5.5	9
Phenylalanine	19	16.8	11
Triptophan	4	1.9	3
Total	328	283.2	293

	Human[4]	% Carbohydrate	Rat[5]
Hexose	11.5	13.1	9.8
Hexosamine	9.0	7.1	9.5
Sialic acid	4.1	8.3	6.4
Fucose	1.5	0.1	2.1
Total	26.5	28.6	27.8

Quoted from: [1]Mickelson *et al.* (1982); [2]Mickelson and Westphal (1979); [3]Favre *et al.* (1984); [4]Muldoon and Westphal (1967); [5]Chader and Westphal (1968).

TABLE 1.22. *Association Constants of Human Corticosterone Binding Globulin with Various Steroids*

Steroids	Association constants $K_a(10^8 \text{ M}^{-1})$	Dissociation rate constants $K_{-1}(\text{S}^{-1})(20°)$
Cortisol	2.4 (4°) 0.9 (20°) 0.2 (37°)	0.031
Corticosterone	9.6 (4°)	0.047
Deoxycorticosterone	6.8 (4°)	0.10
Progesterone	3.4 (4°) 1.2 (20°) 0.2 (37°)	0.16 – –
Prednisolone	3.7 (4°)	–
R-5020	0.05 (4°)	–

Quoted from Chan and Slaunwhite (1977); Stroupe *et al.* (1978); Mickelson *et al.* (1981).

TABLE 1.23. *Physicochemical Properties of Corticosteroid Binding Globulin in Various Species*

Species	Affinity constant $K_a(10^8 \text{ M}^{-1})$	Sedimentation coefficient (S)	Half-life $t_{\frac{1}{2}}$
Mouse	11.0 (4°)	4.25	28 min (4°)
Rat	27.0 (4°)		
	0.3 (37°)	–	23 min (0°)
Guinea-pig	1.0 (37°)	3.2	2 days
Bovine	4.1 (4°)	–	–
Sheep	1.2 (37°)	–	–
Human	(see Table 1.22)	3.2	–

Quoted from Rosner and Hochberg (1972); Fairclough and Liggins (1975); Martin *et al.* (1976); Dalle *et al.* (1980); Raymoure and Kuhn (1980); Lindenbaum and Chatterton (1981); Pearlman *et al.* (1981); Favre *et al.* (1984).

can be explained because proteins synthesized by cell-free systems are not glycosylated, as seen in Table 1.21. Carbohydrates represent 25–30% of the mol. wt of CBG. Tables 1.22 and 1.23 give physicochemical characteristics of CBG in the human and in other animal species.

5. Uteroglobin

Another interesting protein which is found during gestation is uteroglobin. This protein binds specifically progesterone; however, its presence is only limited to rabbit or to other members of the order Lagomorpha. Uteroglobin was discovered in 1967 by Krishnan and Daniel from the uterine fluid of rabbit at early pregnancy. These authors observed that this protein, which was nominated 'blastokinin', could be involved in the mechanism to induce blastulation of the rabbit morula and facilitate blastocyst development. Independently, in 1968, Beier found the same protein, also in uterine fluid of rabbit and named it 'uteroglobin'.

5.1. Physicochemical Properties of Uteroglobin and Binding to Progesterone

Table 1.24 gives the values of different physicochemical properties of uteroglobin obtained from uterine luminal fluid of rabbit. Purification of this protein was obtained after chromatography on Sephadex G-100, Sephacryl S-200 and carboxymethyl cellulose (Nieto *et al.*, 1977). Uteroglobin is a globular protein (Murray *et al.*, 1972) constituted of 70 amino acids, where glutamic acid, leucine and lysine are the most abundant.

The affinity constant for the uteroglobin–progesterone complex was calculated to be $K_A = 3 \times 10^6 \, \text{M}^{-1}$ (0°C) (Beato and Baier, 1975). It is to be remarked that some progesterone derivatives, e.g. 5α-pregnane-3,20-dione and 3β-hydroxy-5α-pregnan-20-one have a relative binding affinity (RBA) significantly higher than progesterone itself (see Table 1.24) and that a synthetic steroid with progesterone properties, norethynodrel, has a RBA three to four times higher than progesterone. The RBA of

TABLE 1.24. *Physicochemical Characteristics of Uteroglobin*

Molecular weight	14–16 000
Sedimentation coefficient ($S_{w,20}$)	1.6
Isoelectric point (pI)	5.4
Stokes radius (Å)	18.4
Number of amino acids	70
Binding specificity (RBA)	
Progesterone	100
5α-Pregnane 3,20-dione	222
5β-Pregnane 3,20-dione	24
3β-Hydroxy-5α-pregnane	160
R-5020	10
Norethynodrel[a]	357
Estradiol-17β	53
Estradiol-17α	1
Estriol	42
Cortisol	0
Corticosterone	0

RBA: Relative binding affinity; [a]Norethynodrel: 17α-Ethinyl-17β-hydroxy-5(10)-estren-3-one.
Quoted from McGaughey & Murray (1972); Beato (1976); Fridlansky & Milgrom (1976); Nieto *et al.* (1977); Ponstingl *et al.* (1978).

estrogens to uteroglobin shows considerable discrepancies. Beato's group give **RBA** values for estradiol of 50% and for estrone 37% related to progesterone (see Table 1.24), whereas Fridlansky and Milgrom (1976) give values of only about 1% for both estrogens.

5.2. Concentration of Uteroglobin during Gestation of the Rabbit

Uteroglobin is mainly of endometrial origin; it appears in the uterine fluid 3 days post-coitum, reaches maximal levels (250–450 μg/ml) at 5–7 days of pregnancy and decreases at 9–11 days (Fig. 1.13).

5.3. Control of Uteroglobin Secretion

The production of uteroglobin in the uterine fluid is principally under the control of progesterone. The secretion of this protein can also be stimulated by different progesterone derivatives: 20α-hydroxy-4-pregnen-3-one; 5α-pregnane-3,20-dione; pregnene derivatives: 3β,20α-dihydroxy-5-pregnene and 3β,17,20α-trihydroxy-5-pregnene (Arthur & Chang, 1974; Chilton *et al.*, 1977). A similar effect was obtained with various synthetic steroids: medroxy-progesterone acetate, chlormadinone acetate and melengestrol acetate (Arthur and Chang, 1974; Bostwick and Britt, 1978). It is notable that norethynodrel which has an affinity (RBA) three to four times that of progesterone for binding to uteroglobin, does not have a significant effect on its production.

The effect of estrogens on uteroglobin induction, is conditioned by the experimental conditions: when estradiol is given alone it produces a dose-dependent increase of uteroglobin secretion and when estradiol is given simultaneously with a constant dose

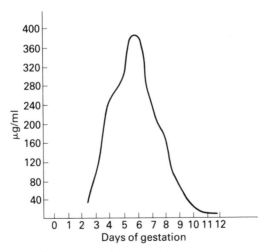

FIG 1.13. Concentration of Uteroglobin in Rabbit Uterine Fluid in the First Period of Gestation.

Quoted from Mayol and Longenecker (1974).

of progesterone, at the smallest dose it increases the effect of progesterone but at a higher concentration provokes a significant decrease in the stimulatory effect induced by progesterone (Janne *et al.*, 1980). Different androgens, testosterone or 5α-dihydrotestosterone are also capable of induced uteroglobin secretion (Feigelson *et al.*, 1977; Torkkeli *et al.*, 1978). Janne *et al.* (1980) suggest that the induction of uteroglobin by the androgens is mediated by the progesterone receptor.

5.4. Biosynthesis of Uteroglobin

The high concentration of uteroglobin in the uterine fluid a few days after conception agrees with the rapid incorporation of labeled amino acids in this protein more than any others (Murray and Daniel, 1973). 'In vitro' studies confirm that the synthesis of uteroglobin is under the control of progesterone or of the combination of progesterone and estradiol (Garcea *et al.*, 1979; Nieto and Beato, 1980).

Treatment of the rabbit with actinomycin D during the first 5 days of pregnancy shows the suppression of uteroglobin (Murray and Whitson, 1974). These authors show also that puromycin does not completely suppress uteroglobin. The data indicate that: 1. new mRNA is necessary for uteroglobin synthesis and 2. uteroglobin formation operates at the transcriptional level. Bullock (1980) demonstrated in the first days of rabbit gestation a correlation of uteroglobin secretion and uteroglobin mRNA production.

Young *et al.* (1981) studied the correlation of uteroglobin mRNA and the levels of nuclear progesterone receptors. The $mRNA_{UG}$ activity was assessed by translation *in vitro* of poly A-rich endometrial RNA and immunoprecipitation of the synthesized peptides using anti-uteroglobin antibodies. They observed that $mRNA_{UG}$ activity reached a maximal on day 4 of gestation and declined thereafter, whereas nuclear progesterone receptors rose on day 2 and then declined. A similar discrepancy between receptor level and the tissue response to progesterone was also found when uteroglobin was induced by exogenous hormone administration. This discrepancy between receptor level and the tissue response to progesterone can be explained by: 1. the possibility that the transient rise of the nuclear receptors triggers synthesis of long-lived mRNA, or 2. the basal levels of nuclear receptors exceeding the threshold required for stimulation of $mRNA_{UG}$ activity (Young *et al.*, 1981). In a quantitative analysis by hybridization, Kumar and Bullock (1982) evaluated at 250 molecules of uteroglobin in RNA per uterine cell in nonpregnant rabbit, and the number increased to 6800 molecules cell on day 4 of pregnancy.

Shen *et al.* (1983) studied the hormonal control of rabbit uteroglobin gene transcription using rabbit endometrial nuclei obtained from ovariectomized rabbits subjected to different hormonal treatments. The isolated nuclei were incubated with [^{3}H]-UTP to assess the synthesis of newly elongated RNA transcripts by the incorporation of [^{3}H]-UMP and the labeled RNA represented by uteroglobin sequences was evaluated by hybridization with cloned uterine DNA. The authors concluded that the action of progesterone on the control of uteroglobin is effective by: 1. exerting a mitogenic effect on the endometrial cells, 2. enhancing total cellular transcriptional activity, and 3. preferential stimulation of uteroglobin gene transcription.

5.5. Uteroglobin in Other Organs

The presence of uteroglobin is not limited only to the uterine fluid but has also been observed in other organs of the rabbit. Kay and Feigelson (1972) reported the presence of this protein in oviduct secretions where it is primarily under the control of estradiol (Goswami and Feigelson, 1974). Beier *et al.* (1975) demonstrated that uteroglobin is present in the rabbit seminal vesicles and El Etreby *et al.* (1983) gave evidence that androgens are the main factor for the induction of uteroglobin in the genital tract of male rabbit.

Uteroglobin was also found in the respiratory tract of the rabbit (Noske and Feigelson, 1976) and Bullock (1977) gave evidence of the presence of a specific mRNA of uteroglobin. In opposition to the reproductive tissues, in the lung, uteroglobin is not controlled by gonadal steroids, but there is evidence that cortisol enhances pulmonary uteroglobin levels (Feigelson *et al.*, 1977).

Conclusions

The different information in which many plasma proteins bind steroid hormones with high affinity suggest that these proteins could be involved in the transportation of the hormone to the target tissues. However, the reality shows that the presence of these proteins which bind specifically to various steroid hormones is very limited to the species: α-fetoprotein only in mouse and rat, progesterone binding globulin (PBG) only in the guinea-pig, uteroglobin only in the rabbit. This led to the general conclusion that despite the fact that steroid hormones can eventually bind specifically and with high affinity to various plasma proteins, the most acceptable hypothesis is that the steroid hormones reach the target tissues by diffusion. The presence and the biological role of these proteins to a small number of species is very intriguing, but it can be suggested that they could be involved in a protective mechanism of the hormone action. The case of uteroglobin is probably different because the data prove that this protein could be related to the process of implantation, however very recent information shows that there is a direct effect on this mechanism. The authors who discovered this protein also consider that the role of uteroglobin is still obscure.

In conclusion, the discovery of plasma proteins which specifically bind steroid hormones has had an enormous impact in advancing the knowledge of the interaction of steroid hormones with macromolecules; however, complementary information is needed to know their physiological function.

References

ABELEV, G. I. (1963) Study of the antigenic structure of tumors. *Acta Unio. Inter. Contra Cancrum* **19:** 80–82.

ABELEV, G. I. (1968) Production of embryonal serum alpha-globulin by hepatomas: a review of experimental and clinical data. *Cancer Res.* **28:** 1344–1350.

ABELEV, G. I., ASSECRITOVA, I. V., KRAEVSKY, N. A., PEROVA, S. D. and PEREVOD-CHIKOVA, N. I. (1967) Embryonal serum of α-globulin in cancer patients: diagnostic value. *Int. J. Cancer* **2:** 551–558.

ABRAMOVICH, D. R., TOWLER, C. M. and BOHN, H. (1978) The binding of sex steroids in human maternal and fetal blood at different stages of gestation. *J. Steroid Biochem.* **9:** 791–794.

ACKLAND, N., HEAP, R. B. and WEIR, B. J. (1979) Progesterone binding plasma proteins of pregnancy in hystricomorph rodents. *Res. Steroids* **8:** 343–345.

ACS, Z. and STARK, E. (1973) The role of transcortin in the distribution of corticosterone in the rat. *Horm. Metab. Res.* **5:** 279–282.

ALIAU, S., MARTI, J. and MORETTI, J. (1978) Bovine alpha-fetoprotein. Isolation and characterization. *Biochimie* **60:** 663–672.

ALIAU, S., MARTI, J. and MORETTI, J. (1980) Levels of fetoproteins in fetal serum and extra embryonic fluids during ontogenesis in the ovine species. *Int. J. Biochem.* **11:** 49–54.

ALIAU, L. D., FERGUSON-SMITH, M. A., DONALD, I., SWEET, E. M. and GIBSON, A. A. M. (1973) Amniotic fluid alpha-fetoprotein in the antenatal diagnosis of spina bifida. *Lancet* **ii:** 522–525.

ALPERT, E., DRYSDALE, J. W., ISSELBACHER, K. J. and SHUR, P. H. (1972) Human α-fetoprotein. Isolation, characterization and demonstration of microheterogeneity. *J. Biol. Chem.* **247:** 3792–3798.

ANDERSON, D. C., LASLEY, B. L., FISHER, R. A., SHEPHERD, J. H., NEWMAN, L. and HENDRICKX, A. G. (1976) Transplacental gradients of sex-hormone binding globulin in human and simian pregnancy. *Clin. Endocrinol.* **5:** 657–669.

ARTHUR, A. T. and CHANG, M. C. (1974) Induction of blastokinin by oral contraceptive steroids: implications for fertility control. *Fertil. Steril.* **25:** 217–221.

ATTARDI, B. and RUOSLAHTI, E. (1977) Alphafetoprotein is not a component of the 8 S estradiol receptor from the immature mouse uterus or brain. *Steroids* **30:** 711–716.

AUSSEL, C. and MASSEYEFF R. (1977) Binding of estrogens to molecular variants of rat alpha-fetoprotein. *FEBS Lett.* **81:** 363–365.

AUSSEL, C. and MASSEYEFF R. (1978) Rat alpha-fetoprotein–estrogen interaction. *J. Steroid Biochem.* **9:** 547–551.

AUSSEL, C. and MASSEYEFF, R. (1983a) Inhibition of rat alpha-fetoprotein-estrogen interaction by adult rat ovarian extracts—role of unsaturated fatty acids. *J. Steroid Biochem.* **19:** 1219–1222.

AUSSEL, C. and MASSEYEFF, R. (1983b) On rat alpha-fetoprotein as a fatty acid carrier. Influence of the structure of fatty acids. *Biochem. Biophys. Acta* **752:** 324–328.

AUSSEL, C., LAFAURIE, M. and STORA, C. (1981a) Rôle physiologique de l'alpha-foetoprotéine (AFP). Effet d'injection d'AFP sur l'activité ovarienne du rat femelle adulte. *C. R. Acad. Sci. (Paris)* **293:** 553–556.

AUSSEL, C., STORA, C. and KREBS, B. (1980) Alpha-fetoprotein and serum hormone levels following liver intoxication with carbon tetrachloride. *Biochem. Biophys. Res. Commun.* **95:** 796–800.

AUSSEL, C., URIEL, J. and MERCIER-BODARD, C. (1973) Rat α-fetoprotein, isolation, characterization and estrogen binding properties. *Biochimie* **55:** 1431–1437.

AUSSEL, C., LAFAURIE, M., MASSEYEFF, R. and STORA, C. (1981b) *In vivo* regulation of ovarian activity by alpha-fetoprotein. *Steroids* **38:** 195–204.

BAKER, M. E., FRECKER, D. G. N. and FANESTIL, D. D. (1982) Inhibition of estrogen binding to rat alpha-fetoprotein by tryptophan *p*-nitrophenyl esters. *J. Steroid Biochem.* **16:** 503–507.

BAKER, M. E., MORRIS, C. S. and FANESTIL, D. D. (1980) Binding of the chymotrypsin substrate, tryptophan methyl ester, by rat α-fetoprotein. *Biochim. Biophys. Acta* **632:** 611–618.

BALLARD, P. L., KITTERMAN, J. A., BLAND, R. D., CLYMAN, R. I., GLUCKMAN, P. D., PLATZKER, A. C. G., KAPLAN, S. L. and GRUMBACH, M. M. (1982) Ontogeny and regulation of corticosteroid binding globulin capacity in plasma of fetal and newborn lambs. *Endocrinology* **110:** 359–366.

BAMMANN, B. L., COULAM, C. B. and JIANG N-S. (1980) Total and free testosterone during pregnancy. *Am. J. Obstet. Gynecol.* **137:** 293–298.

BARDIN, C. W., MUSTO, N., GUNSALUS, G., KOTITE, N., CHENG, S. L., LARREA, F. and BECKER, R. (1981) Extracellular androgen binding proteins. *Ann. Rev. Physiol.* **43:** 189–198.

BARFORD, D. A., DICKERMAN, L. H. and JOHNSON, W. E. (1985) α-Fetoprotein: relationship between maternal serum and amniotic fluid levels. *Am. J. Obstet. Gynecol.* **151:** 1038–1041.

BATRA, S., BENGTSSON, L. P., GRUNDSELL, H. and SJÖBERG N.-O. (1976) Levels of free and protein-bound progesterone to plasma during late pregnancy. *J. Clin. Endocr. Metab.* **42:** 1041–1047.

BEAMER, N., HAGEMENAS, F. and KITTINGER, G. W. (1972) Protein binding of cortisol in the Rhesus monkey (*Macaca mulatta*). *Endocrinology* **90:** 325–327.

BEATO, M. (1976) Binding of steroids to uteroglobin. *J. Steroid Biochem.* **7:** 327–334.

BEATO, M. and BAIER, R. (1975) Binding of progesterone to the proteins of the luminal fluid. Identification of uteroglobin as the binding protein. *Biochim. Biophys. Acta* **392:** 346–356.

BEIER, H. M. (1968) Uteroglobin: a hormone-sensitive endometrial protein involved in blastocyst development. *Biochim. Biophys. Acta* **160:** 289–291.

BEIER, H. M., BOHN, H. and MULLER, W. (1975) Uteroglobin-like antigen in the male genital tract secretions. *Cell Tiss. Res.* **165:** 1–11.

BELANGER, L., FRAIN, M., BARIL, P., GINGRAS, M. C., BARTKOWIAK, J. and SALA-TREPAT, J. M. (1981) Glucocorticoid suppression of alpha-fetoprotein synthesis in developing rat liver. Evidence for selective gene repression at the transcriptional level. *Biochemistry* **20:** 6665–6672.

BENASSAYAG, C., VALLETTE, G., DELORME, J., SAVU, L., NUNEZ, E. A. and JAYLE, M. F. (1977) Rat and human embryo and post-natal sera contain a potent endogenous competitor of estrogen-rat alpha-fetoprotein interactions. *Steroids* **30:** 771–785.

BENASSAYAG, C., SAVU, L., VALLETTE, G., DELORME, J. and NUNEZ, E. A. (1979) Relations between fatty acids and oestrogen binding properties of pure rat alpha$_1$-foetoprotein. *Biochim. Biophys. Acta* **587:** 227–237.

BENNO, R. H. and WILLIAMS, T. H. (1978) Evidencer for intracellular localization of alpha-fetoprotein in the developing rat brain. *Brain Res.* **142:** 182–186.

BERGSTRAND, C. G. and CZAR, B. (1956) Demonstration of new protein fraction in serum from human fetus. *Scand. J. Clin. Lab. Invest.* **8:** 174.

BERGSTRAND, C. G. and CZAR, B. (1957) Paper electrophoretic study of human fetal serum protein with demonstration of a new protein fraction. *Scand. J. Clin. Lab. Invest.* **9:** 277–286.

BERNUTZ, C., HANSLE, W. O., HORN, K., PICKARDT, C. R., SCRIBA, P. C., FINK, E., KOLB, H. and TSCHESCHE, H. (1979) Isolation, characterization and radioimmunoassay of corticosteroid-binding globulin (CBG) in human serum—clinical significance and comparison to thyroxine-binding globulin (TBG). *Acta Endocrinol.* **92:** 370–384.

BHARGAVA, A. S., POGGEL, H. A. and GUNZEL, P. (1979) Diagnostic value of α$_1$-fetoprotein determinations in monitoring pregnancy in Rhesus monkeys. *Toxicol. Lett.* **4:** 163–167.

BOHN, H. (1974) Isolierung, Charakterisierung und quantitative immunologische Bestimmung des Steroid-bindenden β-Globulins. *Blut* **29:** 17–31.

BOSTWICK, E. F. and BRITT, J. H. (1978) Blastokinin secretion, ovarian activity, and embryo survival after melengestrol acetate in rabbits. *Proc. Soc. Exptl. Biol. Med.* **157:** 220–224.

BROCK, D. J. H. (1978) Protein marker in disease (1). Alpha-fetoprotein and the prenatal diagnosis of neural tube defects. *J. R. Coll. Surg. Edinburgh* **23:** 184–192.

BROCK, D. J. H. and SCRIMGEOUR, J. B. (1972) Early prenatal diagnosis of anencephaly. *Lancet* **ii:** 1252–1253.

BROCK, D. J. H. and SUTCLIFFE, R. G. (1972) Alpha-fetoprotein in the antenatal diagnosis of anencephaly and spina bifida. *Lancet* **ii:** 197–199.

BRUMMUND, W., ARVAN, D. A., MENNUTI, M. T. and STARKOVSKY, N. A. (1980) Alpha-fetoprotein in the routine clinical laboratory: evaluation of a simple radioimmunoassay and review of current concepts in its clinical application. *Clin. Chim. Acta* **105:** 25–39.

BULLOCK, D. W. (1977) *In vitro* translation of messenger RNA for a uteroglobin-like protein from rabbit lung. *Biol. Reprod.* **17:** 104–107.

BULLOCK, D. W. (1980) Uterine proteins as markers of progesterone action. In: *Steroid Induced Uterine Proteins*, Beato, M. (Ed.), Elsevier/North-Holland Biomedical Press, Amsterdam, New York, Oxford, pp. 315–318.

BURTON, R. M., HARDING, G. B., ABOUL-HOSN, W. R., MACLAUGHLIN, D. T. and WEST-PHAL, U. (1974) Progesterone binding globulin from the esrum of pregnant guinea pig, a polydis-perse glycoprotein. *Biochemistry* **13**: 3554–3561.

CABALLERO, C., VEKEMANS, M., LOPEZ DEL CAMPO, J. G. and ROBYN, C. (1977) Serum alpha-fetoprotein in adults, in women during pregnancy, in children at birth, and during the first week of life: a sex difference. *Am. J. Obstet. Gynecol.* **127**: 384–389.

CAPUTO, M. J. and HOSTY, T. A. (1972) The presence of the sex binding globulin in amniotic fluid. *Am. J. Obstet. Gynecol.* **113**: 804–811.

CAPUTO, M. J. and HOSTY, T. A. (1974) Further characterization of the sex hormone-binding globulin in amniotic fluid. *Am. J. Obstet. Gynecol.* **118**: 496–498.

CASTELLET, R. and PASQUALINI, J. R. (1973) Etude d'un complexe proteine-progesterone-^{3}H dans le plasma de cobaye en gestation. Application à l'évaluation de la progesterone. *C. R. Acad. Sci., Paris (Serie D)* **276**: 1205–1208.

CHADER, G. J. and WESTPHAL, U. (1968) Steroid-protein interactions. XVIII. Isolation and observations on the polymeric nature of the corticosteroid-binding globulin of the rat. *Biochemistry* **7**: 4272–4282.

CHAN, D. W. and SLAUNWHITE, W. R. Jr. (1977) The chemistry of human transcortin. The effects of pH, urea, salt, and temperature on the binding of cortisol and progesterone. *Arch. Biochem. Biophys.* **182**: 437–442.

CHAUSSAIN, J. L., BRIJAWI, A., GEORGES, P., ROGER, M., DONNADIEU, M. and JOB, J. C. (1978) Variations of serum testosterone estradiol binding globulin (TeBG) binding capacity in infants during the first year of life. *Acta Paediatr. Scand.* **67**: 649–653.

CHENG, S. L., STROUPE, S. D. and WESTPHAL, U. (1976) Steroid-protein interactions. Purification of progesterone-binding globulin by affinity chromatography. *FEBS Lett.* **64**: 380–384.

CHILTON, B. S., DANIEL, J. C. Jr and BOOHER, C. B. (1977) Induction of uterine protein synthesis by synthetic progestins. *Fertil. Steril.* **28**: 269–272.

CLARKE, L. E. (1980) The distribution of rabbit alpha-fetoprotein (RAFP) and its molecular variants throughout gestation. *J. Reprod. Immunol.* **2**: 109–126.

DALLE, M., EL HANI, A. and DELOST, P. (1980) Changes in cortisol binding and metabolism during neonatal development in the guinea-pig. *J. Endocr.* **85**: 219–227.

DAUGHADAY, W. H. (1958a) Binding of corticosteroids by plasma proteins. V. Corticosteroid-binding globulin activity in normal human beings and in certain disease states. *Arch. Intern. Med.* **101**: 286–290.

DAUGHADAY, W. H. (1958b) Binding of corticosteroids by plasma proteins. III. The binding of corticosteroid and related hormones by human plasma and plasma protein fractions as measured by equilibrium dialysis. *J. Clin. Invest.* **37**: 511–518.

DELPRE, G. and GILAT, T. (1978) L'alpha-foeto-protéine. *Gastroenterol. Clin. Biol.* **2**: 87–106.

DE PHILLIP, R. M., FELDMAN, M., SPRUILL, W. A., FRENCH, F. S. and KIERSZENBAUM, A. L. (1982) The secretion of androgen-binding protein and other proteins by rat Sertoli cells in culture: a structural and electrophoretic study. *Ann. N. Y. Acad. Sci.* **383**: 360–371.

DIAMOND, M., RUST, N. and WESTPHAL, U. (1969) High-affinity binding of progesterone, testos-terone and cortisol in normal and androgen-treated guinea pigs during various reproductive stages: relationship to masculinization. *Endocrinology* **84**: 1143–1151.

DUAX, W. L. and NORTON D. A. (1975) *Atlas of Steroid Structure*, Vol. 1, IFI-Plenum, New York.

DUAX, W. L., GRIFFIN, J. F., WEEKS, C. M. and WAWRZAK, Z. (1988) The mechanism of action of steroid antagonists: insights from crystallographic studies. *J. Steroid Biochem. (Proc.)* **4B**: 481–492.

DUBE, J. Y., TERMBLAY, R. R., DIONNE, F. T. and CHAPDELAINE, P. (1979) Binding of androgens in dog prostate cytosol and in plasma. *J. Steroid Biochem.* **10**: 449–458.

DZIEGIELEWSKA, K. M., EVANS, C. A. N., FOSSAN, G., LOR-SCHEIDER, F. L., MALI-NOWSKA, D. H., MØLLGARD, K., REYNOLDS, M. L., SAUNDERS, N. R. and

WILKINSON, S. (1980) Proteins in cerebrospinal fluid and plasma of fetal sheep during development. *J. Physiol* **300**: 441–445.

EL ETREBY, M. F., BEIER, H. M., ELGER, W., MAHROUS, A. T. and TOPERT, M. (1983) Immunocytochemical localization of uteroglobin in the genital tract of male rabbits. *Cell Tis. Res.* **229**: 61–73.

EVANS, J. J., WHITE, F. J. and SIN, I. L. (1981) Concentration and relationship to progesterone of progesterone-binding globulin in pregnant guinea-pigs: measurement by progesterone tracer binding assay. *J. Endocr.* **90**: 331–335.

EVANS, J. J., SIN, I. L. and WHITE, F. J. (1982) Progesterone binding globulin and progesterone in guinea-pigs after ovariectomy, abortion and parturition. *J. Steroid Biochem.* **16**: 171–173.

FAIRCLOUGH, R. J. and LIGGINS, G. C. (1975) Protein binding of plasma cortisol in the foetal lamb near term. *J. Endocr.* **67**: 333–341.

FAVRE, G., LE GAILLARD, F., MATTRET-TURRION, M. H., DUMUR, V. and DAUTREVAUX, M. (1984) Physico-chemical properties and evidence for electrophoretic variants of rat transcortin. *Biochimie* **66**: 361–369.

FEIGELSON, M., NOSKE, J. G., GOSWAMI, A. K. and KAY, E. (1977) Reproductive tract fluid proteins and thier hormonal control. *Ann. N. Y. Acad. Sci.* **286**: 273–286.

FELDMAN, D., MONDON, C. E., HORNER, J. A. and WEISER, J. N. (1979) Glucocorticoid and estrogen regulation of corticosteroid-binding globulin production by rat liver. *Am. J. Physiol.* **237**: E493–E499.

FOREST, M. G., CATHIARD, A. M. and BERTRAND, J. A. (1973) Total and unbound testosterone levels in the newborn and in normal and hypogonadal children: use of a sensitive radioimmunoassay for testosterone. *J. Clin. endocr. Metab.* **36**: 1132–1142.

FOREST, M. G., SIZONENKO, P. C., CATHIARD, A. M. and BERTRAND, J. (1974) Hypophysogonadal function in humans during the first year of life. *J. Clin. Invest.* **53**: 819–828.

FRIDLANSKY, F. and MILGROM, E. (1976) Interaction of uteroglobin with progesterone, 5α-pregnane-3,20-dione and estrogens. *Endocrinology* **99**: 1244–1251.

FUJII, H. and KOTANI, M. (1986) Promoting effect of estrogen on regeneration of the liver transplanted to an ectopic site in mice. *Virchows Arch. (Anat. Pathol.)* **409**: 453–460.

GARCEA, N., CAMPO, S., CARUSO, A., SCOTTO, V. and SICCARDI, P. (1979) Blastokinin. A utero-specific protein induced by progesterone in the rabbit. *Res. Steroids* **8**: 41–46.

GARDNER S., BURTON, B. K. and JOHNSON, A. M. (1981) Maternal serum alpha-fetoprotein screening: a report of the Forsyth County Project. *Am. J. Obstet. Gynecol.* **140**: 250–253.

GITLIN, D. (1975) Normal biology of alpha-fetoprotein. *Ann. N. Y. Acad. Sci.* **259**: 7–16.

GITLIN, D. and BOESMAN, M. (1966) Serum alpha-fetoprotein albumin and pG-globulin in the human conceptus. *J. Clin. Invest.* **45**: 1826–1838.

GITLIN, D. and BOESMAN, M. (1967) Sites of serum α-fetoprotein synthesis in the human and in the rat. *J. Clin. Invest.* **56**: 1010–1016.

GITLIN, D. and PERRICELLI, A. (1970) Synthesis of serum albumin, prealbumin, α-fetoprotein, α_1-antitripsin and transferin by the human yolk sac. *Nature* **228**: 995–997.

GOODMAN, W. G., MICKELSON, K. E. and WESTPHAL, U. (1981) Immunochemical determination of corticosteroid-binding globulin in the guinea-pig during gestation. *J. Steroid Biochem.* **14**: 1293–1296.

GORIN, M. B., COOPER, D. L., EIFERMAN, F., VAN DE RIJN, P. and TILGHMAN, S. M. (1981) The evolution of α-fetoprotein and albumin. I. A comparison of the primary amino acid sequences of mammalian α-fetoprotein and albumin. *J. Biol. Chem.* **256**: 1954–1959.

GOSWAMI, A. and FEIGELSON, M. (1974) Differential regulation of a low-molecular-weight protein in oviductal and uterine fluids by ovarian hormones. *Endocrinology* **95**: 669–675.

GOURDEAU, H. and BELANGER, L. (1983) Guinea-pig α_1-fetoprotein: purification, characterization, development and hormonal regulation, and behavior in diethylnitrosamine hepatocarcinogenesis. *Can. J. Biochem. Cell Biol.* **61**: 1133–1146.

GRIFFIN, J. F., DUAX, W. L. and WEEKS, C. M. (1984) *Atlas of Steroid Structure*, Vol. 2, IFI-Plenum, New York.

HADJIAN, A. J., CHEDIN, M., COCHET, C. and CHAMBAZ, E. M. (1975) Cortisol binding to proteins in plasma in the human neonate and infant. *Pediat. Res.* **9:** 40–45.

HANSSON, V., RITZEN, M. E., FRENCH, F. S., WEDDINGTON, S. C. and NAYFEH, S. N. (1975) Testicular androgen-binding protein (ABP): comparison of ABP in rabbit testis and epididymis with a similar androgen-binding protein (TeBG) in rabbit serum. *Molec. Cell. Endocr.* **3:** 1–20.

HARDING, G. B., BURTON, R. M. STROUPE, S. D. and WESTPHAL, U. (1974) Steroid-protein interactions. XXVIII. The isoelectric point and pH stability of the progesterone binding globulin. *Life Sci.* **14:** 2405–2412.

HASSOUX, R., BERGES, J. and URIEL, J. (1977) Affinity chromatography of mouse alpha-fetoprotein (AFP) on oestradiol-sepharose adsorbents—isolation and properties. *J. Steroid Biochem.* **8:** 127–132.

HEAP, R. B. (1969) The binding of plasma progesterone in pregnancy. *J. Reprod. Fert.* **18:** 546–548.

HEAP, R. B. (1970) Dynamic aspects of progesterone metabolism. *J. Reprod. Fert.* **22:** 189–190.

HEAP, R. B. and DEANESLY, R. (1967) The increase in plasma progesterone levels in the pregnant guinea-pig and its possible significance. *J. Reprod. Fert.* **14:** 339–341.

HEAP, R. B. and ILLINGWORTH, D. V. (1974) The maintenance of gestation in the guinea-pig and other hystricomorph rodents: changes in the dynamics of progesterone metabolism and the occurrence of progesterone-binding globulin (PBG). *Symp. Zool. Soc. Lond.* **34:** 385–415.

HEAP, R. B., ACKLAND, N. and WEIR, B. J. (1981) Progesterone-binding proteins in plasma of guinea pigs and other hystricomorph rodents. *J. Reprod. Fert.* **63:** 477–489.

HELGASON, S., DAMBER, J.-E., DAMBER, M.-G., VON SCHOULTZ, B., SELSTAM, G. and SODERGARD, R. (1982) A comparative longitudinal study on sex hormone binding globulin capacity during estrogen replacement therapy. *Acta Obstet. Gynecol. Scand.* **61:** 97–100.

HEYNS, W. (1977) The steroid-binding β-globulin of human plasma. *Adv. Steroid Biochem. Pharmacol.* **6:** 59–79.

IDO, E. and MATSUNO, T. (1982) Purification and physicochemical and immunological analysis of chicken alpha-fetoprotein. *Jap. J. Med. Sci. Biol.* **35:** 87–96.

ILLINGWORTH, D. V., HEAP, R. B. and PERRY, J. S. (1970) Changes in the metabolic clearance rate of progesterone in the guinea pig. *J. Endocr.* **48:** 409–417.

ILLINGWORTH, D. V., ACKLAND, N., HEAP, R. B. and WEIR, B. J. (1973) Progesterone-binding proteins: occurrence, capacity and binding affinity in hystricomorph rodents. *J. Endocr.* **58:** ii.

JANNE, O., HEMMINKI, S., ISOMAA, V., ISOTALO, H., KOPU, H., ORAVA, M. and TORKKELI, T. (1980) Uteroglobin synthesis and its relationship to changes in progesterone receptors, RNA polymerases and poly(A) polymerases in the rabbit uterus. In: *Steroid-induced Uterine Proteins*, Beato, M. (Ed.), Elsevier/North-Holland Biomedical Press, Amsterdam, New York, Oxford, pp. 319–340.

JANZEN, R. M., MABLY, E. R., TAMAOKI, T., CHURCH, R. B. and LORSCHEIDER, F. L. (1982) Synthesis of alpha-fetoprotein by the pre-implantation and post-implantation bovine embryo. *J. Reprod. Fert.* **65:** 105–110.

JUDGE, S. M., SALTZMAN, A. G. and LIAO, S. (1983) Alpha-protein: a marker for androgen action in the rat ventral prostate. In: *Gene Regulation by Steroid Hormones*, II, Roy, A. K. and Clark, J. H. (Eds), Springer Verlag, New York, pp. 267–275.

KAY, E. and FEIGELSON, M. (1972) An estrogen modulated protein in rabbit oviducal fluid. *Biochim. Biophys. Acta* **271:** 436–441.

KEEL, B. A. and ABNEY, T. O. (1984) The kinetics of estrogen binding to rat α-fetoprotein. *Experientia* **40:** 503–505.

KEKOMAKI, M., SEPPALA, M., EHNHOLM, C., SCHWARTZ, A. L. and RAIVIO, K. (1971) Perfusion of isolated human fetal liver: synthesis and release of α-fetoprotein and albumin. *Int. J. Cancer* **8:** 250–258.

KERCKAERT, J. P., BAYARD, B., DEBRAY, H., SAUTIERES, P. and BISERTE, G. (1977) Rat α-fetoprotein heterogeneity. Comparative chemical study of the two electrophoretic variants and their ricinus lectin binding properties. *Biochim. Biophys. Acta* **493**: 293–303.

KIOUSSIS, D., EIFERMAN, F., VAN DE RIJN, P., GORIN, M. B., INGRAM, R. S. and TILGH-MAN, S. M. (1981) The evolution of α-fetoprotein and albumin. II. The structures of the α-fetoprotein and albumin genes in the mouse. *J. Biol. Chem.* **256**: 1960–1967.

KOBLINSKY, M., BEATO, M., KALIMI, M. and FEIGELSON, P. (1972) Glucocorticoid-binding proteins of rat liver cytosol. II. Physical characterization and properties of the binding proteins. *J. Biol. Chem.* **247**: 7897–7904.

KOGA, K., O'KEEFE, D. W., IIO, T. and TAMAOKI, T. (1974) Transcriptional control of α-fetoprotein synthesis in developing mouse liver. *Nature* **252**: 495–497.

KOMISSARENKO, V. P., MIKOSHA, A. S. and KRAVCHENKO, V. I. (1969) Transcortin content in the plasma of rats given corticosteroids. *Prob. Endokrinol.* **15**: 54–58.

KOTANI, M., FUJII, H., TERAO, K., HAYAMA, T., TAGAH and HIRAI H. (1987) The effect of estriol on the production of alpha-fetoprotein by the liver in adult mice. *Virchows Arch. A.* **411**: 1–4.

KOVARU, F., MARES, V., KOVARU, H. and MULLER, L. (1985) Alpha-fetoprotein in the thymus and brain of embryonic pigs. *Histochem. J.* **17**: 576–578.

KRISHNAN, R. S. and DANIEL, J. C. Jr (1967) "Blastokinin": inducer and regulator of blastocyst development in the rabbit uterus. *Science* **158**: 490–492.

KRULIK, R. and SVOBODOVA, J. (1969) The binding of corticosteroids by plasmatic proteins in cattle. *Physiol. Bohemoslov.* **18**: 141–146.

KUMAR, N. M. and BULLOCK, D. W. (1982) Hybridization analysis of steady-state levels of uteroglobin mRNA in rabbit uterus and lung during pregnancy. *J. Endocr.* **94**: 407–414.

LAI, P. C. W., MEARS, G. J., VAN PETTEN, G. R., HAY, D. M. and LORSCHEIDER, F. L. (1978) Fetal-maternal distribution of ovine alpha-fetoprotein. *Am. J. Physiol.* **235**: E27–E31.

LARDINOIS, R., ANAGNOSTAKIS, D., ORTEXZ, M. A. and DELISLE, M. (1972) Human α₁-foetoglobulin during the last trimester of gestation. *Clin. Chim. Acta* **37**: 81–90.

LAURENT, C., DE LAUZON, S., CITTANOVA, N., NUNEZ, E. and JAYLE, M. F. (1975) The comparative specificity of three oestradiol-binding proteins. Rat α-foetoprotein, rat liver 17β-hydroxysteroid dehydrogenase and anti-(oestradiol-6-carboxymethyloxime-bovine serum albumin) anti-serum. *Biochem. J.* **151**: 513–518.

LEA, O. A. (1973) Isolation and characterization of a progesterone- and testosterone-binding globulin from pregnant guinea-pig serum. *Biochim. biophys. Acta* **317**: 351–363.

LEA, O. A., BESSESEN, A. and STØA, K. F. (1976) Progesterone-binding globulin and testosterone-binding activity in guinea pig serum during pregnancy: relationship to progesterone and oestrogens. *Acta endocr. (Copenh.)* **81**: 367–378.

LINDENBAUM, M. and CHATTERTON, R. T., Jr (1981) Interaction of steroids with dexamethasone-binding receptor and corticosteroid-binding globulin in the mammary gland of the mouse in relation to lactation. *Endocrinology* **109**: 363–375.

LINKIE, D. M. and LA BARBERA, A. R. (1979) Serum estrogen binding proteins in tissues of the immature rat: quantitation by radioimmunoassay. *Proc. Soc. Exp. Biol. Med.* **161**: 7–12.

MACLAUGHLIN, D. T. and WESTPHAL, U. (1974) Steroid-protein interactions. XXX. A progesterone-binding protein in the uterine cytosol of the pregnant guinea-pig. *Biochim. Biophys. Acta* **365**: 372–388.

MAHOUDEAU, J. A. and CORVOL, P. (1973) Rabbit testosterone-binding globulin. I. Physico-chemical properties. *Endocrinology* **92**: 1113–1119.

MARTIN, B., FOUCHET, C. and THIBIER, M. (1976) Steroid-protein interactions in bovine plasma. *J. Reprod. Fert.* **46**: 143–149.

MARUYAMA, Y., AOKI, N., SUZUKI, Y., OHNO, Y., IMAMURA, M., SAIKA, T., SINOHARA, H. and YAMAMOTO, T. (1987) Sex-steroid-binding plasma protein (SBP), testosterone, oestradiol and dehydroepiandrosterone (DHEA) in prepuberty and puberty. *Acta Endocrinol.* **114:** 60–67.

MASOPUST, J., KITHIER, K., RADL, J., KOVTECKY, J. and KOTAL, L. (1968) Occurrence of fetoprotein in patients with neoplasms and non-neoplastic diseases. *Int. J. Cancer* **3:** 364–373.

MAYOL, R. F. and LONGENECKER, D. E. (1974) Development of a radioimmunoassay for blastokinin. *Endocrinology* **95:** 1534–1542.

MCGAUGHEY, R. W. and MURRAY, F. A. (1972) Properties of blastokinin: amino acid composition, evidence for subunits, and estimation of isoelectric point. *Fertil. Steril.* **23:** 399–404.

MEARS, G. J., LAI, P. C. W., VAN PETTEN, G. R. and LORSCHEIDER, F. L. (1981) Fetal-maternal transfer and catabolism of ovine ^{125}I-labeled α-fetoprotein. *Am. J. Physiol.* **240:** E191–E196.

MERCIER, C., ALFSEN, A. and BAULIEU, E. E. (1966) A testosterone binding globulin. *Excerpta Med. Intern. Congr. Ser.* N° 101, p. 212.

MERCIER-BODARD, C., RENOIR, J-M. and BAULIER E-E. (1979) Further characterization and immunological studies of human sex steroid binding plasma protein. *J. Steroid Biochem.* **11:** 253–259.

METZ, DEB, MICOUIN, C. and CHAMBAZ E. M. (1977) Origine placentaire de la proteine de la liaison de la progesterone chez le cobaye gravide: étude immunohistologique. *C. R. Acad. Sci., Paris (Serie D)* **285:** 937–940.

MICKELSON, K. E. and WESTPHAL, U. (1979) Purification and characterization of the corticosteroid-binding globulin of pregnant guinea pig serum. *Biochemistry* **18:** 2685–2690.

MICKELSON, K. E., FORSTHOEFEL, J. and WESTPHAL, U. (1981) Steroid-protein interactions. Human corticosteroid-binding globulin: some physicochemical properties and binding specificity. *Biochemistry* **20:** 6211–6218.

MICKELSON, K. E., HARDING, G. B., FORSTHOEFEL, M. and WESTPHAL, U. (1982) Steroid-protein interactions. Human corticosteroid-binding globulin: characterization of dimer and electrophoretic variants. *Biochemistry* **21:** 654–660.

MILGROM, E., ALLOUCH, P., ATGER, M. and BAULIEU, E.-E. (1973) Progesterone-binding plasma protein of pregnant guinea pig. Purification and characterization. *J. Biol. Chem.* **248:** 1106–1114.

MILLET, A. and PASQUALINI, J. R. (1978) Liaison specifique de la ^{3}H-progesterone a une proteine du plasma du foetus de cobaye. *C. R. Acad. Sci., Paris (Serie D)* **287:** 1429–1432.

MILUNSKY, A., ALPERT, E., NEFF, R. K. and FRIGOLETTO, F. D. (1980) Prenatal diagnosis of neural tube defects. IV. Maternal serum alpha-fetoprotein screening. *Obstet. Gynecol.* **55:** 60–66.

MIURA, K., LAW, S. W. T., NISHI, S. and TAMAOKI, T. (1979) Isolation of α-fetoprotein messenger RNA from mouse yolk sac. *J. Biol. Chem.* **254:** 5515–5521.

MIZEJEWSKI, G. J., VONNEGUT, M. and JACOBSON, H. I. (1983) Estradiol-activated α-fetoprotein suppresses the uterotropic response to estrogens. *Proc. Natl. Acad. Sci. U.S.A.* **80:** 2733–2737.

MOLLGARD, K., JACOBSEN, M., JACOBSEN, G. K. and CLAUSEN, P. P. (1979) Immunohistological evidence for an intracellular localization of plasma proteins in human foetal choroid plexus and brain. *Neurosci. Lett.* **14:** 85–90.

MORO, R. and URIEL, J. (1981) Early localization of alpha-fetoprotein in the developing nervous system of the chicken. *Oncodevelop. Biol. Med.* **2:** 391–398.

MULDOON, T. G. (1967) Isolation and characterization of corticosteroid-binding globulin (transcortin) from human plasma. University of Louisville: Doctoral dissertation.

MULDOON, T. G. and WESTPHAL, U. (1967) Steroid-protein interactions. XV. Isolation and characterization of corticosteroid-binding globulin from human plasma. *J. Biol. Chem.* **242:** 5636.

MURRAY F. A. and DANIEL, J. C. Jr (1973) Synthetic pattern of proteins in rabbit uterine flushings. *Fertil. Steril.* **24:** 692–697.

MURRAY, F. A. and WHITSON, G. L. (1974) Effects of actinomycin D and puromycin on blastokinin synthesis by the rabbit uterus. *Biol. Reprod.* **11**: 421–428.

MURRAY, F. A., McGAUGHEY, R. W. and YARUS, M. J. (1972) Blastokinin: its size and shape, and an indication of the existence of subunits. *Fert. Steril.* **23**: 69–77.

NGUYEN B.-L., HATIER, R., JEANVOINE, G., ROUX, M., GRIGNON, G. and PASQUALINI, J. R. (1988) Effect of estradiol on the progesterone receptor and on morphological ultrastructures in the fetal and newborn uterus and ovary of the rat. *Acta Endocr. (Copenh.)* **117**: 249–259.

NIETO, A. and BEATO, M. (1980) Synthesis and secretion of uteroglobir in rabbit endometrial explants cultured *in vitro*. *Molec. Cell. Endocr.* **17**: 25–39.

NIETO, A., PONSTINGL, H. and BEATO, M. (1977) Purification and quaternary structure of the hormonally induced protein uteroglobin *Arch. Biochem. Biophys.* **180**: 82–92.

NISHI, S. (1970) Isolation and characterization of human fetal α-globulin from the sera of fetuses and a hepatoma patient. *Cancer Res.* **30**: 2507–2513.

NISHI, S. (1975) Chemical and immunological properties of α-fetoprotein. *Taisha* **12**: 3–8.

NOMURA, M., IMAI, M., TAKAHASHI, K., KUMAKURA, T., TACHIBANA, K., AOYAGI, S., USUDA, S., NAKAMURA, T., MIYAKAWA, Y. and MAYUMI, M. (1983) Three-site sandwich radioimmunoassay with monoclonal antibodies for a sensitive determination of human alpha-fetoprotein. *J. Immunol. Meth.* **58**: 293–300.

NØRGAARD-PEDERSEN, B. and AXELSEN, N. H. (1978) Carcinoembryonic proteins. Recent progress. *Scand. J. Immunol.* Suppl. **Vol. 8**: 1–683.

NØRGAARD-PEDERSEN, B., ALBRECHTSEN, R. and TEILUM, G. (1975) Serum alpha-fetoprotein as a marker for endodermal sinus tumor (yolk sac tumor) or a vitelline component of terato-carcinoma. *Acta Pathol. Microbial. Scand.* **83**: 573–589.

NOSKE, I. G. and FEIGELSON, M. (1976) Immunological evidence of uteroglobin (blastokinin) in the male reproductive tract and in nonreproductive ductal tissues and their secretions. *Biol. Reprod.* **15**: 704–713.

NUNEZ, E., ENGELMANN, F., BENASSAYAG, C. and JAYLE, M. F. (1971a) Identification et purification préliminaire de la foetoprotéine liant les oestrogènes dans le sérum de rats nouveau-nés. *C. R. Acad. Sci. (Paris) (Serie D)* **273**: 831–834.

NUNEZ, E., SAVU, L., ENGELMANN, F., BENASSAYAG, C., CREPY, O. and JAYLE, M. F. (1971b) Origine embryonnaire de la protéine sérique fixant l'oestrone et l'oestradiol chez la ratte impubère. *C. R. Acad. Sci. (Paris) (Série D)* **273**: 242–245.

NUNEZ, E. A., BENASSAYAG, C., SAVU, L., VALLETTE, G. and JAYLE, M. F. (1976) Serum binding of some steroid hormones during development in different animal species. Discussion on the biological significance of this binding. *Ann. Biol. Anim. Bioch. Biophys.* **16**: 491–501.

OAKEY, R. E. (1975) Serum cortisol binding capacity and cortisol concentration in the pregnant baboon and its fetus during gestation. *Endocrinology* **97**: 1024–1029.

OBIEKWE, B. C., MALEK, N., KITAU, M. J. and CHARD, T. (1985) Maternal and fetal alphafetoprotein (AFP) levels at term. Relation to sex, weight and gestation of the infant. *Acta Obstet. Gynecol. Scand.* **64**: 251–253.

PASQUALINI, J. R. and NGUYEN, B.-L. (1980) Progesterone receptors in the fetal uterus and ovary of the guinea pig: evolution during fetal development and induction and stimulation in estradiol-primed animals. *Endocrinology* **106**: 1160–1165.

PASQUALINI, J. R., SUMIDA, C. and GELLY, C. (1976) Cytosol and nuclear [^{3}H]oestradiol binding in the foetal tissues of guinea pig. *Acta Endocr. (Copenh)*. **83**: 811–828.

PASQUALINI, J. R., SUMIDA, C., GELLY, C. and NGUYEN, B.-L. (1977) A general view of the quantitative evaluation of cytosol and nuclear steroid hormone receptors in the fetal compartment of guinea-pig. *J. Steroid Biochem.* **8**: 445–451.

PEARLMAN, W. H., SKRZYNIA, C., HAMPEL, M. R., PENG, L.-H. and BERKO, R. M. (1981) The levels of corticosterone-binding proteins in rat milk and coincidental serum, and the dissociation rates of the corticosterone-protein complexes. *Endocrinology* **108:** 741–746.

PEDERSEN, K. O. (1944) Fetuin, a new globulin isolated from serum. *Nature (London)* **154:** 575.

PEDERSEN, K. O. (1947) Ultracentrifugal and electrophoretic studies of fetuin. *J. Phys. Colloid. Chem.* **51:** 164–171.

PERRIN, F. M. and FOREST, M. G. (1975) Time course of the effect of adrenalectomy on transcortin binding characteristics: appraisal of different methods of calculation. *Endocrinology* **96:** 869–878.

PERROT, M. and MILGROM, E. (1978) Immunochemical studies of guinea pig progesterone-binding plasma protein. *Endocrinology* **103:** 1678–1685.

PERROT-APPLANAT, M. and DAVID-FERREIRA, J. F. (1982) Immunocytochemical localization of progesterone-binding protein (PBP) in guinea-pig placental tissue. *Cell Tissue Res.* **223:** 627–639.

PERROT-APPLANAT, M. and MILGROM, E. (1979) Messenger ribonucleic acid for corticosteroid-binding globulin. Translation and preliminary characterization. *Biochemistry* **18:** 5732–5737.

PERROT-APPLANAT, M., DAVID-FERREIRA, J. F. and DAVID-FERREIRA, K. L. (1981) Immunocytochemical localization of corticosteroid-binding globulin (CBG) in guinea pig hepatocytes. *Endocrinology* **109:** 1625–1633.

PETERSON, R. E., NOKES, G., CHEN, P. S. and BLACK, R. L. (1960) Estrogens and adrenocortical function in man. *J. Clin. Endocr. Metab.* **20:** 495–514.

PETRA, P. H., STANCZYK, F. Z., SENEAR, D. F., NAMKUNG, P. C., NOVY, M. J., ROSS, J. B. A., TURNER, E. and BROWN, J. A. (1983) Current status of the molecular structure and function of the plasma sex steroid-binding protein (SBP). *J. Steroid Biochem.* **19:** 699–706.

PIHKO, H. and RUOSLAHTI, E. (1973) High level of alpha-fetoprotein in sera of adult mice. *Int. J. Cancer* **12:** 354–360.

PINEIRO, A., OLIVITO, A.-M. and URIEL, J. (1979) Fixation d'acides gras polyinsaturés par l'alphafoetoprotéine et la sérum albumine de rat. Comparaison avec l'accumulation de ces acides dans le cerveau au cours du développement post-natal. *C. R. Acad. Sci. (Paris) (Série D)* **289:** 1053–1056.

PINEIRO, A., CALVO, M., IGUAZ, F., LAMPREAVE, F. and NAVAL, J. (1982) Characterization, origin and evolution of alpha-fetoprotein and albumin in postnatal rat brain. *Int. J. Biochem.* **14:** 817–823.

PONSTINGL, H., NIETO, A. and BEATO, M. (1978) Amino acid sequence of progesterone-induced rabbit uteroglobin. *Biochemistry* **17:** 3908–3912.

PUTNAM, F. W. (1965) Structure and function of the plasma proteins. In: *The Proteins. Composition, Structure and Function*, Vol. III, Neurath, H. (Ed.), Academic Press, New York, pp. 153–267.

RAYMOURE, W. J. and KUHN, R. W. (1980) Steroid-binding proteins in guinea pig milk and plasma. *Endocrinology* **106:** 1747–1754.

RAYMOURE, W. J. and KUHN, R. W. (1983) A homologous radioimmunoassay for rat corticosteroid-binding globulin. *Endocrinology* **112:** 1091–1097.

RAYNAUD, J.-P. (1973) Influence of rat oestradiol binding plasma protein (EBP) on uterotrophic activity. *Steroids* **21:** 249–258.

RAYNAUD, J.-P., MERCIER-BODARD, C. and BAULIEU, E. E. (1971) Rat estradiol binding plasma protein (EBP). *Steroids* **18:** 767–788.

RENOIR, J. M., MERCIER-BODARD, C. and BAULIEU E-E. (1980) Hormonal and immunological aspects of sex steroid-binding plasma protein of primates. *J. Reprod. Fertil., Suppl.* **28:** 113–119.

RIVAROLA, M. A., FOREST, M. G. and MIGEON, C. J. (1968) Testosterone, androstenedione and dehydroepiandrosterone in plasma during pregnancy and at delivery: concentration and protein binding. *J. Clin. Endocr. Metab.* **28:** 34–40.

ROSENBAUM, W., CHRISTY N. P. and KELLY W. G. (1966) Electrophoretic evidence for the presence of an estrogen-binding β-globulin in human plasma. *J. Clin. Endocr. Metab.* **26:** 1399–1403.

ROSENTHAL, H. E., SLAUNWHITE, W. R. Jr. and SANDBERG, A. A. (1969) Transcortin: a corticosteroid-binding protein of plasma. X. Cortisol and progesterone interplay and unbound levels of these steroids in pregnancy. *J. Clin. Endocr. Metab.* **29:** 352–367.

ROSNER, W. and DARMSTADT, R. A. (1973) Demonstration and partial characterization of a rabbit serum protein which binds testosterone and dihydrotestosterone. *Endocrinology* **92:** 1700–1707.

ROSNER, W. and HOCHBERG, R. (1972) Corticosteroid-binding globulin in the rat: isolation and studies of its influence on cortisol action 'in vivo'. *Endocrinology* **91:** 626–632.

RUOSLAHTI, E. and SEPPALA, M. (1971) Studies of carcinoma-fetal proteins: physical and chemical properties of human α-fetoprotein. *Int. J. Cancer* **7:** 218–225.

RUOSLAHTI, E., HIRAI, H., BELANGER, L., KJESSLER, B., KOHN, J., MASSEYEF, R., NISHI, S., NØRGAARD-PEDERSEN, B., NUNEZ, E. A., SEPPALA, M., TALERMAN, A., and URIEL, J. (1978) Alpha-foetoprotein. *Scand. J. Immunol.* **8** (Supp. 8): 3–26.

SARCIONE, E. J. and BIDDLE, W. (1987) Elevated serum alpha fetoprotein levels in postmenopausal women with primary breast carcinoma. *Disease Markers* **5:** 75–79.

SARCIONE, E. J. and HART, D. (1985) Biosynthesis of alpha-fetoprotein by MCF-7 human breast cancer cells. *Int. J. Cancer* **35:** 315–318.

SAVU, L., CREPY, O., GUERIN, M. A., NUNEZ, E. A., ENGELMANN, F., BENASSAYAG, C. and JAYLE, M. F. (1972) Etudes des constantes de liaison entre les oestrogènes et l'α_1-protéine de rat. *FEBS Lett.* **22:** 113–116.

SAVU, L., NUNEZ, E. A. and JAYLE, M. F. (1974a) Haute affinité du sérum d'embryon de souris pour les oestrogénes. *Biochim. Biophys. Acta* **359:** 273–281.

SAVU, L., VALLETTE, G., NUNEZ, E., AZRIA, M. and JAYLE, M. F. (1974b) Etude comparative de la liaison entre les protéines sériques et les oestrogénes libres au cours du développement de diverses espèces animales. In: *Colloque sur l'Alpha-foetoprotéine, Monographies de l'INSERM*, Nice, France, pp. 75–83.

SCHACHTER, B. S. and TORAN-ALLERAND, C. D. (1982) Intraneuronal α-fetoprotein and albumin are not synthetized locally in developing brain. *Develop. Brain Res.* **5:** 93–98.

SCHILLER, H. S., KULCHINSKI, L. and LUTHY, D. A. (1978) Radioimmunoassay of alpha-fetoprotein, with special reference to iodination and purification techniques. *Clin. Chem.* **24:** 275–279.

SELL, S. (1974) In: *Alpha-fetoprotein*, Masseyeff, R. (Ed.), INSERM, Paris, pp. 365–381.

SELL, S. and ALEXANDER, D. (1974) Rat alpha-fetoprotein. V. Catabolism and fetal-maternal distribution. *J. Natl. Cancer Inst.* **52:** 1483–1489.

SELL, S., LEFFER, H. L., SHINOZUKA, H., LOMBARDI, B. and GOCHMAN, N. (1981) Rapid development of large numbers of alpha-fetoprotein-containing "oval" cells in the liver of rats fed N-2-fluorenyl-acetamide in a choline-devoid diet. *Gann* **72:** 479–487.

SEPPALA, M. (1975) Fetal pathophysiology of human alpha-fetoprotein. *Ann. N. Y. Acad. Sci.* **259:** 59–73.

SEPPALA, M. and RUOSLAHTI, E. (1972) Radioimmunoassay of maternal serum alpha-fetoprotein during pregnancy and delivery. *Am. J. Obstet. Gynecol.* **112:** 208–212.

SEPPALA, M. and RUOSLAHTI, E. (1976) Alpha-fetoprotein. *Contr. Gynec. Obstet.* **2:** 143–186.

SHEN, X. Z., TSAI, M. J., BULLOCK, D. W. and WOO, S. L. C. (1983) Hormonal regulation of rabbit uteroglobin gene transcription. *Endocrinology* **112:** 871–876.

SLADE, B. and MILNE, J. (1978) The ontogeny of alpha-foetoprotein in the chicken. *Experientia* **34:** 520–522.

SLAUNWHITE, W. R., Jr and SANDBERG, A. A. (1959) Transcortin: a corticosteroid-binding protein of plasma. *J. Clin. Invest.* **38:** 384–

SMITH, K. M., LAI, P. C. W., ROBERTSON, H. A., CHURCH, R. B. and LORSCHEIDER, F. L. (1979) Distribution of alpha$_1$-fetoprotein in fetal plasma, allantoic fluid, amniotic fluid and maternal plasma of cows. *J. Reprod. Fert.* **57:** 235–238.

SOLOFF, M. S., CREANGE, J. E. and POTTS, G. O. (1971) Unique estrogen-binding properties of rat pregnancy plasma. *Endocrinology* **88:** 427–432.

SOLOFF, M. S., SWARTZ, S. K., PEARLMUTTER, F. A. and KITHIER, K. (1976) Binding of
17β-estradiol by variants of AFP in rat amniotic fluid. *Biochim. Biophys. Acta* **427**: 644–651.

SOWERS, S. G., REISH, R. L. and BURTON, B. K. (1983) Fetal sex-related differences in maternal serum α-fetoprotein during the second trimester of pregnancy. *Am. J. Obstet. Gynecol.* **146**: 786–789.

STREL'CHYONOK, O. A., SURVILO, L. I., TSAPELIK, G. Z. and SVIRIDOV, O. V. (1983)
Purification and physicochemical properties of the sex steroid-binding globulin of human blood
plasma. *Biokhimiya* **48**: 756–762.

STROUPE, S. D. and WESTPHAL, U. (1975a) Conformational changes in the progesterone binding
globulin-progesterone complex. *Biochemistry* **14**: 3296–3300.

STROUPE, S. D. and WESTPHAL, U. (1975b) Steroid-protein interactions. XXXIII. Stopped-flow
fluorescence studies of the interaction between steroid hormones and progesterone-binding globulin. *J.
Biol. Chem.* **250**: 8735–8739.

STROUPE, S. D., HARDING, G. B., FORSTHOEFEL, M. H. and WESTPHAL, U. (1978) Kinetic
and equilibrium studies on steroid interaction with human corticosteroid-binding globulin. *Biochemistry*
17: 177–182.

SUZUKI, Y. and SINOHARA, H. (1984) Subunit structure of sex-steroid binding plasma proteins from
man, cattle, dog, and rabbit. *J. Biochem.* **96**: 751–759.

SUZUKI, Y., ITAGAKI, E., MORI, H. and HOSOYA, T. (1977) Isolation of testosterone-binding
globulin from bovine serum by affinity chromatography and its molecular characterization. *J. Biochem.*
81: 1721–1731.

SUZUKI, Y., OKUMURA, Y. and SINOHARA, H. (1979) Purification and characterization of
testosterone-binding globulin of canine serum. *J. Biochem.* **85**: 1195–1203.

SWARTZ, S. K. and SOLOFF, M. S. (1974) The lack of estrogen binding by human α-fetoprotein. *J.
Clin. Endocr. Metab.* **39**: 589–591.

SYKES, S. and DENNIS, P. M. (1977) Electroradioimmunoassay: a sensitive method for the quantitation
of alpha-fetoprotein. *Clin. Chim. Acta* **79**: 309–316.

TATARINOV, Y. S. (1965) Content of embryospecific α-globulin in the blood serum of human fetus,
newborn, and adult man in primary cancer of liver. *Vopr. Med. Khim.* **11**: 20–24.

TORKKELI, T., KRUSIUS, T. and JANNE, O. (1978) Uterine and lung uteroglobins in the rabbit.
Two similar proteins with differential hormonal regulation. *Biochim. Biophys. Acta* **544**: 578–592.

TROJAN, J. and URIEL, J. (1979) Localisation intracellulaire de l'alpha-foetoprotéine et de la sérumal-
bumine dans le systeme nerveux central du rat au cours du développement foetal et postnatal. *C. R.
Acad. Sci. (Paris) (Série D)* **289**: 1157–1160.

TROJAN, J. and URIEL, J. (1980) Immunochemical localization of alphafetoprotein in the developing
rat brain. *Oncodevelop. Biol. Med.* **1**: 107–111.

TROJAN, J. and URIEL, J. (1986) Localisation de l'alpha-foetoprotéine (AFP) au cours de l'ontogenèse
in vivo et *in vitro*. In: *Binding proteins of Steroid Hormones, Colloque INSERM*, Vol. 149, pp. 483–496.

TUCZECK, H. V., FRITZ, P., WAGNER, T., BRAVN, V., GRAW, A. and WEGNER, G. (1981)
Synthesis of alpha-fetoprotein (AFP) and cell proliferation in regenerating livers of NMRI mice after
partial hepatectomy. An immunohistochemical and autoradiography study with [^{3}H]-thymidine.
Virchows Arch. (Cell Pathol.) **38**: 229–237.

TULCHINSKY, D. and OKADA, D. (1975) Hormones in human pregnancy. IV. Plasma progesterone.
Am. J. Obstet. Gynecol. **121**: 293–299.

URIEL, J., DE NECHAUD, B. and DUPIERS, M. (1972) Estrogen-binding properties of rat, mouse and
man foeto-specific serum protein. Demonstration by immuno-autoradiographic methods. *Biochem.
Biophys. Res. Commun.* **46**: 1175–1180.

URIEL, J., AUSSEL, C., BOUILLON, D., DE NECHAUD, B. and LOISILLIER, F. (1973) Localization of rat liver alpha-foetoprotein by cell affinity labelling with tritiated oestrogens. *Nature New Biol.*
244: 190–192.

URIEL, J., DUPIERS, M., RIMBAUT, C. and BUFFE, D. (1981A) Maternal serum levels of sex steroid-binding protein during pregnancy. *Brit. J. obstet. Gynaecol.* **88:** 1229–1232.

URIEL, J., FAIVRE-BAUMAN, A., TROJAN, J. and FOIRET, D. (1981B) Immunocytochemical demonstration of alpha-fetoprotein uptake by primary cultures of fetal hemispher cells from mouse brain. *Neurosci. Lett.* **27:** 171–175.

VALLETTE, G. (1986) Alpha-foetoproteine et reponse immunitaire. In: *Binding Proteins of Steroid Hormones, Colloque INSERM,* Vol. 149, pp. 441–451.

VALLETTE, G., BENASSAYAG, C. SAVU, L., DELORME, J., NUNEZ, E. A., DOUMAS, J., MAUME, G. and MAUME, B. F. (1980) The serum competitor of oestrogen-rat alpha-foetoprotein interaction. Identification as a mixture of non-esterified fatty acids. *Biochem. J.* **187:** 851–856.

VAN BAELEN, H., VANDOREN, G., and DE MOOR, P. (1977a) Concentration of transcortin in the pregnant rat and its foetuses. *J. Endocr.* **75:** 427–431.

VAN BAELEN, H., ADAM-HEYLEN, M., VANDOREN, G. and DE MOOR, P. (1977b) Neonatal imprinting of serum transcortin levels in the rat. *J. Steroid Biochem.* **8:** 735–736.

VERMEULEN, A., VERDONCK, L., VAN DER STRAETEN, M. and ORIE, N. (1969) Capacity of the testosterone-binding globulin in human plasma and influence of specific binding of testosterone on its metabolic clearance rate. *J. Clin. Endocr. Metab.* **29:** 1470–1480.

VERSEE, V. and BAREL, A. O. (1978a) Rat alpha-foetoprotein. Purification, physicochemical characterization, oestrogen-binding properties and chemical modification of the thiol group. *Biochem. J.* **175:** 73–81.

VERSEE, V. and BAREL, A. O. (1978b) Characterization of the binding properties of rat alpha-fetoprotein (AFP). *FEBS Lett.* **96:** 155–158.

VEYSSIERE, G., BERGER, M., CORRE, M., JEAN-FAUCHER, C., DETURCKHEIM, M. and JEAN, C. (1979) Percentage binding of testosterone and dihydrotestosterone and unbound testosterone and dihydrotestosterone in rabbit maternal and fetal plasma during sexual organogenesis. *Steroids* **34:** 305–317.

VILLACAMPA, M. J., LAMPREAVE, F., CALVO, M., NAVAL, J., PINEIRO, A. and URIEL, J. (1984) Incorporation of radiolabelled alphafetoprotein in the brain and other tissues of the developing rat. *Develop. Brain. Res.* **12:** 77–82.

WATABE, H. (1974) Purification and chemical characterization of α-fetoprotein from rat and mouse. *Int. J. Cancer* **13:** 377–388.

WEISS, P. A. M., PURSTNER, P., LICHTENEGGER, W. and WINTER, R. (1978) Alpha-fetoprotein content of amniotic fluid in normal and abnormal pregnancies. *Obstet. Gynecol.* **51:** 582–585.

WESTPHAL, U. (1958) Diffusion of progesterone and deoxycorticosterone into nitrocellulose (Lusteroid): a potential source of error in ultracentrifugation. *J. Lab. Clin. Med.* **51:** 473–478.

WESTPHAL, U. (1966) Steroid-protein interactions. XII. Distribution of progesterone and corticosteroid hormone among serum proteins. *Hoppe-Seylers Z. physiol. Chem.* **346:** 243–256.

WESTPHAL, U. (1971) Steroid-Protein Interactions. In: *Monographs on Endocrinology,* Gross, F., Labhart, A., Mann, T., Samuels, L. T. and Zander J. (Eds), Vol. 4. Springer-Verlag, Berlin, Heidelberg, New York.

WESTPHAL U. (1986) Steroid protein interactions II. In *Monographs on Endocrinology,* Gross F., Grumbach M. M., Labhart A., Lipsett M. B., Mann T., Sumuels L. T. and Zander J. (Eds), Springer-Verlag, Berlin, Heidelberg, New York, Tokyo.

WESTPHAL, U., STROUPE, S. D. and CHENG, S.-L. (1977a) Progesterone binding to serum proteins. *Ann. N. Y. Acad. Sci.* **286:** 10–28.

WESTPHAL, U., STROUPE, S. D., KUTE, T. and CHENG, S.-L. (1977b) Steroid interactions with progesterone-binding globulin. *J. Steroid Biochem.* **8:** 367–374.

WOLF, G., ARMSTRONG, E. R. and ROSNER, W. (1981) Synthesis 'in vitro' of corticosteroid-binding globulin from rat liver messenger ribonucleic acid. *Endocrinology* **108:** 805–811.

WONG, P. Y., DORAN, T. A., HO, F. F. K. and MEE, A. V. (1979) Evaluation of four "kit" immunoassay methods for determination of alpha-fetoprotein in serum during pregnancy. *Clin. Chem.* **25:** 1905–1908.

WOODS, J. A. (1983) Cellular immunolocalization of α-fetoprotein in rat liver. *Histochem. J.* **15:** 1021–1028.

WU, C. H., MENNUTI, M. T. and MIKHAIL, G. (1979) Free and protein-bound steroids in amniotic fluid of mid-pregnancy. *Am. J. Obstet. Gynecol.* **133:** 666–672.

YACHNIN, S., HSU, R., HEINRIKSON, R. L. and MILLER, J. B. (1977) Studies on human α-fetoprotein. Isolation and characterization of monomeric and polymeric forms and amino-terminal sequence analysis. *Biochim. Biophys. Acta.* **493:** 418–428.

YAMAMOTO, S. and OHSAWA, N. (1976) Effects of dexamethasone on the levels of plasma corticosteroid binding globulin in rat and monkeys. *Biochem. Biophys. Res. Commun.* **72:** 489–498.

YAMAMOTO, R., KIMURA, S., MATSUURA, A., FUKUDA, Y., HAYAKAWA, T. and KATO, K. (1986) Two-site enzyme immunoassay for α-fetoprotein involving column chromatography. *J. Immunol. Meth.* **87:** 197–201.

YANG CHOU, J. and SAVITZ, A. J. (1986) Alpha-fetoprotein synthesis in transformed fetal rat liver cells. *Biochem. Biophys. Res. Commun.* **135:** 844–851.

YANNONE, M. E., MUELLER, J. R. and OSBORN, R. H. (1969) Protein binding of progesterone in the peripheral plasma during pregnancy and labor. *Steroids* **13:** 773–781.

YOSHA, S., LONGCOPE, C. and BRAVERMAN, L. E. (1984) The effect of D- and L-thyroxine on sex hormone-binding globulin in rabbits. *Endocrinology* **115:** 1446–1450.

YOUNG, C. E., SMITH, R. G. and BULLOCK, D. W. (1981) Uteroglobin mRNA and levels of nuclear progesterone receptor in endometrium. *Molec. Cell. Endocr.* **22:** 105–112.

ZIMMERMAN, E. F., BOWEN, D., WILSON, J. R. and MADAPPALLY, H. M. (1976) Developmental microheterogeneity of mouse alpha-proteins: purification and partial characterization. *Biochemistry* **15:** 5534–5543.

2

Receptors, Mechanism of Action and Biological Responses of Hormones in the Fetal, Placental and Maternal Compartments

Contents

Introduction

Steroid Hormone Receptors: Historical Background and Present Concepts

The idea that hormones, in analogy to drugs, bind to components in tissues which respond biologically to the hormonal signal goes back as far as the beginning of this century when Langley (1905) and later Ehrlich (1913) proposed that drugs act by first binding to 'receptors'. Considerable work and effort have been devoted over the years to the demonstration of a particular hormone–target tissue interaction which would later determine the biological changes observed in the target tissue in response to hormone treatment.

During the 1950s, Szego and Roberts (1953) and Mueller *et al.* (1958) in their study of the action of estrogens, hypothesized that the interaction of estrogens with some tissue component was the initial step in the mechanism of action of the hormone. However, proof of this interaction remained elusive; methods and reagents available at the time required injection of pharmacological amounts of estrogens due to the low specific radioactivity of the ^{14}C-labelled compounds used (Twombly, 1951; Twombly and Schoenewaldt, 1951; Hanahan *et al.*, 1953; Budy, 1955). Under these conditions, it was generally observed that estrogens did not accumulate in specific target organs.

What was necessary was a method permitting the detection of very small doses of hormone, preferably in the physiological range, to demonstrate selective localization in hormone sensitive tissues. This became available when Glascock and Hoekstra in 1959 and Jensen and Jacobson in 1960 used tritium-labelled compounds of higher specific activity to show for the first time that a synthetic compound with estrogenic properties ($[^{3}H]$-diethylstilbestrol) and the natural estrogen ($[^{3}H]$-estradiol), were selectively accumulated and retained by organs known to respond to estrogens (uterus, vagina, pituitary). These observations have triggered a whole body of continuing research on the nature of the binding components responsible for this selective affinity and their role in the mechanism of action of hormones (among numerous reviews, see King and Mainwaring, 1974; Clark and Peck, 1979; Muldoon, 1980; Grody *et al.*, 1982; Clark and Markaverich, 1988).

The tenet that receptors mediate steroid hormone action has served as the basis for studies not only on estrogen receptors but also for receptors of other steroid hormones which have since been characterized and widely studied: glucocorticoids (Munck and

Brinck-Johnsen, 1968); androgens (Fang *et al.*, 1969); progesterone (Sherman *et al.*, 1970) and mineralocorticoids (Herman *et al.*, 1968).

The term 'receptor' has been applied to designate the intracellular or membrane proteins to which steroid and polypeptide hormones bind and which mediate their biological effects. Receptors provide the underlying specificity and sensitivity for hormone activity. Although the term is sometimes loosely interpreted for reasons of facility, it excludes other macromolecules such as serum proteins to which hormones can also bind (see Chapter 1). Steroid hormone receptors are intracellular proteins that interact directly with hormone-responsive elements of the genome to induce transcription. As will be seen in the following section, peptide hormone receptors are integral cell membrane proteins that trigger a cascade of events mediated by signal transducers that modulate post-translational changes of proteins or regulate transcription.

In 1964, Talwar *et al.* and, in 1966, Toft and Gorski established some of the characteristics which now describe steroid hormone receptor macromolecules in general. The estrogen receptor studied was a protein found in the cytosol fraction after homogenization of the rat uterus, sedimenting at 8.5–9 S in low ionic strength sucrose density gradients and having a high affinity for estradiol. The binding sites were saturable and specific for estrogens. After binding to the hormone, the receptor was shown to undergo a transformation in its conformation to a form with higher affinity for nuclear acceptor sites which could be recognized by a decrease in its sedimentation coefficient to 4–5 S in high ionic strength sucrose density gradients. Besides having these characteristics, receptors are also preferentially found in hormone target organs or cells, and the binding of a hormone to its receptor should be correlated with a biological response.

It was previously thought that the unoccupied receptor resided in the cytoplasmic compartment of the cell and that upon binding to its specific hormone, the receptor underwent a translocation from the cytoplasm to nuclear acceptor sites. However, recent lines of evidence are more consistent with the idea that the receptor is localized mainly in the nucleus. In the absence of hormone, the receptor is so loosely associated with nuclear elements that it is extractable during homogenization. After binding the hormone, the receptor develops a stronger affinity for DNA. Sheridan *et al.* observed in 1979 by autoradiography under 'non-translocating' conditions that most of the estrogen receptor was already in the nucleus. In cytochalasin B-enucleated cells, the concentration of estrogen receptor was found to be low in cytoplasts, and there was no evidence that removing most of the cytoplasm of the cell removed any of the unoccupied receptor (Welshons *et al.*, 1985). Immunohistochemical studies with specific monoclonal antibodies to the estrogen receptor detected antibody binding predominantly in the nucleus, not in the cytoplasm, even in the absence of hormone (King and Greene, 1984). Similar observations have also been made for the mammalian progesterone receptor (Perrot-Applanat *et al.*, 1985) and for the androgen receptor (Tan *et al.*, 1988). However, some controversy still exists as to the subcellular localization of estrogen receptors (Clark and Markaverich, 1988).

Unlike the sex hormone receptors, the ligand-free glucocorticoid receptor (and probably the mineralocorticoid receptor as well (Krozowski *et al.*, 1989)) is largely localized in the cytoplasm (Antakly and Eisen, 1984; Wikström *et al.*, 1987; Picard and Yamamoto, 1987) although conflicting data also exist for the glucocorticoid receptor (Welshons, *et al.*, 1985).

The availability of specific monoclonal antibodies to receptor proteins has opened new perspectives in receptor research since it is now possible to detect receptors by their antigenic sites instead of by radioactive ligand binding. Monoclonal antibodies have greatly promoted the development of techniques for the purification of steroid hormone receptors and the subsequent advance in the knowledge of steroid receptor structure and the different aspects of the molecular biology of receptor–gene interactions.

Functional analyses have shown that steroid hormone receptors act as transcriptional enhancer factors. They interact with inducible regulatory sequences (hormone-responsive elements situated upstream of specific hormone-inducible genes) that regulate biological processes through modulation of transcription of these genes (Payvar *et al.*, 1981; Jost *et al.*, 1985; Green and Chambon, 1988).

Steroid hormone receptor genes have been cloned, and great progress has been made in elucidating their structure and their functional domains (Green *et al.*, 1986; Green and Chambon, 1988; Evans, 1988). cDNAs for all known steroid receptors have been isolated and sequenced (Hollenberg *et al.*, 1985; Green *et al.*, 1986; Jeltsch *et al.*, 1986; Arriza *et al.*, 1987; McDonnell *et al.*, 1987; Chang *et al.*, 1988). Site-directed mutagenesis has permitted the identification of domains of the receptor proteins responsible for ligand binding, DNA binding, *trans* activation of transcription, dimerization and immunogenicity, and the amino acid sequences have been deduced from the nucleotide sequences (Green and Chambon, 1988).

The ligand-binding domain is situated at the carboxyl terminus of the protein and contains a large number of hydrophobic amino acids. Hormone binding is thought to dissociate the 90 000 Da heat shock protein from the hormone-binding domain, to lead to conformational changes in receptor structure and to unmask the DNA-binding domain. Receptor dimers are then formed that bind tightly to the hormone-responsive element. Hormone-responsive elements are 15 base pair palindromes that show great structural similarity, much as the DNA binding domains of the receptor proteins. The DNA-binding domain, located about 330 residues from the carboxyl end of the molecule, is rich in cysteines and basic amino acids and is highly conserved among steroid receptors. Between the ligand-binding and DNA-binding domains there exists a short region, highly variable in both composition and length, that is thought to act as a hinge facilitating folding of the ligand-binding domain onto the DNA-binding region. Towards the amino terminus of the protein is a region of comparatively low homology which is highly variable in length between receptors. This region represents the immunogenic domain and is largely responsible for the differences observed in molecular size between steroid receptors (Godowski *et al.*, 1987; Kumar *et al.*, 1987; Pratt, 1987; Green and Chambon, 1988; Denis *et al.*, 1988).

The steroid hormone receptors belong to a superfamily of ligand-activated transcription factors with structural similarities that also includes thyroid hormone, vitamin D_3 and retinoic acid (vitamin A-related metabolite) receptors (Evans, 1988). Furthermore, sequence analysis of the receptors has revealed that they are related to the product of the v-erb-A oncogene of avian erythroblastosis virus and the c-erb-A proto-oncogene (Weinberger *et al.*, 1985, 1986; Green *et al.*, 1986; Sap *et al.*, 1986). This relationship indicates that these molecules may all be part of a superfamily of regulatory proteins that have arisen over evolutionary time.

Polypeptide Hormone Receptors

Like the steroid hormones, the first step in peptide hormone action is the specific binding to receptors. Binding sites for peptide hormones are localized almost exclusively at the surface of their target cells in the plasma membrane fraction. Polypeptide hormone receptors are integral transmembrane proteins with the specific hormone binding site at the extracellular amino terminus and an intracellular domain at the carboxyl terminus that possesses intrinsic tyrosine kinase activity.

Polypeptide hormone membrane receptors can only be extracted by procedures that extensively disrupt the membrane, but nonionic detergents such as Triton X-100 solubilize the receptor while preserving its binding properties (Cuatrecasas, 1972). Polypeptide hormone membrane receptors have been purified and their structure and function are being studied (Jacobs and Cuatrecasas, 1981; Van Obberghen and Gammeltoft, 1986; Dufau and Kusuda, 1987; Hazum and Conn, 1988). These receptors are glycoproteins, and phospholipids appear to be important components of a number of membrane receptors.

Antibodies have been developed against some purified peptide hormone receptors. Antibodies have been raised against the purified GnRH (gonadotropin-releasing hormone) receptor that appear to recognize domains of the receptor other than the hormone binding site (Hazum *et al.*, 1987). A series of monoclonal antibodies has been produced against the human insulin receptor that recognizes either the intracellular protein kinase domain (Morgan and Roth, 1986) or the extracellular ligand binding domain of the receptor (Soos, *et al.* 1986). A polyclonal antibody has been prepared against highly purified rat luteal LH/CG receptor whose epitope is not in the ligand binding domain (Rosemblit *et al.*, 1988).

The presence of specific receptors for LH (luteinizing hormone) in the ovary and testis was first demonstrated by autoradiographic localization of radioiodinated LH or hCG (human chorionic gonadotropin) (DeKrester *et al.*, 1969, 1971) and by the ability of these tissues to bind preferentially labeled LH or hCG *in vitro* (Catt *et al.*, 1971; Dufau and Catt, 1978). Results from numerous studies have clearly demonstrated that receptors for LH are localized in the plasma membrane of target cells (Catt *et al.*, 1972). FSH (follicle-stimulating hormone) receptors have also been demonstrated in the testis, particularly in plasma membrane fractions from the seminferous tubule (Means and Vaitukaitis, 1972).

In rat luteal cells the majority of LH/hCG binding sites are localized along regions of the cell surface facing capillaries, which is characterized by microvillus folds, whereas the basolateral surfaces of the luteal cells are characterized by junctional complexes and contain very few binding sites (Anderson *et al.*, 1979). Not only are receptors for LH localized in the plasma membrane, they also appear to be concentrated in specific regions of the membrane and not distributed uniformly over the entire cell surface.

Binding sites with high specificity and affinity for prolactin and other lactogenic hormones have been demonstrated in the mammary gland (Posner *et al.*, 1974). Analysis of the binding properties of prolactin receptors has shown considerable overlap with the behavior of growth hormone receptors, in particular with that of human growth hormone (hGH) (Posner, 1976). Human growth hormone also interacts with specific receptors present in human cells that do not interact with other growth hormones or prolactin (Lesniak *et al.*, 1973; Carr and Friesen, 1976). The location of the prolactin receptors is predominantly at the plasma membrane (Shiu and Friesen, 1974b) but intracellular sites in the Golgi apparatus have also been demonstrated (Nolin and Witorsch, 1976).

The binding of polypeptide hormones to their specific receptors at the cell surface initiates a chain of intracellular events, mediated by second messenger signal transducers (Rozengurt, 1986). The final result of this chain of events is the appropriate biological response by the target cell to the hormone.

The receptor for LH is linked biochemically to the enzyme adenylate cyclase and binding of LH to this receptor results in activation of adenylate cyclase (Marsh, 1975; Dufau and Catt, 1978). Intracellular cAMP that is produced binds to the regulatory subunit of the cAMP-dependent protein kinase (Flockhard and Corbin, 1982) and activates this enzyme to phosphorylate endogenous protein substrates which results in altered activity of these biological regulators leading to a response. It is generally accepted that all of the intracellular effects of cAMP are mediated via the cAMP-dependent protein kinase (Kuo and Greengard, 1969).

The activity of cAMP-dependent protein kinase is enhanced in steroidogenic tissue and the increase in protein kinase activity and steroid secretion are highly correlated. Besides the post-translational phosphorylation of proteins, protein kinases may influence nuclear events, gene expression and protein synthesis (Jungmann and Hunzicker-Dunn, 1978). Cyclic AMP-dependent protein kinase can phosphorylate proteins in the cytoplasm or act through cAMP response elements in the promoter regions of cAMP-regulated genes (Waterman *et al.*, 1985; Comb *et al.*, 1986; Short *et al.*, 1986; Hoeffler *et al.*, 1989).

Other mediators also serve as transducers of the hormonal stimulus. Calcium and its intracellular receptor calmodulin and Ca^{2+}-phospholipid dependent protein kinase C are probably involved as signal transducers of GnRH action (Conn, 1986; Hazum and Conn, 1988). An increase in transmembrane Ca^{2+} flux in response to GnRH could be measured (Clapper and Conn, 1985). Calmodulin, after binding Ca^{2+}, alters the activity of several enzymes and cytoskeletal proteins implicated in the secretory process (Chafouleas *et al.*, 1982) and has been found to localize in association with the GnRH receptor after GnRH treatment (Jennes *et al.*, 1985). GnRH has also been shown to produce rapid increases in 1,2-diacylglycerol (Andrews and Conn, 1986) that activates protein kinase C activity (Nishizuka, 1986).

The intrinsic receptor protein kinase activity represents another means of transducing the hormonal signal. The binding of insulin to its receptor activates the receptor protein tyrosine kinase. Receptor protein kinase activity leads to autophosphorylation of the receptor and also leads to increased phosphorylation of other cellular proteins (Herrera and Rosen, 1987). Receptor kinase activity then triggers a cascade of events resulting in the final hormone effects. Phosphorylation is reversible so that receptor function is regulated in a positive as well as a negative manner.

Many laboratories have shown an association of several polypeptide hormones with nuclei of target cells (Burwen and Jones, 1987). This evidence requires that an alternative transport pathway exists, resulting in delivery of endocytosed polypeptide to the nucleus instead of lysosomes. Polypeptides may exert at least some of their biological effects directly at the nuclear level.

Upon binding to its membrane receptor, the polypeptide hormone is internalized into the target cell by receptor-mediated endocytosis. The newly formed endocytic vesicles

provide the structural basis for the subsequent vesicular transport of the receptor–
ligand complexes to the lysosomal compartment of the target cell. Lysosomal degradation of the receptor–ligand complexes accounts for the down-regulation of receptors
and the self-limiting response of the target cell to hormone-induced stimulation.
Physiological increases in endogenous hormone positively regulates membrane receptors
but major elevations in circulating hormone often cause down-regulation of LH
receptors and desensitization in target cells (Dufau and Catt, 1978; Dufau *et al.*, 1984).

Receptors in the Fetal, Maternal and Placental Compartments

During gestation in most animal species, the different hormones increase very
sharply, particularly after mid-gestation. For instance, estrogens in human pregnancy
reach values 100–1000 times higher than in the nonpregnant states, and progesterone
increases 10–100 times (see Volume I, Chapter 2). The biological role of these higher
quantities of the hormone produced and circulating in both the fetal and maternal
compartments is not very well established. However, with the discovery in the early
1970s of the presence of estrogen receptors in the fetal brain (Pasqualini and Palmada,
1971) and in the fetal uterus (Pasqualini and Nguyen, 1976), and of mineralocorticoid
receptors in the fetal kidney (Pasqualini and Sumida, 1971) of guinea-pigs, as well as
the demonstration of a correlation of estrogen receptors with biological responses, an
important step was reached in a better understanding of hormone action during fetal
life. Subsequently, the presence of other steroid and polypeptide hormones was demonstrated in different fetal target organs and in the placenta of various species. This
chapter will deal with the ontogeny of the structure and function of some receptor
systems in a variety of organs during gestation. Wherever possible, the presence of
receptors will be discussed in relation to their biological activity. Comparisons will be
made between receptors, biological action and the large changes in hormonal milieu
which occur during gestation. It will be shown that receptors for several different
hormones co-habitate in the same tissues and one hormone can also have several
'target' organs where its receptor has been found to be localized. Changes taking place
concomitantly in the fetal and maternal compartments will be evoked.

A. ESTROGEN RECEPTORS

1. In the Fetal Compartment

1.1. Guinea-pigs

The mammalian fetus for which the most ample information exists on estrogen
receptors during gestation is the guinea-pig (for review see Pasqualini *et al.*, 1983b;
Sumida and Pasqualini, 1985; Pasqualini and Sumida, 1986). The guinea-pig fetus has
proven to be an excellent model system for several reasons: 1. the length of gestation
of this rodent is very long (59–72 days), fascilitating studies at many stages of
development; 2. four of the natural hormones present are the same as in the human
(estradiol, estriol, progesterone and cortisol); 3. a major part of the plasma estrogen
in the guinea-pig fetus is in the form of sulfo-conjugates; 4. estrogens do not bind in

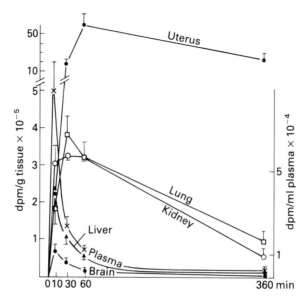

FIG 2.1. Concentration of ^{3}H-Estradiol (Expressed as dpm/g Tissue) in the Fetal
Organs and Plasma of the Guinea-pig, as a Function of Time, after Subcutaneous
Injection of ^{3}H-Estradiol to the Fetus.
Mean values ±SD. Quoted from Gulino and Pasqualini (1980).

a significant fashion to plasma proteins. The study of estrogen receptor binding in fetal
rats is hampered by the presence of α-fetoprotein, a plasma protein with high affinity
for estradiol in rats and mice (see Chapter 1). The fetal guinea-pig uterus has been
studied extensively because it was possible not only to demonstrate the presence of
specific estrogen receptors in this tissue very early in fetal development but also to
correlate receptors with the biological activity of estrogens in the fetal uterus. Estrogen
receptors have also been found in other reproductive organs (vagina, ovary, testes) and
in other organs such as the brain, thymus, kidney and lung.

The presence of a macromolecule with high affinity and specificity for ^{3}H-estradiol in
uterine cytosol and nucleus of fetal guinea-pigs was shown by Pasqualini and Nguyen
in 1976. Other data also indicated that the fetal guinea-pig uterus selectively retains
^{3}H-estradiol as compared to other fetal organs after injection of ^{3}H-estradiol to the fetus
(Fig. 2.1) (Gulino and Pasqualini, 1980) and, by autoradiography, a higher density of
silver grains corresponding to radioactive estradiol injected to the fetus was shown to be
localized in the fetal uterus (Pasqualini et al., 1978a).

1.1.1. UTERUS

1.1.1.1. Physicochemical Properties of the Estrogen Receptor

The physicochemical characteristics of the estrogen receptor in the fetal guinea-pig
uterus which are shown in Table 2.1 are similar to those of the receptor present in

immature or mature uteri of other animal species (for review see King and Mainwaring, 1974) except for the remarkably high concentration of binding sites per cell. With the technique used, most ($>90\%$) of these binding sites are found in the cytosol fraction and about 90% are not occupied by endogenous hormone (Sumida and Pasqualini, 1979a). As seen in Table 2.2, the subcellular distribution of estrogen receptor reflects the relatively low circulating unconjugated estrogen concentrations, and the concentration of binding sites already occupied by endogenous hormone corresponds well with the amount of estradiol plus estrone actually present in the whole uterine tissue itself. The large quantities of high affinity estrogen receptor sites in the uterus enable the fetus to concentrate estrogens in the uterus in the face of relatively low concentrations of circulating estradiol and estrone, the uterus containing 3–20 times more of these estrogens than other tissues studied (lung, kidney and brain) (Gelly *et al.*, 1981).

The estrogen receptor in fetal uterus also binds ^{3}H-estriol and ^{3}H-estrone with high affinity so that the physiological significance of other estrogens cannot be neglected. Estrone and estriol competitively inhibit ^{3}H-estradiol binding to macromolecules in fetal uterine cytosol. The relative binding affinities are 40% for estrone and 20% for estriol (Pasqualini *et al.*, 1980a; Lanzone *et al.*, 1983). Estriol and estrone dissociate more

TABLE 2.1. *Physicochemical Properties of Cytosol Estrogen Receptor in Fetal Guinea-pig Uterus (55–65 Days of Gestation)*

Number of sites	12–19 pmol/mg DNA
	1–2 pmol/mg protein
	40–100 pmol/g tissue
	4–7 pmol/uterus
	40 000–70 000 sites/cell
$K_d{}^a$ ($\times 10^{-9}$ M), 4° C	0.4
$k_{+1}{}^b$ ($\times 10^5$ M^{-1} sec^{-1}), 4° C	0.5
$k_{-1}{}^c$ ($\times 10^{-6}$ sec^{-1}), 4° C	2.2
$k_{-1}{}^c$ ($\times 10^{-4}$ sec^{-1}), 25° C	1.9
Binding specificity	Estradiol > estrone > estriol
	No binding of nonestrogens
Sedimentation coefficient (S)	8 S in low salt
	4 S in high salt
Isoelectric point (pI)	6.1–6.2
DEAE chromatography	Elutes at 0.15–0.2 M KCl
Ammonium sulfate precipitation	36%
Proteolysis	Destroyed
Thermal stability	Labile at 37° C
Immunorecognition	Binds to monoclonal antibody against human estrogen receptor

[a]dissociation constant; [b]association rate constant; [c]dissociation rate constant. Quoted from Pasqualini and Nguyen (1976); Pasqualini and Cosquer-Clavreul (1978); Sumida and Pasqualini (1979a,b); Gulino *et al.* (1981); Giambiagi and Pasqualini (1982); Gulino and Pasqualini (1982); Screpanti *et al.* (1982); Giambiagi *et al.* (1984).

TABLE 2.2. *Comparison of the Subcellular Distribution of Estrogen Receptor in the Uterus and Endogenous Unconjugated Estrogens of the Fetal Guinea-pig*

Estrogen receptor (pmol/mg tissue)				Estrogen concentrations			
				Tissue concentration		Plasma concentration	
		Total cytosol + nuclear					
Cytosol	Nuclear	Unoccupied sites	Occupied sites	Estradiol Estrone (pmol/mg tissue)		Estradiol Estrone (pmol/ml plasma)	
75.0 ± 10.5	5.0 ± 2.3	70.9 ± 9.3	9.1 ± 3.5	4.6 ± 0.2	5.5 ± 0.9	0.09 ± 0.02	0.35 ± 0.08

Unoccupied and occupied receptor binding sites are the sum of cytosol and nuclear binding. The receptor concentrations and endogenous hormone levels in fetal plasma and whole fetal uterine tissue are from fetuses at the end of gestation (55–65 days). Means $\pm$ SE
Quoted from Sumida and Pasqualini (1979a); Gelly *et al.* (1981).

rapidly from the receptor as indicated by their higher dissociation rate constants $(k_{-1}(\times 10^{-4} \, \text{sec}^{-1})$ at 25° C: 1.9 ± 0.2 (SE) for estradiol; 6.0 ± 0.5 for estriol and 16 ± 0.7 for estrone (Pasqualini *et al.*, 1980b; Gulino *et al.*, 1981; Lanzone *et al.*, 1983).

The fetal estrogen receptor becomes more tightly bound in the nucleus when exposed to estradiol, either by whole tissue incubation *in vitro* or when administered transplacentally *in vivo* (Sumida and Pasqualini, 1979a; Sumida and Pasqualini, 1980). Retention of the receptor in the nucleus *in vitro* is specific for estrogens or other compounds (anti-estrogens) which bind to cytosol estrogen receptor and is temperature-, time- and concentration-dependent. However, under either *in vivo* or *in vitro* conditions, conversion of the receptor from a form easily extractable during homogenization to the form strongly retained in the nucleus is never stoichiometric or complete and, eventually, exposure to estradiol leads to a loss of receptor, similar to the mechanism of receptor 'processing' described by Horwitz and McGuire (1978) in human breast cancer cells in culture. Studies on the immunorecognition of the fetal guinea-pig estrogen receptor by a monoclonal antibodies developed against a human estrogen receptor have aided in further characterizing the estrogen receptor in the fetal guinea-pig uterus.

1.1.1.2. Immunorecognition of the Fetal Uterine Estrogen Receptor by Various Monoclonal Antibodies Obtained against the Human Estrogen Receptor

A specific monoclonal antibody (D547 Spγ) raised against estrogen receptor partially purified from the cytosol fraction of MCF-7 human breast cancer cells (Greene *et al.*, 1980) according to the method of Köhler and Milstein (1975) is able to recognize the uterine estrogen receptor from the fetal guinea-pig and has been used to study the conformation of the fetal estrogen receptor (Giambiagi and Pasqualini, 1982). With the use of this monoclonal antibody, in the cytosol fraction of the fetal uterus of guinea-pig, two forms of estrogen receptor were revealed on sucrose density gradients in high ionic

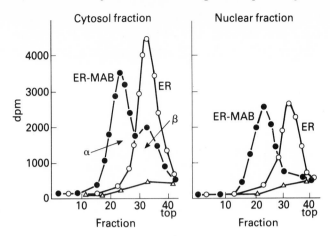

Fig 2.2. Immunorecognition of the Estrogen Receptor of the Fetal Guinea-pig
Uterus by a Monoclonal Antibody.
Estrogen receptor complexes with and without the monoclonal antibody (MAB)
were centrifuged in high salt sucrose density gradients. Adapted from Giambiagi and
Pasqualini (1982).

strength buffer (Fig. 2.2); only one of these forms (the α-form) which corresponds
to the activated receptor, binds to the monoclonal antibody. The nonbinding form
was called the β-form and represented the nonactivated receptor (Giambiagi *et al.*,
1984). Only 40–60% of the total cytosol estrogen receptor binds to the monoclonal
antibody while 90–100% of the receptor retained in the nucleus is bound to the
antibody (Fig. 2.2). It is possible to follow the disappearance of the α-form from the
cytosol (the β-form is not affected) and the appearance of estrogen receptor–monoclonal antibody complex in the nucleus. The transfer depends on incubation time and
temperature, but is never complete, both forms persisting in the cytosol even after
30 min at 25° C (Giambiagi *et al.*, 1984). The experimental conditions which lead to
increased activation of the cytosol receptor (i.e. increased binding to DNA cellulose)
also increase its binding to the monoclonal antibody. During the process, the β-form is
converted to the α-form (Giambiagi and Pasqualini, 1985). These observations indicate
that the epitope of the monoclonal antibody D547 is completely masked in the
nonactivated receptor.

Incubation of the receptor with RNAase A increases the binding of the receptor to
DNA-cellulose by 100%, but it does not increase the binding to the monoclonal
antibody (Giambiagi and Pasqualini, 1987). Although RNAase A treatment increases
the affinity of the estrogen receptor for DNA-cellulose, it does not cause a dissociation
of the oligomeric native form of the receptor into the monomeric (or dimeric) forms
normally associated with the activated form of the receptor. However RNA, which also
provokes an increase in the binding of the receptor to DNA cellulose, induces the
dissociation of the nonactivated receptor into forms that are recognized by the
monoclonal antibody D547 (Giambiagi and Pasqualini, 1989). The data suggest that
the mechanism of the receptor activation by RNAase is different from that provoked by
temperature, time, salt concentration or RNA.

(a)

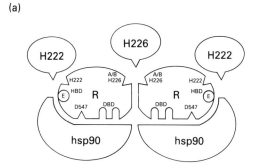

(b)

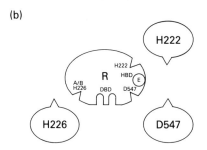

(c)

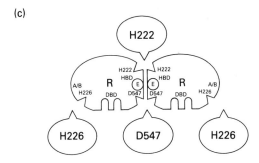

FIG 2.3. Hypothetical Model for the Conformation of the Oligomer, Monomer, and Dimer Estrogen Receptor of the Fetal Uterus of Guinea-pig and their Interaction with the Three Monoclonal Antibodies (D547, H222, H226).

(a) In the nonactivated oligomeric form of the estrogen receptor of fetal uterus of guinea-pig. The epitope for the monoclonal antibody D547, between the hormone-binding (HBD) and the DNA binding (DBD) domains are completely masked. H222 epitope is totally exposed and the H226 epitope partially; (b) in the hypothetical intermediate monomeric receptors the three epitopes are exposed; (c) in the activated dimeric receptors the epitopes for the monoclonal antibody H222 are totally exposed (A/B region) and that for the H222 epitope (hormone-binding domain, HBD) and for D547 epitope (intermediate region) partially masked. E: estrogen; R: hormone binding unit; HSP: heat shock protein; A/B: NM$_2$-terminal region of the receptor. Quoted from Giambiagi and Pasqualini (1990), with permission of *Endocrinology*.

The use of two other monoclonal antibodies (H222 and H226) whose epitopes are located on other domains of the estrogen receptor structure has permitted further study of the changes in conformation of the estrogen receptor during the process of activation. One of these antibodies (H222) has an epitope that is situated near the hormone binding region of the receptor and is well exposed in the nonactivated and the activated forms of the receptor. The epitope of the other antibody (H226) is located closer to the DNA binding domain and is partially masked in the nonactivated form of the receptor (Giambiagi and Pasqualini, 1988).

Thus, monoclonal antibodies to the human estrogen receptor that also recognize the fetal guinea-pig estrogen receptor have become very useful. This is particularly the case in the study of the changes in the conformation of the receptor during the process of activation of the receptor using these monoclonal antibodies. Activation of the estrogen receptor induces dissociation of the heat shock protein (HSP) and releasing of the activated (DNA-binding) monomer receptor which associate to yield the activated (hormone-responsive element-binding) homo-dimer. Alternatively, activation may induce dissociation of the HSP and releasing of the activated dimer receptor with further rearrangement of the estradiol-binding subunits. A hypothetical model for the tertiary structure of the different forms of the estrogen receptor with the three monoclonal antibodies (D547, H222 and H226) are presented in Fig. 2.3 (Giambiagi and Pasqualini, 1990).

1.1.1.3. Ontogeny of the Estrogen Receptor in the Fetal and Neonatal Uterus

During fetal development in the guinea-pig, estrogen receptors appear very soon (from at least 34–35 days of gestation) after differentiation of the gonads and reach maximal levels between 55 and 60 days of gestation before declining (Fig. 2.4). During this period, the fetal guinea-pig uterus differentiates from an organ having only a pseudostratified high columnar epithelium surrounded by relatively undifferentiated stromal cells at 44 days (Fig. 2.5(a)) to a uterus with an external layer of circular and longitudinal muscle by the end of gestation (Fig. 2.5(b)) (Gulino *et al.*, 1984). Uterine glands only develop after birth. Since the circulating levels of estrogens are relative low and remain constant in fetal guinea-pig plasma (Fig. 2.4) (Gelly *et al.*, 1981), the developmental increase and decline appear to be independent of endogenous estrogens (the actual tissue concentrations during development remain to be explored). The total circulating estrogens do not vary significantly during the perinatal period while the concentrations of the estrogen receptors fall (Table 2.3). The proportion of receptor more tightly bound in the nucleus increases from 7% in the fetus and 1-day-old neonate to 18% in the 8-day-old animal. Estradiol itself does not stimulate synthesis of estrogen receptor in the fetus since animals treated with estradiol show decreased concentrations of uterine receptor. Replenishment of receptor only occurs five days after an acute treatment with no net increase in receptor concentration (Sumida and Pasqualini, 1980; Gulino *et al.*, 1981). However, in the neonatal guinea-pig uterus, a net increase of 60% over basal receptor levels can be observed 48 h after treatment (Gulino and Pasqualini, 1983). This may indicate that as the uterus matures, estrogens begin to induce the synthesis of their own receptor but the part of the receptor population that is estrogen-independent may be a component of the uterine cells.

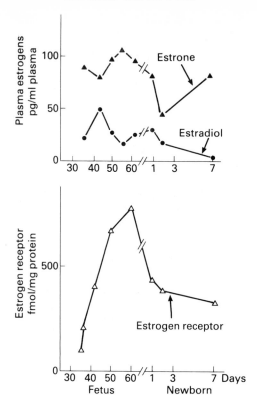

FIG 2.4. Ontogeny of Cytosol Estrogen Receptors in the Fetal and Neonatal Guinea-pig Uterus and Plasma Estradiol and Estrone Concentrations. Means ±SD. Adapted from Pasqualini *et al.* (1976b).

TABLE 2.3. *Changes in Subcellular Distribution of Estrogen Receptors in the Perinatal Guinea-pig Uterus*

| | Estrogen receptor (pmol/mg DNA) | | | | Plasma concentration (pg/ml plasma) | |
| | | | Total cytosol + nuclear | | | |
	Cytosol	Nuclear	Unoccupied Sites	Occupied Sites	Estradiol	Estrone
Fetuses	17.9 ± 3.3	1.3 ± 0.6	16.7 ± 2.9	2.4 ± 1.0	25 ± 6	94 ± 21
Newborns						
1 day old	7.8 ± 1.5	0.5 ± 0.1	7.7 ± 1.4	0.1 ± 0.1	31 ± 11	82 ± 15
8 day old	6.2 ± 1.4	1.3 ± 0.3	5.5 ± 0.9	0.7 ± 0.5	ND	80 ± 13

Mean ± SE

Quoted from Sumida and Pasqualini (1979a); Gelly *et al.* (1981).

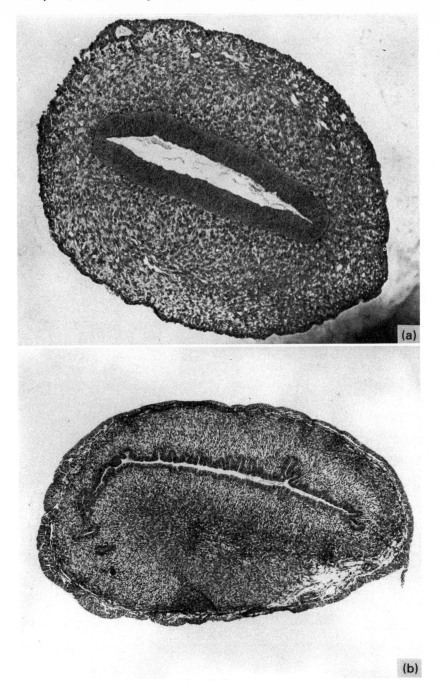

FIG 2.5. Cross Sections of Fetal Uteri of Guinea-pig.
(a) Uterus of a 44-day-old fetus (magnification: ×96); (b) uterus of a 63-day-old fetus (magnification: ×38). Quoted from Gulino *et al.* (1984).

1.1.1.4. Ontogeny of Estrogen Responsiveness

The estrogen receptor found in the fetal guinea-pig uterus has the physicochemical characteristics of a receptor protein and also its functional properties since its presence can be correlated with some estrogen-inducible responses in the fetus. In the fetal guinea-pig, two parameters of estrogen action have been studied: 1. the induction of the progesterone receptor and 2. the uterotrophic effect.

Under normal physiological conditions in the fetus, detectable levels of progesterone receptor only appear 10–15 days after the estrogen receptor (Pasqualini *et al.*, 1980c) (Fig. 2.6). This observation suggests that endogenous estrogens, in the presence of sufficient quantities of estrogen receptor, are capable of exerting a hormonal effect in a fetal tissue. Since the circulating levels of estrogens are relatively low and remain constant in fetal guinea-pig plasma (Gelly *et al.*, 1981), the appearance of progesterone receptor seems to be independent of abrupt changes in endogenous estrogens and may, therefore, depend on the estrogen receptor concentrations. It is possible that before 50 days of gestation, the estrogen receptor concentrations are not sufficient to induce progesterone receptor synthesis in the face of such low levels of circulating estrogens. A

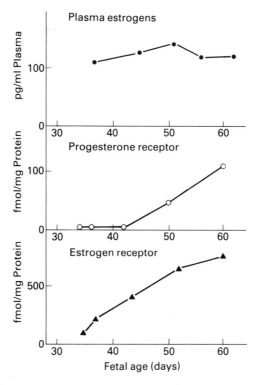

FIG 2.6. Comparison of Fetal Plasma Estrogen Levels, Progesterone Receptor and Estrogen Receptor Concentrations in the Fetal Uterus of the Guinea-pig during Development.
The values of plasma estrogens (estradiol plus estrone) are quoted from Gelly *et al.* (1981). Receptor data are adapted from Pasqualini *et al.* (1976b).

sufficiently high concentration of estrogen receptors may be a prerequisite for the action of endogenous estrogens in the fetal guinea-pig uterus.

1.1.1.5. Ontogeny of Responsiveness to Exogenous Estrogens

(a) *Unconjugated Estrogens*

Administration of estradiol transplacentally to the fetus causes an increases in the wet and dry weights of the fetal uterus (Gulino *et al.*, 1981) which is proportionally the same regardless of fetal age (Sumida and Pasqualini, 1980) (Fig. 2.7). This trophic effect is represented by an increase in the overall size of the uterine horns and in the width of the stromal and myometrial layers with a 95% increase in the height of the luminal epithelial cells (Gulino *et al.*, 1984).

Treatment of the fetuses with estradiol also causes a seven to ten-fold increase in progesterone receptor concentrations even at a gestational age when progesterone receptors are barely detectable in the fetal uterus (Fig. 2.8) (Pasqualini and Nguyen, 1979a,b; 1980).

Estrone treatment also leads to a similar wet weight gain and increase in the concentrations of progesterone receptors as estradiol treatment (Lanzone *et al.*, 1983). It has been suggested that, in the fetal guinea-pig uterus, estrone itself exerts a biological action since no significant metabolic conversion to estradiol was observed in the fetal uterus (Lanzone *et al.*, 1983).

Daily administration of estriol for three days to pregnant guinea-pigs also causes the same increases in dry and wet weights of the fetal uterus and concentrations of

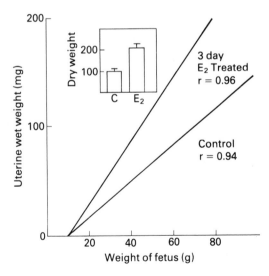

FIG 2.7. Effect of Estradiol Treatment on Wet Weights and Dry Weights of Fetal Guinea-pig Uteri.
Fetal body weight is indicated as the measure of fetal age. Inset represents the ratio of estradiol-treated to control dry weights as a percentage. Quoted from Pasqualini *et al.* (1983) with permission from University Park Press.

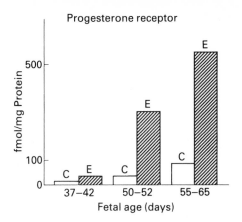

FIG 2.8. Ontogeny of Progesterone Receptor Stimulation by Exogenously Administered Estradiol in Uteri of the Guinea-pig Fetus.
C = uteri from untreated animals; E = uteri from fetuses treated for 3 days with
estradiol. Adapted from Pasqualini *et al.* (1980b).

progesterone receptors as estradiol and estrone (Gulino *et al.*, 1981). Therefore, estriol
can be a potent estrogen when present in a high enough concentration. This is a
significant observation since estriol is quantitatively the most important estrogen
circulating during human pregnancy.

(b)   *Estrogen Sulfates*

Estrogen sulfates with the sulfate on the C_3 position which is susceptible to enzymatic
hydrolysis provoke both a uterine weight gain and a stimulation of the progesterone
receptor when injected transplacentally to the fetus (Pasqualini *et al.*, 1982). On the
other hand, estrogens with the sulfate on the C_{17} position that is not hydrolyzed show
very little or no biological effect (Pasqualini *et al.*, 1982). Figure 2.9 shows the effect of
various estrogen sulfates on the weight of the fetal uterus after administration to
pregnant guinea-pigs. Estrogen sulfates which also circulate in high amounts in human
pregnancy can also be considered as potentially active estrogens and may serve as a
form of storage.

1.1.1.6. Correlation of Biological Responses with Nuclear
Retention of Estrogen Receptors

The uterotrophic effect can be correlated with long-term retention of estrogen
receptor in the nucleus which can be seen when the uterotrophic effects of estradiol and
estriol are compared (Fig. 2.10). Estriol was used because of its known 'weak' agonist
uterotrophic effect (Clark *et al.*, 1977b) which has been explained by the short retention
time of the estriol receptor complex in uterine nuclei (Anderson *et al.*, 1975). The
weight gain provoked by estradiol is maintained as long as estrogen receptor remains in
the nucleus (Fig. 2.10), but when estriol is administered, uterine weight regresses after
two days in conjunction with the loss of estriol receptor complexes from the nucleus.

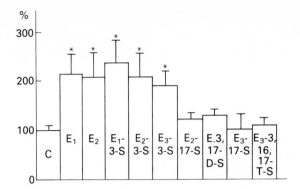

FIG 2.9. Effect of Seven Different Estrogen Sulfates, as well as Unconjugated Estrone and Estradiol on the Weight of the Fetal Uterus of Guinea-pig.

Pregnant guinea-pigs (days 55–65 of gestation) were injected s.c. with 1 mg/kg/day of estrone (E_1), estradiol (E_2) or with 1.4–2.1 mg/kg/day of the following sulfates: estrone-3-sulfate (E_1-3-S), estradiol-3-sulfate (E_2-3-S), estriol-3-sulfate (E_3-3-S), estradiol-17-sulfate (E_2-17-S), estriol-17-sulfate (E_3-17-S), estradiol-3,17-disulfate (E_2-3,17-DS), estriol-3,16,17-trisulfate (E_3-3,16,17-TS) (dissolved in 20% v/v ethanol-saline solution) for three days and sacrificed on day 4. Uteri were excised, stripped of adhering fat and weighted. Control (C) animals received the vehicle alone. Values represent the mean $\pm$SD of 5–21 determinations. *$p < 0.001$ (p calculated vs nontreated animals). Quoted from Pasqualini *et al.* (1982), with the permission of *Acta Endocrinologica*.

Changes in nuclear retention of the estrogen receptor precede the appearance of the progesterone receptor response (Fig. 2.11) (Gulino *et al.*, 1981). After a single injection of estradiol, estrogen receptors are retained in the nucleus for as long as seven days. However, despite the continuing presence of estrogen receptor in the nucleus, the progesterone receptor concentration diminishes after two days (Fig. 2.11). After a single injection of estriol, similar kinetics of the induction and disappearance of progesterone receptors are observed, but the estriol receptor complex is only retained in the nuclei for one day. This difference does not seem to influence the fate of the progesterone receptor which apparently also depends on factors other than the estrogen receptor system.

The fetal guinea-pig uterus is an estrogen-responsive organ, but the role of the estrogen receptor depends on the parameter studied. Although the uterotrophic effect shows a good correlation with estrogen receptor kinetics, progesterone receptor stimulation is not directly dependent on the estrogen receptor system.

1.1.1.7. Induction of Progesterone Receptor in the Fetal Uterus in Culture

Progesterone receptors can also be induced *in vitro* in organ culture of fetal uterine explants and in monolayer culture of cells from the fetal uterus. In the organ culture system, the increase in progesterone receptor concentrations in the explants over three days of culture is due to *de novo* synthesis of the receptor protein; it occurs spontaneously in the absence of any hormonal stimulus (Sumida *et al.*, 1983). In the cell cultures,

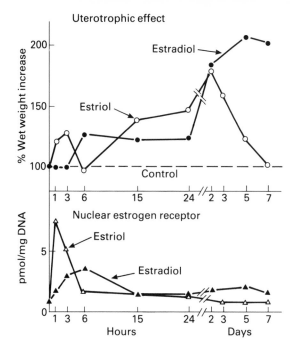

FIG 2.10. Comparative Kinetics of the Uterotrophic Response to Estradiol and
Estriol in the Fetal Guinea-pig Uterus.
The uterine wet weights of treated animals are expressed as a percent of the average
weight of untreated uteri of the same age. Adapted from Gulino *et al.* (1981).

progesterone receptor is increased by the addition of estradiol to the medium although
the cells show no growth response to estradiol (Sumida *et al.*, 1988).

1.1.1.8. Other Biological Effects of Estrogens in the Fetal Uterus

Other manifestations of estrogen action in the fetal guinea pig uterus can be
mentioned although their correlation with estrogen receptors has not yet been elucidated.

(a) *RNA Polymerase I and II*

Administration of estradiol to the pregnant guinea-pig leads to four-fold increases in
RNA polymerase I and II activities by 2 h (Lauré and Pasqualini, 1983).

(b) *Protein Synthesis*

Administration of estradiol also increases 20-fold the incorporation of ^{3}H-leucine into
fetal uterine proteins by 24 h (Sumida and Pasqualini, 1981).

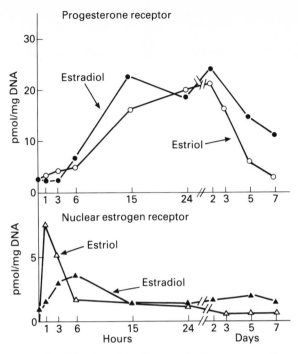

FIG 2.11. Comparative Kinetics of the Increase in Progesterone Receptor Concentrations in the Fetal Guinea-pig Uterus in Response to Estradiol and Estriol Treatments.
Pregnant guinea-pigs (55–64 days of gestation) were injected with 1 mg estradiol or estriol/kg b.w. and progesterone and estrogen receptors were measured in the fetal uteri. Quoted from Gulino *et al.* (1981).

(c) *Acetylation of Histones and Proteins of the High Mobility Group (HMG)*

The acetylation of histones and high mobility group proteins involves conformational changes in chromatin that lead to increased DNA template activity and transcription (Allfrey, 1980). When estradiol is injected directly to the fetus, only 10 min later there is already a seven to ten-fold increase in the acetylation of nuclear histones $H_2 + H_3$ and H_4 (Pasqualini *et al.*, 1981). Estradiol treatment of fetuses also leads to a 33% stimulation of the acetylation of high mobility group proteins (HMG) $1 + 2$ and a 126% increase in the acetylation of HMG $14 + 17$. Studies carried out with 2-day-old guinea-pigs show that estradiol provokes a selective increase in the acetylation of the HMG-14 proteins (Pasqualini *et al.*, 1989).

1.1.2. VAGINA

1.1.2.1. Physicochemical Properties of the Estrogen Receptor

It is well known that vaginal tissues in different animal species, including human, respond to the action of endogenous or exogenous estrogens. Estrogen receptors have

TABLE 2.4. *Physicochemical Properties of Cytosol Estrogen Receptor in Fetal Guinea-pig Vagina (62–64 Days of Gestation)*

Number of sites	~7 pmol/mg DNA
	290 fmol/mg protein
	15–16 pmol/g tissue
	1.3–1.4 pmol/vagina
	~4000 sites/cell
K_d ($\times 10^{-9}$ M), 4° C	0.13
Binding specificity	Estradiol = estrone = estriol
	= ethynylestradiol =
	diethylstilbestrol
Sedimentation coefficient	8–9 S in low salt
	4.5 S in high salt
Immunorecognition	Binds to monoclonal antibody
	against human estrogen receptor

Quoted from Nguyen *et al.* (1986).

been reported in vaginal tissues of rabbits (Payne and Katzenellenbogen, 1980), mice (Cunha *et al.*, 1982) and humans (Wiegerinck *et al.*, 1980). The receptors are also present in the vagina during fetal life in the guinea-pig (Nguyen *et al.*, 1986). As seen in Table 2.4, the specific binding of [^{3}H]-estradiol in the cytosol fraction of the fetal vagina has a high affinity, and the concentration of binding sites is relatively high. Binding is specific for natural and synthetic estrogens. On low salt sucrose density gradients containing molybdate, the [^{3}H]-estradiol-receptor complex sediments as an 8–9 S peak, which is similar to the sedimentation behavior of the fetal uterine estrogen receptor (Nguyen *et al.*, 1986). The vaginal receptor is also recognized by the same monoclonal antibody developed against the human estrogen receptor that also binds to the fetal uterine estrogen receptor. As in the uterus, the concentration of estrogen receptor in the vagina decreases considerably after birth to approximately 1 pmol/ mg DNA in the 5-day-old neonate (Nguyen *et al.*, 1986).

1.1.2.2. Responses to Estrogen in the Fetal Vagina

After a 12-day treatment of estradiol to pregnant guinea-pigs, the fetal vagina wet weight increases three-fold compared to untreated fetuses of the same gestational age (Nguyen *et al.*, 1986). Progesterone receptor concentrations increase approximately ten times in the vagina of these estradiol-treated fetuses.

Histological studies showed drastic morphological alterations in the epithelial cells. Similarly, the ultrastructural examination with transmission electron microscopy showed the alteration of mitochondria, the development of the rough endoplasmic reticulum, and the formation of numerous vacuoles and secretory granules.

1.1.3. MALE REPRODUCTIVE ORGANS

Specific [^{3}H]-estradiol receptors are present in the fetal testis of the guinea-pig from 34 to 50 days of gestation. The levels are relatively low (30–56 fmol/mg protein),

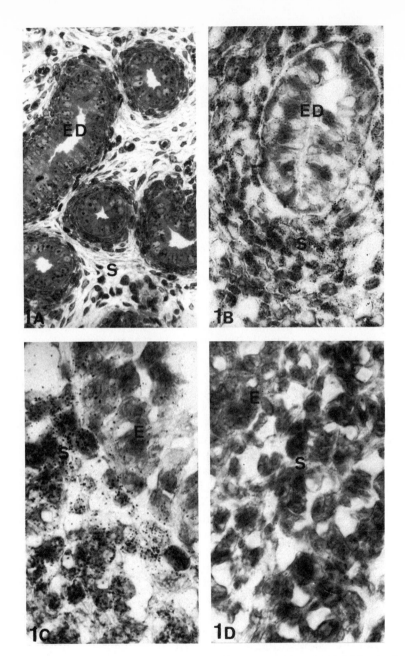

FIG 2.12. Autoradiographic Localization of [^{3}H]-Estradiol in the Epididymis, Seminal Vesicle and Prostate of Fetal Guinea-pig.

(a) General view of the traverse semithin section of the epididymis (control) of the 50-day-old fetuses of guinea-pig. ED: epididymal duct; S: stroma; ($\times$320); (b) Autoradiography of the fetal epididymis after s.c. injection of 150 μCi of [^{3}H]estradiol to 50-day-old fetuses. The silver grains are concentrated mainly in the nuclei of the stroma cells (S) ($\times$500); (c) Autoradiography of the epididymis of 60-day-old fetuses. E: epithelium; S: stroma; ($\times$760); (d) Autoradiography of the fetal epididymis after injection of 150 μCi of [^{3}H]-estradiol plus an excess of 100-fold unlabeled estradiol ($\times$790). All exposures: 7 months. Quoted from Hatier *et al.* (1990), with the permission of the *International Journal of Andrology.*

especially when compared to the concentrations found in the fetal uterus (Pasqualini *et al.*, 1976c).

Recent data, using autoradiography methods, show that in 50–60-day-old fetuses there is a selective localization of [^{3}H]-estradiol in the epididymis, seminal vesicles and prostate. The retention of the radioactivity is present in the stroma cells of these fetal organs, whereas the epithelium does not exhibit any, or very little, location of silver grains (Fig. 2.12) (Hatier *et al.*, 1990). The data suggest that the mesenchymal stroma of these male fetal reproductive organs might be considered as a target tissue for the estrogen response.

1.1.4. BRAIN

Pasqualini and Palmada (1972) described a protein showing saturable binding of ^{3}H-estradiol of high affinity in whole brain cytosols which sedimented in the 8.5–9 S region of a low salt sucrose density gradient. In a high salt gradient, two other components of 6–6.5 S and 4–5 S appeared. Tardy *et al.* (1983), using the tritiated synthetic estrogen ^{3}H-moxestrol (R2858) which has little affinity for plasma proteins, were able to confirm the presence of an 8.6 S macromolecule whose binding of ^{3}H-moxestrol could be suppressed by unlabeled R2858 and estradiol but not by progesterone or testosterone.

The concentration of specific ^{3}H-estradiol binding in brain cytosol increases from 3.4 fmol/mg protein or 8 fmol/mg DNA between 29 and 35 days of gestation to 15.5 fmol/mg protein or 125 fmol/mg DNA by 49 to 50 days of gestation and remain at this level until at least one day after birth (Pasqualini *et al.*, 1978b). No statistically significant differences were observed between male and female fetal brains. The dissociation constant of this binding component is 3.2 ± 0.8 (SD) $\times 10^{-10}$ M but a second population of binding sites of lower affinity and higher capacity was also evident from Scatchard plots of the binding data (Pasqualini *et al.*, 1978b).

Contradictory results were reported by Plapinger *et al.* (1977) who were not able to detect any 8-S specific estrogen binding component in cytosols of whole fetal guinea-pig brains of 40 days gestation. Only a 4-S ^{3}H-estradiol binding component which was not suppressible by either unlabeled estradiol or R2858 was seen and ascribed to nonspecific blood contaminants. However, in the hypothalamic–preoptic area–amygdala (HPA), an estrogen specific macromolecule sedimenting in the 8–9 S region was detected. According to this report, a large proportion of the estradiol binding observed in fetal brain cytosol represents the second population of lower affinity binding sites which are saturable by estradiol but not by R2858 and are measurable by Sephadex G25 gel filtration but not by sucrose density gradient centrifugation. A putative estrogen receptor in fetal guinea-pig brain would appear to be located more precisely in the HPA region of the brain.

Complementary observations from autoradiographic studies of ^{3}H-estradiol taken up and retained by fetal guinea-pig brain tend to confirm the localization of radioactivity in cell nuclei of the arcuate nucleus and preoptic area of the hypothalamus (Tardy and Pasqualini, 1983). Moreover, autoradiography combined with immunohistochemistry has demonstrated the simultaneous presence of ^{3}H-estradiol and GnRH (gonadotrophin releasing hormone) in the cell body of neurons of the arcuate nucleus and preoptic area (Tardy and Pasqualini, 1983), areas known to be implicated in the estradiol modulation of the release of GnRH (Knobil, 1974; Goodman, 1978). The presence of putative estrogen receptors in fetal guinea-pig brain would thus suggest their role in sexual differentiation of the brain whose critical period occurs prenatally in this animal species (Phoenix *et al.*, 1959; Goy *et al.*, 1967; Brown-Grant and Sherwood, 1971) and the possible functioning of the hypothalamo–pituitary–gonadal axis in the guinea-pig fetus.

1.1.5. THYMUS

In the human, the thymus already begins to play a role in the maturation and control of immune functions in utero (Asantila *et al.*, 1974; Gill and Repetti, 1979). Gonadal steroids have been shown to affect immune functions (Luster *et al.*, 1980) and thymic morphology (Sobhon and Jirasattham, 1974) in adult animals, and estrogen administration during the perinatal period can impair thymus-derived immune functions (Kalland *et al.*, 1979; Luster *et al.*, 1979; Kalland, 1980), an observation with consequences for the fetal thymus considering the large increase in circulating estrogens during human pregnancy. The direct effect of estrogens on the developing and differentiating thymus, possibly by an estrogen receptor-mediated mechanism, can thus be postulated.

1.1.5.1. Properties of the Estrogen Receptors in the Fetal Thymus

Saturable, high affinity binding sites for ^{3}H-estradiol have been found in the cytosol and nucleus of fetal guinea-pig thymus from at least 36 days of gestation (Screpanti *et al.*, 1982). Some physicochemical properties of these binding sites are summarized in Table 2.5. The receptor characteristics resemble those described for the fetal uterine

TABLE 2.5. *Physicochemical Properties of Cytosol Estrogen Receptor in Fetal Guinea-pig Thymus (End of Gestation)*

Number of sites	31 fmol/mg protein
	57 fmol/mg DNA
	1300 fmol/g tissue
	520 fmol/thymus
K_d ($\times 10^{-9}$ M), 4° C	0.18
k_{+1}[a] ($\times 10^5$ M^{-1} sec^{-1}), 4° C	1.0
k_{-1}[b] ($\times 10^{-6}$ sec^{-1}), 4° C	4.4
k_{-1}[b] ($\times 10^{-4}$ sec^{-1}), 26° C	3.3
Binding specificity	Estradiol > estrone = diethyl-stilbestrol > R2858 > estriol
	No binding of other steroids
Sedimentation coefficient	8 S in low salt
	4 S in high salt
DEAE chromatography	Elutes at 0.15–0.2 M KCl

[a]Association rate constant; [b]dissociation rate constant.
Quoted from Screpanti *et al.* (1982); Gulino *et al.* (1983).

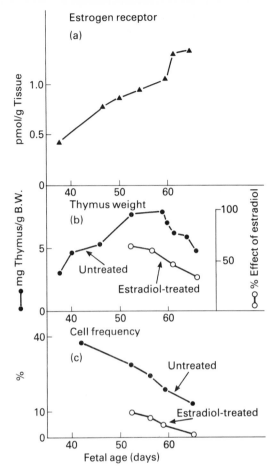

FIG 2.13. Ontogeny of Cytosol Estrogen Receptors and Estrogen Responsiveness in
the Thymus of the Fetal Guinea-pig.
(a) Cytosol estrogen receptor concentrations; (b) weight of fetal thymus (mg/g b.w.)
and effect of 6 daily injections of 1 mg estradiol/kg b.w. to pregnant guinea-pigs
expressed as percent of weights of thymuses from untreated fetuses of the same age;
(c) frequency of large lymphoid cells in the subcapsular cortex of thymi from
untreated and estradiol-treated fetuses. Quoted from Gulino *et al.* (1983).

estrogen receptor except that the concentration of binding sites is lower. When exposed
to estradiol, the cytosol receptor acquires a higher affinity for nuclear elements in a
temperature-dependent manner (Screpanti *et al.*, 1982) where it can be extracted by
0.4 M KCl-containing buffer and sediments at 5 S in a high salt sucrose density
gradient. The concentration of receptor increases from 10 fmol/mg protein at 36 days of
gestation to 39 fmol/mg protein at the end of gestation with no significant sex
differences (Fig. 2.13(a)) (Screpanti *et al.*, 1982).

High affinity ^{3}H-estradiol binding ($K_d = 0.5 \pm 0.02$ (SE) $\times 10^{-9}$ M) was further
demonstrated to be present in the thymocytes isolated from the fetal guinea-pig thymus

(Gulino *et al.*, 1985). Further separation of the thymocytes into two populations of large lymphoblastoid cells and small, high density cells revealed a much higher concentration of estrogen receptors in the lymphoblastoid cells: 1002 ± 200 (SE) sites per cell vs 61 ± 6 (SE) sites per cell in the small lymphocytes. Estrogen receptors in the thymus thus appear to be related to the stage of maturation of the lymphoid cells.

1.1.5.2. Estrogen Responsiveness of the Fetal Thymus

The presence of estrogen binding sites in the fetal thymus could be involved in the expression of some biological responses provoked by transplacental administration of estradiol to the fetuses. After three or six daily injections of 1 mg estradiol/kg b.w. to the pregnant guinea-pig, a 50% decrease in weight of the fetal thymus was observed (Fig. 2.13(b)), representing a reduction in size of thymic lobules and a decrease in width of the cortical lymphoid area. Already by 24 h after injection of estradiol, a selective decrease in the number of the large lymphoid cells (the more highly proliferating lymphocytes) in the subcapsular cortex was observed (Fig. 2.13(c)), which is also related to an estradiol-induced reduction in the incorporation of ^{3}H-thymidine into DNA (Screpanti *et al.*, 1982; Gulino *et al.*, 1983).

During fetal development, the progressive increase in estrogen receptor concentrations in the cytosol of fetal thymus is accompanied by an intensification of the response of the thymus to estrogen treatment. At all ages, from 60 to 70% of the receptor complexes are retained in the nucleus in response to estrogen treatment. The growth of the fetal thymus slows and the frequency of large lymphoid cells decreases with increasing fetal age, corresponding to the periods of both maximal cytosol estrogen receptor levels and maximal estrogen responsiveness (Figs 2.13(a,b,c)). These observations indicate that the fetal thymus responds to estrogens via mechanisms which seem to involve the presence and development of an estrogen receptor system.

1.1.6. KIDNEY

Estrogen receptors have also been found in fetal kidney (Pasqualini *et al.*, 1973). Although at first glance this particular receptor may appear to be ubiquitous, this is in fact due to the multiplicity of possible actions of this group of hormones in a wide variety of tissues. In 1939, Taylor *et al.* observed that a relationship existed between estrogens and sodium and potassium balance at the end of pregnancy, and in 1970, Johnson and co-workers showed the effect of estrogens on electrolyte balance in normal dogs, so that the finding of estrogen receptors in the fetal kidney could be of biological significance.

High affinity, saturable binding of ^{3}H-estradiol was demonstrated in fetal guinea-pig kidney cytosol and nucleus both after *in vivo* administration of ^{3}H-estradiol directly to the fetus and after *in vitro* incubation of ^{3}H-estradiol with kidney cell suspensions at 37°C (Pasqualini *et al.*, 1974b). In the cytosol fraction, two populations of binding sites are present, the one with a higher affinity and lower capacity having a dissociation constant (K_d) of 2.5×10^{-10} M at 4° C and the second population having a K_d of 7.7×10^{-9} M (Pasqualini *et al.*, 1974b). Binding in both the cytosol and nuclear fractions is specific for estrogens (estradiol, estrone, estriol) with no competition by testosterone, cortisol or aldosterone (Pasqualini *et al.*, 1976b; Sumida *et al.*, 1978). The retention of ^{3}H-estradiol complexes in the nucleus *in vitro* is temperature-dependent (Pasqualini *et al.*, 1974b). A particular of the kidney which merits comment is the greater conversion of estrone to estradiol in this organ compared to the other fetal organs studied (Pasqualini *et al.*, 1974b; 1976b). Although the estrogen binding sites have an equivalent affinity for estradiol and estrone, when fetal kidney tissue is exposed either *in vivo* or *in vitro* to ^{3}H-estrone, a greater percentage of the bound radioactivity is in the form of ^{3}H-estradiol even when compared to the fetal uterus whose receptor has a slightly higher affinity for estradiol than estrone (Pasqualini *et al.*, 1974b; Lanzone *et al.*, 1983).

During fetal development, the concentrations of cytosol and nuclear estrogen receptors rise from 51 fmol/g tissue at 34–35 days of gestation, 337 fmol/g tissue at 37–38 days, 449 fmol/g tissue at 49–50 days and to 1070 fmol/g tissue at 60–65 days (Pasqualini *et al.*, 1976c; Pasqualini and Sumida, 1980). It remains to be shown that these estrogen binding sites in fetal kidney are functional receptors with physiological significance.

1.1.7. LUNG

A possible role of estrogens in the maturation of the human lung has been suggested by the relationship observed between low concentrations of estrogens in the urine of infants and the incidence of respiratory distress syndrome (Dickey and Robertson, 1969). Estrogens have also been found to increase surfactant biosynthesis both *in vivo* and *in vitro* in fetal lungs (Gross *et al.*, 1979; Khosla and Rooney, 1979; Khosla *et al.*, 1980; Khosla *et al.*, 1983). Although the estrogen receptor mechanism has not been proven to mediate these estrogenic effects, it is significant that estrogen receptors have been found in fetal lung tissue of different animals, including the guinea-pig.

Specific binding of ^{3}H-estradiol was demonstrated in the cytosol and nucleus of fetal guinea-pig lung tissue both *in vivo* and *in vitro* (Pasqualini *et al.*, 1976b; Sumida *et al.*, 1978). In the cytosol, the dissociation constant of ^{3}H-estradiol binding is between 4 and 8×10^{-10} M and binding is specific for estrogens (Sumida *et al.*, 1978; Pasqualini and Sumida, 1980). An important feature of estrogen binding in fetal guinea-pig lung is that, in contrast to the other fetal tissues which show specific estrogen binding sites, fetal lung preferentially takes up and retains estrone rather than estradiol (Pasqualini *et al.*, 1976b). Analysis of the radioactivity bound to cytosol macromolecules after *in vivo* administration of ^{3}H-estradiol to the fetuses showed that 71% was in the form of ^{3}H-estrone (Pasqualini *et al.*, 1976b). The concentrations of estrogen binding sites in cytosol and nucleus of fetal lung are considerably higher than in fetal kidney, rising progressively from 254 fmol/g tissue at 34–35 days of gestation to 2830 fmol/g tissue at 60–65 days (Pasqualini *et al.*, 1976c).

To summarize what is happening to the estrogen receptor simultaneously in the different fetal tissues studied, Fig. 2.14 shows the ontogeny of estrogen receptor concentrations in the guinea-pig fetus. The absolute values of receptor concentrations vary greatly among the tissues, being the highest in the uterus, but such differences should not be overemphasized. The tissues are composed of very heterogeneous cell types and information is lacking on the precise location of estrogen receptors and estrogenic responsiveness within these fetal tissues. Estrogen receptors would be expected to be found in estrogen responsive cell types which may represent only a fraction

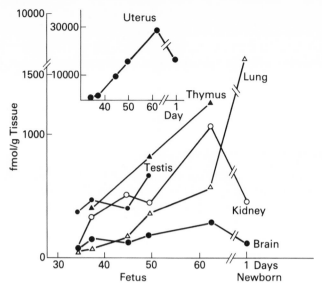

FIG 2.14. Ontogeny of Estrogen Receptor Concentrations in Tissues of the Guinea-pig Fetus and Newborn.
The values represent the sum of cytosol and nuclear binding. The values for estradiol binding in the uterus are indicated in the inset. Adapted from Pasqualini and Sumida (1986).

of the whole organ. The example of the fetal brain has already been pointed out where estrogen receptors are localized mostly in the hypothalamus and not in the cortex. What is apparent is that in all the tissues studied the estrogen receptor concentrations tend to increase with fetal age. Concomitantly, no significant variations occur in the concentrations of unconjugated estradiol and estrone circulating in fetal guinea-pig plasma (see Figure 2.4) (Gelly *et al.*, 1981). Whether estrogen receptors could be a limiting factor in fetal response to estrogens depends on the tissue since in the fetal thymus estrogen responsiveness increases with increasing estrogen receptor concentrations while in the fetal uterus the trophic response to estrogen treatment is the same regardless of age and receptor concentration. Estrogen receptors do appear to be distributed in many fetal tissues and the specificity of the response would derive from the tissue, implying influence from other factors, hormonal or otherwise.

1.2. Rats

1.2.1. UTERUS

The use of tritiated diethylstilbestrol and R2858 (moxestrol), two synthetic estrogens with very weak affinity for α-fetoprotein, has made it possible to measure more accurately estrogen receptor binding in rat tissues during the perinatal period. A cytosol estrogen receptor having a sedimentation coefficient of 8 S in a low salt sucrose density gradient is present in the Müllerian ducts of 20-day-old rat fetuses (Sömjen *et al.*, 1976).

In contrast, kidneys from fetal rats of the same age bind ^{3}H-diethylstilbestrol but only in the 4 S region of the gradient. Kimmel and Harmon (1980) have also demonstrated specific estrogen binding in fetal rat uterine cytosol. In addition, the same group found that estrogens (estradiol, ethynyl estradiol and diethylstilbestrol) are capable of stimulating the activity of ornithine decarboxylase, an enzyme which is involved in polyamine synthesis, thus showing that the fetal rat uterus is estrogen responsive (Kimmel *et al.*, 1981).

1.2.1.1. Characteristics of the Fetal Estrogen Receptor

A study by Nguyen *et al.* (1988) has characterized the estrogen receptor in the fetal rat uterus by using ^{3}H-R2858 as specific ligand. As seen in Table 2.6, the results confirm the presence of specific estrogen binding sites in the fetal rat uterus at the end of gestation. These sites have a very high affinity and specificity for estrogens. However, the number of binding sites is very low compared to that in the neonatal uterus, showing that estrogen receptors increase postnatally in the rat.

1.2.1.2. Estrogen Responses in the Fetal Rat Uterus

The fetal rat uterus responds to exogenously administered estradiol by a seven to eight-fold increase in progesterone receptors at 20 days of fetal age whereas there is no significant response at 18 days (Nguyen *et al.*, 1988). Estradiol increases the size of the lumen and the size of the uterine horn in the fetus but an increase in height of the epithelial cells was observed only in the estradiol-treated uteri from 1-day-old animals (Nguyen *et al.*, 1988).

TABLE 2.6. *Physicochemical Properties of Cytosol Estrogen Receptor in the Uterus of Fetal and Neonatal Rats*

	Fetal		Neonatal	
	18 days	20 days	1 day	5–6 days
Number of sites				
pmol/mg DNA	0.05	0.12	0.28	2.8
fmol/mg protein	10	20	40	980
fmol/uterus	0.4	1.6	4.2	80
sites/cell	200	400	1000	10000
K_d, 4° C	7×10^{-11} M*		1–3×10^{-10} M**	3×10^{-9} M***
Binding specificity	Natural and synthetic estrogens			
Sedimentation coefficient	8 S in low salt			8 S in low salt 4 S in high salt

*Specific binding of [^{3}H]-R2858; **Specific binding of [^{3}H]-DES; ***Specific binding of [^{3}H]-estradiol
Quoted from Clark and Gorski (1970); Sömjen *et al.* (1974); Kimmel and Harmon (1980); Medlock *et al.* (1981); Nguyen *et al.* (1988).

The synthetic estrogens, ethynylestradiol and diethylstilbestrol, stimulate ornithine decarboxylase activity in the fetal rat uterus when administered to pregnant rats on day 20 of gestation (Kimmel *et al.*, 1981).

1.2.1.3. Estrogen Receptors in the Neonatal Uterus

Because the rat uterus progressively acquires the capacity to fully respond to estrogens during postnatal life, in contrast to the guinea-pig, brief mention will be made here of the characteristics of the estrogen receptor system in the neonatal rat uterus.

The uteri of the 20-day-old fetal rat and the 5-day-old neonate are very similar in that both consist of a cuboidal to low columnar luminal epithelium with an undifferentiated stroma. Uterine glands only appear from day 9 as invaginations of the luminal epithelium into the stroma. The number of glands increases to day 15 (Branham *et al.*, 1985; Nguyen *et al.*, 1988).

Table 2.6 shows a comparison of the physicochemical characteristics of the fetal and neonatal estrogen receptors. Figure 2.15 shows the postnatal increase in estrogen receptors in rat parallel to the rise in serum estradiol. Estrogen binding peaks at 10 days. Nuclear receptors could also be detected in nontreated neonates with concentrations of 0.18 pmol/mg DNA at 5 days of age to 0.2–0.3 pmol/mg DNA at 10 to 12 days which gradually continue to rise (Medlock *et al.*, 1981; Sheehan *et al.*, 1981). Ovariectomy of 2-day-old rats does not prevent the post-natal rise in cytosol receptors although

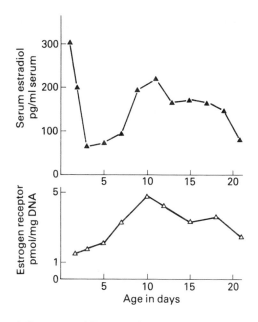

Fig 2.15. Post-natal Ontogeny of Estrogen Receptors in the Rat Uterus and Serum Estradiol Concentrations.
Serum estradiol in female rats was measured by radioimmunoassay (Döhler and Wuttke, 1975). Cytosol estrogen receptor concentrations in the rat uterus adapted from Clark and Gorski (1970) and Medlock *et al.* (1981).

extra-ovarian sources of estrogen were not eliminated (Clark and Peck, 1979). The adrenals are a good potential source of estrogens, as seen by the almost complete disappearance of plasma 'estradiol' 24 h after ovariectomy plus adrenalectomy of 20-day-old rats (Rabii and Ganong, 1976). Ovariectomy alone of 5-day-old rats decreases the plasma 'estradiol' by only about half the values of intact animals.

When exposed to estrogen, the estrogen receptors are capable of being more tightly retained in the nucleus, at least from day 3 of postnatal age (Sömjen *et al.*, 1973; Peleg *et al.*, 1979; Medlock *et al.*, 1981). Recycling and replenishment of receptors occurs in a similar fashion from at least day 6 to day 20 postnatally although a net increase in receptors above initial levels was only observed on day 25 (Peleg *et al.*, 1979). As in the fetal guinea-pig uterus, estrogen-induced synthesis of its own receptor may depend on maturation of the uterus but estrogen-independent receptor synthesis may be a constitutive property of the uterine cells.

1.2.1.4. Action of Estrogens in the Newborn Rat Uterus

Synthetic estrogens such as diethylstilbestrol or moxestrol (R2858) that are not sequestered by binding to α-fetoprotein provoke a 30% increase in uterine wet weight and a 1.6-fold stimulation of DNA synthesis in 5-day-old rats 24 h after a single injection (Raynaud, 1973; Lyttle *et al.*, 1979; Stack and Gorski, 1983). However, the uterotrophic response to estrogens increases with age, suggesting that the developing uterus is capable of responding to estrogens by a rapid, initial increase in wet weight, but the response matures with age.

Endogenous estrogens could be exerting an effect very early in post-natal life since ovariectomy combined with adrenalectomy of 6-day-old rats lower uterine wet weights of 10-day-old rats (Sheehan *et al.*, 1982). Injection of specific anti-estradiol serum over four-day periods also effectively reduces uterine wet weights only 18 h after the last injection even in the neonates treated between two and five days after birth (Reiter *et al.*, 1972).

Ornithine decarboxylase activity is stimulated by estrogens in the fetal rat uterus and can be maximally induced in the 5-day-old rat (Olson *et al.*, 1983), making this enzyme the most precocious in the series of estrogen-inducible proteins studied in the neonatal rat uterus. Other induced proteins follow, such as the BB isozyme of creatine kinase (IP) (Katzenellenbogen and Greger, 1974) and the progesterone receptor (Raynaud *et al.*, 1980).

Both estradiol and R2858 elicit a seven-fold increase in progesterone receptors in the 4-day-old rat uterus (Raynaud *et al.*, 1980). As in the guinea-pig, responsiveness decreases with age in the rat. Unlike the uterotrophic response, the progesterone receptor response either decreases in sensitivity with age or depends on multiple factors extrinsic to the developing uterus (for reviews see Pasqualini *et al.*, 1983b and Pasqualini and Sumida, 1986).

1.2.2. OVARY

The fetal rat ovary has been shown to contain specific binding sites for the tritiated synthetic estrogen R2858. At 20 days of fetal age, the ovary has more than five times the concentration of sites found in the uterus (~ 0.5 pmol/mg DNA in the cytosol and nuclear fractions combined) (Nguyen *et al.*, 1988). At 18 days of gestation, the fetal ovary contains ∼0.1 pmol/mg DNA of binding sites. While the concentrations of estrogen binding sites increase in the uterus postnatally, there is no difference between the 20-day-old fetal and the 1-day-old neonatal ovaries.

Unlike the fetal uterus, progesterone receptor concentrations can already be stimulated more than three times by exogenously administered estrogen in the fetal ovary by 18 days of gestation. At 20 days of gestation, the effect is about the same as that produced in the uterus (Nguyen *et al.*, 1988).

1.2.3. BRAIN

Estrogen receptors are present in fetal rat brains from as early as seven days before birth (Vito and Fox, 1982). The equilibrilium dissociation constant (K_d) for the binding of ^{3}H-estradiol in the cytosol in brains of 21-day-old fetuses is 10^{-10} M (MacLusky *et al.*, 1979). Estrogen receptor concentrations increase from 5 fmol/mg cytosol protein on day 21 of gestation to 12 fmol/mg protein on post-natal day 5 (MacLusky *et al.*, 1979). Receptors are localized predominantly in the limbic brain (hypothalamus, preoptic area, amygdala) and in the cerebral cortex (MacLusky *et al.*, 1979; Vito and Fox, 1982). Nuclear retention of estrogen receptor complexes can be detected in the limbic brain of male but not of female fetuses, suggesting that the presence of testicular androgen in the circulation and the conversion of testosterone to estradiol by aromatizing enzymes in the limbic brain lead to binding of estradiol to its receptor in this region of the fetal brain (MacLusky *et al.*, 1979).

Sexual differentiation of the rodent brain involves steroid hormones acting during a critical period that could begin during late fetal and early postnatal life (McEwen, 1983). This differentiation depends on the conversion of testosterone secreted by the testes of the developing male to estradiol within the brain itself (McEwen *et al.*, 1977; Christensen and Gorski, 1978).

1.2.4. OTHER FETAL TISSUES

Little is known of estrogen receptor binding in other tissues of fetal rats. An estrogen-binding component (other than α-fetoprotein) has been studied in the cytosol of lung tissues from 20-day fetuses (Mendelson *et al.*, 1981). On polyacrylamide gel electrophoresis, the binding component in lung cytosol could be distinguished from plasma estrogen binding protein by the great difference in electrophoretic mobility. This binder is a heat labile protein with a sedimentation coefficient of 4.5 S on low salt sucrose density gradients, even in the presence of sodium molybdate (the adult uterine estrogen receptor sediments as an 8 S protein). Estrone and estradiol compete equally well for ^{3}H-estradiol binding to this protein but diethylsilbestrol has lower affinity. Estriol does not bind to lung cytosol protein while it does have the same affinity as diethylstilbestrol for plasma protein. The concentration of binding sites was found to be extremely high, 10 000 fmol/mg protein with a dissociation constant of 1.7×10^{-8} M. After birth (5-day neonates), the concentration of receptors decreases to 600 fmol/mg protein. Lung cytosol estrogen complexes could not be translocated into the nucleus. An even greater concentration of estrogen binding sites is found in fetal kidney at 19 days of gestation and even fetal heart shows the same amount of binding as fetal lung. Both of these tissues do not bind estriol (Mendelson *et al.*, 1981).

Although these results suggest the presence of an estrogen binding protein in fetal rat lung, kidney and heart differing from the plasma binding protein by some physico-chemical characteristics, it is clear that, overall, this protein does not correspond to the generally accepted criteria for a receptor protein. The observation that fetal rat lung is an estrogen-responsive tissue by its increase in phosphatidylglycerol synthesis in response to estrogen treatment (Gross *et al.*, 1979) provocatively suggests the presence of a functional estrogen receptor system in the fetal rat lung. However, it is still not clear how fetal lung maturation is regulated by estrogen and whether the mechanism depends on estrogen receptors, especially in view of the observation that cytosol from fetal rabbit lung (which is also estrogen-responsive) also shows binding capacity (in the order of 40 fmol/mg protein) for estradiol and estrone but not for diethylstilbestrol or ethynyl estradiol, two biologically potent estrogens (Khosla *et al.*, 1983). Moreover, this binder does not have strong affinity for nuclear binding sites. Although the estrogen binding component from fetal guinea-pig lung cytosol appears to correspond more closely to the physicochemical criteria for an estrogen receptor protein, the effect of estrogens on lung physiology in this animal species has not been studied, thus making it difficult to invoke species-related differences in the mechanism of estrogen action in the lung.

A study of the ontogeny of the concentrations of endogenous nuclear-specific estradiol binding sites in the liver has shown that the number of binding sites per nucleus is higher during the perinatal period (∼ 1500 sites/nucleus) than at any other period, with no sex-dependent variations (Lax *et al.*, 1983). However, when rats are treated with ethynyl estradiol, no further increase in nuclear receptors can be detected before the onset of puberty.

1.3. Mice

1.3.1. GENITAL TRACT

Indications of estrogen 'receptors' in the genital tract of fetal mice derive from the localization by autoradiographic techniques of tritiated diethylstilbestrol in fetal tissues (Stumpf *et al.*, 1980). Pregnant mice (day 16 of gestation) were injected with 0.5 or 2.0 μg/100 g b.w. of ^{3}H-diethylstilbestrol and fetuses were removed from 80 min to 6 h afterwards. Strong nuclear labeling was observed in the mesenchyme surrounding the Mullerian and Wolffian ducts and the urogenital sinuses and mesenchyme in gubernacula of the testes. In the genital tract, the mesenchymal cells surrounding the epithelial primordia showed the highest concentration of radioactivity; the epithelial primordia itself was not labeled. Only weak nuclear labeling was seen in the interstitial cells of the testes and no nuclear localization of radioactivity occurred in the ovary. Although radioactivity could be found in many fetal tissues, higher concentrations were localized preferentially in estrogen target tissues: primordia of male and female reproductive organs, brain, pituitary and mammary glands. Autoradiography does not prove specific binding of high affinity by the cells where radioactivity is localized but the use of a synthetic radioactive estrogen like ^{3}H-diethylstilbestrol which has very little affinity for α-fetoprotein and the localization of the radioactivity mostly in the nucleus rather than the cytoplasm suggests receptor-like binding.

Autoradiographic studies have also been performed on developing genital tracts of neonatal female mice after injection of either ³H-estradiol or ³H-moxestrol (R2858). Radioactivity was found in the nuclei of cells of the genital tract and labeling could be abolished by exposure to a 600-fold excess of radioinert estradiol but not by nonestrogens (Cunha *et al.*, 1982). From 1–15 days post-partum, nuclear localization of radioactive estrogen in the vagina, cervix and uterus was limited completely to cells in the stroma; epithelial cells only began to show nuclear labeling on day 18 or 20 post-partum. However, the vaginal and uterine epithelia of the 4-day-old mouse responds to exogenous estrogen *in vivo* by an increased rate of proliferation, even in the continued absence of estrogen receptors (Cunha *et al.*, 1985). The finding that only the mesenchyme of the developing female genital tract retains radioactive estrogen suggests that during morphogenesis the mesenchyme mediates hormonal as well as teratogenic effects while the epithelium becomes functionally important in the mature animal (Cunha *et al.*, 1980a,b,c, 1981, 1982, 1985; Cunha and Fujii, 1981).

Estrogen binding was also measured by biochemical assay in the cytosol fraction of the uterus of the fetal mouse using the synthetic estrogen ³H-ORG-2058 as specific ligand. The results showed that the uterus of the 18-day-old fetal mouse contains 140 fmol/mg cytosol protein of estrogen receptor but no progesterone receptor (Hochner-Celnikier *et al.*, 1986). No receptors were detected in the heart, lung, brain, liver or limbs of these fetal mice. Further biochemical studies have shown that uterine horns from 1–5-day-old neonatal mice contain a ³H-estradiol binding component in the cytosol sedimenting in the 8 S region on a low salt sucrose density gradient (Eide *et al.*, 1975) which could be competed for with radioinert estradiol and could not be detected in thigh muscle cytosol nor with the use of ³H-dihydrotestosterone. These results complement the autoradiographic observations demonstrating the presence of putative estrogen receptors in fetal and neonatal mouse uterus.

Injection of a high dose of estradiol (20 μg per mouse) on the day of birth significantly increases the cell proliferation index one day later, although uterine weight and DNA content are not yet affected (Ogasawara *et al.*, 1983). An increase in DNA is only observed on day 3. However, adrenalectomy plus ovariectomy has no significant effect on the cell proliferation index or on uterine weight (Ogasawara *et al.*, 1983).

1.3.2. MAMMARY GLAND

Mammary glands develop by a process of growth, differentiation, development of secretory activity and regression with differences between female and male mammary gland primordia. Although destruction of the fetal ovaries by irradiation does not affect the normal development of the mammary gland (Raynaud and Frilley, 1949), estradiol administered to the female fetus provokes the precocious development of the nipples (Raynaud, 1955). This observation suggests estrogen responsiveness of this fetal tissue, especially since in the mature animal both estrogen and progesterone are required for maximal epithelial cell proliferation and lobuloalveolar differentiation (Lyons *et al.*, 1958; Nandi, 1958; Bresciani, 1965).

Once again, evidence for specific uptake, retention and binding of estrogens in the fetal mouse mammary gland comes only from autoradiographic localization of radioactivity in cells of the mammary gland primordia after injection of ^{3}H-diethylstilbestrol to the mother (16 days of gestation) (Narbaitz *et al.*, 1980). In both female and male fetuses, the nuclei of the mesenchymal cells surrounding the epithelial primordium are more heavily labeled. On the other hand, from actual measurements of specific estrogen receptor binding postnatally, receptors were found to be undetectable before 2 weeks of age but increased 10-fold between 2 and 4 weeks (Hunt and Muldoon, 1977; Muldoon, 1979).

The localization of estrogen in the mesenchyme again emphasizes its importance in differentiation and its influence on the epithelial cells previously alluded to concerning the mouse genital tract (Cunha *et al.*, 1982). In 1949, Balinsky observed that the formation of the epithelial mammary Anlage may be induced by specialized underlying mesenchyme and Kratochwil (1969, 1972) showed that mesenchymal factors control the formation of the ductal branching pattern of the mammary gland. As for the embryonic mouse genital tract, these observations seem to point to the mesenchyme as the primary site of hormonal action in the embryonic mammary gland.

1.3.3. BRAIN

In the mouse, estrogen receptors are present in the fetal brain, particularly in the hypothalamus-preoptic area (Vito and Fox, 1979; 1982). Binding of the synthetic tritiated estrogen, R2858 (moxestrol), in the cytosol fraction, is of high affinity ($K_d = 4 \times 10^{-10}$ M) (Friedman *et al.*, 1983). Fetal hypothalamus (16–18 days of fetal age) contains 45 fmol estradiol bound per g tissue, and fetal brain (minus the hypothalamus) contains only 10 fmol per g tissue, determined by the retention of ^{3}H-estradiol receptor complexes to DNA-cellulose. Using the DNA-cellulose method of measuring receptor binding to compare the estrogen receptors in mouse and rat brains, the concentration of estrogen receptors in fetal mouse hypothalamus-preoptic area is already high at the earliest prenatal age studied (3 days before birth) while the rat hypothalamic estrogen receptor increases at the end of gestation and after birth (Vito and Fox, 1982). The measurement of binding of ^{3}H-moxestrol (R2858) in the cytosol fraction of mouse hypothalamus shows a steady increase in receptor capacity from fetal day 15 to post-natal day 9 (Friedman *et al.*, 1983). Gerlach and co-workers (1983) found a similar ontogenic profile using radioautography. Cells labeled with ^{3}H-moxestrol could not be seen in the hypothalamus and preoptic area of day 13 fetuses but were evident on day 15, with marked increases occurring between fetal day 15 and 18, both in number of labeled cells and in intensity of labeling per cell.

1.4. Humans

1.4.1. BRAIN AND PITUITARY

High affinity, specific binding of ^{3}H-estradiol is present in the cytosol fraction of pituitary, hypothalamus, cortex, and limbic system of both male and female human fetuses (Davies *et al.*, 1975). Binding is specific for natural and synthetic estrogens and androgens or cortisol do not bind. Binding of estradiol by limbic and cortical tissue is greater than by pituitary and hypothalamus.

1.4.2. KIDNEY AND LUNG

Estrogen binding has been reported to occur in cytosol fractions of lung and kidney obtained from human abortuses during the second trimester (Mendelson *et al.*, 1980). Although having characteristics slightly different from those of plasma sex hormone binding globulin or α-fetoprotein, the cytosol estrogen binding protein does not resemble a classical estrogen receptor. The macromolecule binds estrogen with low affinity ($K_d = 10^{-7}$ M), sediments as a 4 S entity in low salt sucrose density gradients and exhibits little or no affinity for diethylstilbestrol. It is interesting to compare these observations with those found by Khosla *et al.* (1983) for estrogen binding in rabbit fetal lung which shares similar characteristics (i.e. relatively low affinity, no binding to diethylstilbestrol or ethynyl estradiol). Moreover, in rabbit fetal lung there was little correlation between estrogen binding and function as measured by estrogen-induced increase in the rate of choline incorporation into phosphatidylcholine, the major component of pulmonary surfactant. Therefore, it appears that the binding components in human fetal lung and kidney as well as in the rabbit fetal lung do not present the characteristics of a receptor protein.

1.4.3. PANCREAS

Pancreatic tissue was obtained from five abortuses (12–14 weeks) which were separated into two pools. High affinity ($K_d = 1.2$–1.3×10^{-9} M) ^{3}H-estradiol binding was detected in the cytosols of fetal pancreas (157 and 175 fmol/mg protein for each of the two pools) and of pancreatic carcinomas (430–1900 fmol/mg protein) but not in normal adult pancreas (Greenway *et al.*, 1981). The authors suggest that a phenomenon of de-repression of fetal genes may occur during the neoplastic process.

1.5. Primates

1.5.1. BRAIN AND PITUITARY

Estrogen receptors are present in brain and anterior pituitaries of fetal rhesus monkeys (*Macaca mulatta*) (135–162 days of fetal age) (Pomerantz *et al.*, 1985). Binding is highest in the anterior pituitary (6 fmol/mg protein), intermediate in the hypothalamus-preoptic area/amygdala (0.8 fmol/mg protein) and lowest in the cerebral cortex (0.1 fmol/mg protein). These receptors may be involved in the action of estrogens on sexual differentiation in primates similar to their role in the rodent brain. The retention of radioactive estradiol in fetal monkey brain after injection of ^{3}H-testosterone to the fetus suggests that estradiol from the aromatization of testosterone binds to existing estrogen receptors in the primate fetal brain (Michael *et al.*, 1989).

1.5.2. UTERUS

Estrogen receptors have been studied by Kimmel *et al.* (1983) and Hochner-Celnikier *et al.* (1986). Specific binding of ^{3}H-R2858 was demonstrated in the uterus of the last third of gestation in cynomolgus monkey fetuses (Hochner-Celnikier *et al.*, 1986). The value of the dissociation constant was 0.2×10^{-10} M, the number of estrogen binding sites 90 fmol/mg protein. No estrogen binding was detected in fetal lung, heart, brain, liver, kidney, adrenal, pituitary, skin, muscle or bone.

In the study by Kimmel and co-workers (1983), in tissue obtained from rhesus monkey fetuses near term (153–157 days of gestation), specific binding of ^{3}H-estradiol was demonstrated in the cytosol fraction. Binding of ^{3}H-estradiol was inhibited by both natural and synthetic estrogens but not by progesterone. The range of concentrations of binding sites was 110–270 fmol/mg protein with a dissociation constant of 0.3–1.0 nM. On low salt sucrose density gradients the ^{3}H-estradiol complexes sedimented at 6–7 S.

1.6. Other Mammals

It is interesting to mention here a study performed on estradiol binding kinetics in the uterus from 2-week-old newborn rabbits because of the undifferentiated state of the lower reproductive tract at this age (Chilton *et al.*, 1987). Moreover, serum estradiol concentrations are extremely low (1.8 ± 0.4 (SD) pg/ml). Lower concentrations of estrogen receptors were found in juvenile uteri compared with adult uteri. Juvenile estrogen receptor showed a faster dissociation rate of steroid from receptor (and a decrease in association constant) and a reduced estrogen receptor activation as measured by binding of estradiol-receptor complex to DNA cellulose. The authors suggested that these factors would limit the biological effect of estradiol on this immature tissue (Chilton *et al.*, 1987).

2. In the Maternal Compartment and During Lactation

2.1. Rats and Mice

2.1.1. UTERUS

The process of nidation in the rat requires synchrony between the action of progesterone and estradiol which leads to endometrial receptivity, decidualization and implantation and nidation (Nelson and Pfiffner, 1930; Yochim and DeFeo, 1962; Zeilmaker, 1963; Yoshinaga *et al.*, 1969; Glasser and Clark, 1975; Psychoyos 1973a,b, 1976). In the rat, the initiation of the egg implantation process occurs on day 5 and can be seen by local endometrial increases in vascular permeability accompanied by stromal edema (Psychoyos, 1960).

For the rat endometrium to enter an ovo-receptive state, the endometrium must have been previously primed with progesterone for at least 48 h before being potentiated by estradiol (Psychoyos, 1973a,b; Glasser and Clark, 1975). It has been proposed that the mammalian blastocyst itself secretes the estradiol or, at least, accumulates the estradiol which provides the stimulus whose effect could be mediated by estrogen receptors at the implantation sites (Perry *et al.*, 1973; Dickmann *et al.*, 1975 and 1976; Borland *et al.*, 1977; George and Wilson, 1978; Singh and Booth, 1979). Studies in rats have not clearly determined whether the blastocyst is implicated or how receptors may be involved but due to the numerous studies using this model, a survey of the literature will give us an idea of how, where and when receptors may be involved in nidation and pregnancy in one animal species.

2.1.1.1. Estrogen Receptors During Implantation and Early Pregnancy

Feherty and co-workers (1970) showed that ^{3}H-estradiol binding in supernatants of pregnant rat uterus was higher in the first week of pregnancy than in the uterus of the nonpregnant animal at any stage of the estrous cycle (Table 2.7). On days 7 and 9, when binding in the conceptus was measured separately from the surrounding uterine wall, binding in the implant areas was five to six times higher than in the uterine wall. Estradiol binding was localized in the developing placenta at 10 days and declined thereafter. Binding was found to be of high affinity in all tissues studied, the K_d at 30° C ranging from 1.5×10^{-10} M in placenta to 4.2×10^{-10} M in whole uterus on day 4.

Subsequent studies have concentrated efforts on the critical period of the first five days of pregnancy when blastocyst implantation occurs in the rat. Peripheral blood levels of estradiol in the pregnant rat increase between day 1 and 4 with a peak on days 3–4 (see Fig. 2.16) (Watson *et al.*, 1975). The rise is accompanied by increases in

TABLE 2.7. *Concentration of Estradiol Binding Sites in the Pregnant Rat Uterus*

Physiological State	Tissue	pmol/mg Tissue
Days of pregnancy		
0	Whole uterus	7.9
1	Whole uterus	7.9
2	Whole uterus	8.6
3	Whole uterus	7.0
4	Whole uterus	8.7
5	Whole uterus	6.9
7	Implantation area	12.7
	Uterine wall	3.3
9	Implantation area	10.8
	Uterine wall	2.0
10	Fetus + membranes	0.5
	Placenta	7.2
	Uterine wall	3.0
13	Fetus	0
	Fetal placenta	0
	Maternal placenta	1.7
	Uterine wall	2.8
18	Placenta	0
	Uterine wall	4.0
Stage of cycle		
Estrus	Whole uterus	1.0 ± 0.3 (SD)
Metestrus	Whole uterus	1.7 ± 0.3 (SD)
Diestrus I	Whole uterus	1.8 ± 0.2 (SD)
Diestrus II	Whole uterus	4.7 ± 1.0 (SD)
Proestrus	Whole uterus	4.9 ± 1.0 (SD)

Pregnancy was determined on the morning after mating by the presence of sperm in the vaginal smears (day 0). Means of at least 3 experiments
Quoted from Feherty *et al.* (1970).

cytoplasmic and nuclear estrogen receptors in the oviduct and the uterus. In the oviduct, high affinity estrogen binding in the nucleus peaks during day 4 of pregnancy at the time of the peak in plasma estradiol concentration in this study, just prior to the transfer of ova from the oviduct to the uterus (Fuentealba *et al.*, 1982).

Mester *et al.* (1974) found higher receptor concentrations in the endometrium than in the myometrium during the first days of gestation. The endometrial cytoplasmic

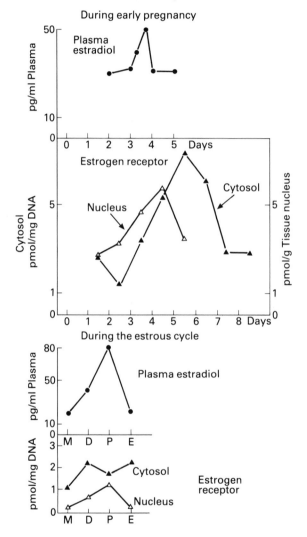

FIG 2.16. Comparison of Cytosol and Nuclear Estrogen Receptors in the Uterus and Plasma Estradiol Concentrations in the Rat during Early Pregnancy and the Estrous Cycle.

Day 1 of pregnancy was the morning on which sperm was first observed in the vaginal smear. Plasma estradiol values are taken from Butcher *et al.* (1974) and Watson *et al.* (1975). Estrogen receptor concentrations are adapted from Mester *et al.* (1974), Glasser and Clark (1975) and Clark *et al.* (1972). M = metestrus; D = diestrus; P = proestrus; E = estrus.

TABLE 2.8. *Estrogen Receptor Concentrations in the Endometrium and Myometrium of the Rat During Early Pregnancy (pmol/mg DNA)*

Day of pregnancy	Endometrium	Myometrium
1	2.66 ± 0.96	0.89
2	1.41 ± 0.37	0.81 ± 0.44
3	3.40 ± 0.59	1.63 ± 0.71
4	5.33 ± 0.89	1.78 ± 0.59
5	7.40 ± 0.52	2.22 ± 0.59
6	6.22 ± 0.22	1.78 ± 0.41
7	2.81 ± 0.74	1.33 ± 0.44
8	2.74 ± 0.52	1.92 ± 0.29

Means $\pm$ SD
Quoted from Mester *et al.* (1974).

estrogen receptor concentration increases up to day 5 and declines during days 7 and 8 (Table 2.8). The equilibrium dissociation constants are $3-5 \times 10^{-10}$ M for the endometrium and $6-9 \times 10^{-10}$ M for the myometrium. The divergence in the concentrations of endometrial and myometrial estrogen receptors during implantation could be explained by the findings of Martel and Psychoyos (1978) that in ovariectomized rats, progesterone treatment increases estrogen receptor levels in the endometrium while having no effect on myometrial receptors. However, in the myometrium, progesterone inhibits the estrogen-induced increase in estrogen receptors.

Circadian variations in nuclear estrogen receptor concentrations of the rat endometrium were reported by Martel and Psychoyos (1976) in both the high salt-extractable and insoluble nuclear fractions, with surges occurring nightly from day 2 to day 5 of pregnancy (cytosol receptors only increased on day 5). By day 6, nuclear receptor levels plateaued at minimal values, which was not the case for the cytosol receptor (see Table 2.8). The last nightly surge on day 4 coincides with the period of implantation in rats, but the increases are not sufficiently well correlated with the pattern of plasma estradiol and progesterone levels. Glasser and Clark (1975) observed only a transient increase in the nuclear estrogen receptor in the whole uterus between days 3 and 4 which declined on day 5. Despite the varying observations, it is clear that the pregnant rat uterus and oviduct contain estrogen receptors whose concentrations seem to vary in a physiological manner with the increases in plasma estradiol or progesterone at a period when the uterus is sensitive to an estrogen stimulus.

2.1.1.2. Estrogen Receptor Concentrations at the Implantation Sites

Receptor concentrations have been compared at the actual implantation sites and the inter-implantation segments of the endometrium of the rat. Logeat *et al.* (1980) found increased nuclear estradiol receptors at the implantation sites (day 6) (Table 2.9) while

TABLE 2.9. *Estrogen Receptors in Implantation and Nonimplantation Segments of the Rat Endometrium*

	Estrogen receptor (pmol/mg DNA)	Reference
Ovx-pregnant controls		
Cytosol	7.31 ± 0.52	Martel and Psychoyos (1981)
Nuclear	0.06 ± 0.04	
Ovx-pregnant-		
P + E-treated[a]		
Implantation sites		
Cytosol	3.40 ± 0.43	
Nuclear	0.03 ± 0.01	
Nonimplantation sites		
Cytosol	7.25 ± 0.61	
Nuclear	0.06 ± 0.10	
6-day Pregnant[b]		
Implantation sites		Logeat *et al.* (1980)
Cytosol	11.33 ± 1.73	
Nuclear	8.83 ± 0.34	
Nonimplantation sites		
Cytosol	12.11 ± 1.05	
Nuclear	4.65 ± 0.33	
Pseudopregnant		
Decidualized horn		Logeat *et al.* (1980)
Cytosol	1.23 ± 0.12	
Nuclear	1.43 ± 0.14	
Nondecidualized horn		
Cytosol	1.33 ± 0.17	
Nuclear	1.38 ± 0.16	

[a]Pregnant rats were ovariectomized on day 3 and treated with 4 mg of progesterone daily. On day 8, implantation was induced by an injection of estradiol (0.25 µg per rat). Implantation sites were visualized by injecting Evans blue;
[b]Six-day pregnant rats were injected with Trypan blue to reveal implantation sites.
Means $\pm$ SE

the cytosol receptor concentrations were not different between the implantation and nonimplantation sites. De Hertogh *et al.* (1986) observed significantly lower estrogen receptor concentrations in cytosols of the endometrium at the implantation sites but confirmed the results of Logeat *et al.* (1980) that the number of nuclear receptors is increased. Both groups thus agree that the nuclear-to-cytosol receptor ratios are significantly higher in the endometrium obtained from implantation sites. No differences were observed between the two sites in the myometrium (De Hertogh *et al.*, 1986).

It should be noted that one study found conflicting results (Martel and Psychoyos, 1981). Delayed implantation rats were used, i.e. pregnant rats ovariectomized on day 3 of pregnancy and treated daily with 4 mg of progesterone. Implantation was induced on day 8 by injecting estradiol (0.25 μg per rat); the rats were sacrificed 24 h later. Implantation segments were visualized by staining with Evans blue dye as in the study by De Hertogh *et al.* (1986), and estrogen receptors were measured in the endometrium. Cytosol and nuclear estrogen receptors were significantly lower at the implantation sites compared to the nonimplantation sites where receptor concentrations were similar to those of the control animals (Table 2.9).

Since dramatic changes occur in vascularization and in uterine cell morphology during the process of decidualization, the receptor data could reflect these changes. For this reason, observations in rats made pseudopregnant by uterine trauma where decidualization occurs in the absence of blastocyst implantation, are useful comparisons and are also included in Table 2.9. Nuclear estrogen receptors are not increased in the decidualized horn of the uterus so that the authors (Logeat *et al.*, 1980) concluded that it is the blastocyst itself that furnishes the steroids which affect the intracellular distribution of receptor. Moreover, since the receptors in the myometrium are unaffected, it is suggested that the estrogenic effect is highly localized at the implantation site of the blastocyst.

Figure 2.16 summarizes the cytosol and nuclear receptor distribution and the plasma estradiol levels during early pregnancy and also indicates the receptor levels found in the uterus during the rat estrous cycle. The results tend to indicate that between days 3 and 4 of gestation in the rat, rising titers of circulating estradiol lead to retention of the estrogen receptor in the nucleus, analogous to the situation prevailing during the estrous cycle. This peak in nuclear binding capacity precedes the implantation period which occurs on day 5 in the rat and, moreover, nuclear receptor concentrations are actually declining at this critical period while cytosol receptor levels are rising. However, at this point, the interaction of the blastocyst with the uterus in the process of decidualization probably enters into play since nuclear estrogen receptors at the implantation site appear to increase.

It is tempting to conclude that the prenidatory increase in estrogen leads to retention of estrogen receptor in the nucleus (much as during the estrous cycle) where it mediates metabolic events crucial for implantation of the blastocyst which itself also contributes an estrogen stimulus which initiates a localized effect on the intracellular distribution of estrogen receptor at the implantation site. Definite proof will depend on further studies on both the estrogen- and progesterone-responsive cell populations and their interactions within the complex organ which is the uterus.

Nidation is a very complex process which involves chemical and physical factors. The physical factors include membrane permeability which is a consequence of the pH change in the environment of nidation. This is correlated with biochemical mechanisms which include antiproteases and a series of other factors such as prostaglandins (particularly $PGF_2\alpha$) and estrogens. The role of estrogens is not very clear and, at the moment, the correlation of the presence of estrogen receptors at the implantation site with the different biochemical steps involved in this process remains to be clarified. In addition, during the nidation period new proteins are synthesized in this environment which include pregnancy associated protein A (PASA) whose role is also to be explored.

2.1.1.3. At Parturition and During Lactation

At the approach of parturition and during lactation, changes occur in estrogen receptor concentrations in the rat uterus. Cytosol estrogen receptors have been measured using techniques which account for both available and endogenous estrogen-occupied estrogen binding sites. Figure 2.17 shows that there is a decrease in estrogen receptor concentration (specific binding of ^{3}H-estradiol at 30° C) before parturition followed by a sharp rise at the time of parturition. Receptor values return to preparturition levels by day 1 post-partum and steadily increase to about day 15 post-partum (Leung *et al.*, 1976; Mohla *et al.*, 1981; Yu and Leung, 1982). The myometrium, which undergoes extensive degradation after delivery, shows a similar decrease from 108 fmol/mg protein to only 25 fmol/mg protein on day 1 post-partum with a significant rise on day 12 (Geyer *et al.*, 1982). The dissociation constants (K_d at 4° C) do not vary significantly throughout the period studied (3.7 ± 0.6 (SE) $\times 10^{-10}$ M) (Yu and Leung, 1982) although an earlier study from the same laboratory seemed to indicate a four-fold increase in K_d between days 1–11 of lactation and days 14–21 (Leung *et al.*, 1976). The uterine estrogen receptor was found to sediment in the 8 S region of sucrose density gradients both pre- and post-partum and during lactation (Leung *et al.*, 1976; Mohla *et al.*, 1981; Yu and Leung, 1982).

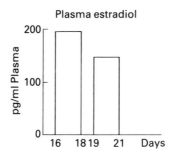

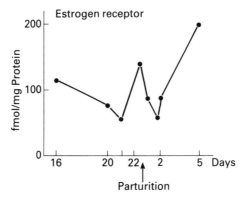

Fig 2.17. Cytosol Estrogen Receptors in the Maternal Rat Uterus before and after Parturition and Plasma Estradiol in the Pregnant Rat.
Plasma estradiol values adapted from de Lauzon *et al.* (1974) and cytosol estrogen receptor data taken from Yu and Leung (1982).

Estrogen receptor levels in the pre- and post-partum uterus are probably regulated by the changes in the hormonal environment occurring at the time of parturition and during lactation which include the sharp increase in estrogens at parturition (Fig. 2.17), the continuous increase in the release of prolactin (Bast and Melampy, 1972; Simpson *et al.*, 1973) and the decrease in progesterone biosynthesis (Fajer and Barraclough, 1967; Leung and Sasaki, 1973; Koligian and Stormshak, 1977). This interplay could contribute to estrogen sensitization of the uterus during the time of parturition.

2.1.1.4. Estrogen Action in the Uterus During Implantation

Estrogen-induced changes in the preimplantation endometrium have been observed that are associated with uterine receptivity to the blastocyst. Estrogen stimulates proliferation of the luminal then the glandular epithelium (Martin and Finn, 1968). Pretreatment with progesterone inhibits this estrogen effect (Finn and Martin, 1973). Neither hormone alone affects the mitotic activity in the stroma but progesterone stimulates stromal mitosis after estrogen-priming (Finn and Martin, 1970). These experimental observations may be related to the hormonal changes that occur during the peri-implantation period. The ovulatory peak in plasma estrogens provokes epithelial proliferation followed by the glandular epithelium. The rise in plasma progesterone conditions the stroma to proliferate in preparation for implantation. Morphological, cytological and metabolic changes can also be provoked by estrogen and progesterone treatment that resemble those associated with the peri-implantation uterus (for a review, see Weitlauf, 1988). The presence of estrogen receptors at the implantation sites of the uterus during this period may be one prerequisite for estrogen activity, but the molecular basis of the complex process involved in endometrial sensitivity and receptivity has not yet been elucidated.

2.1.2. MAMMARY GLAND

During pregnancy and lactation, the differentiation of the mammary gland is under hormonal stimulus and control by prolactin, estrogens, progesterone and other steroid hormones. Numerous studies are described in the literature on the occurrence of estrogen receptors and estrogen action in the rat and mouse mammary glands (for a review see Shyamala, 1985).

The mammary gland of the ovariectomized C3H mouse has been shown to concentrate and retain ^{3}H-estradiol (Puca and Bresciani, 1969) and in an autoradiographic study of mammary glands of lactating mice (post-partum days 11–14) and rats (post-partum day 21), radioactivity was concentrated in nuclei of epithelial cells of alveoli and ducts. Mammary glands of pregnant rats (days 7 and 13 of gestation) showed weak nuclear concentration of radioactivity in some epithelial cells (Sar and Stumpf, 1976). Estrogen receptors were quantitated in the lactating mammary gland of mice and rats as early as 1972 (Shyamala and Nandi, 1972; Wittliff *et al.*, 1972) and in the pregnant mammary gland (Hunt and Muldoon, 1977) and have since led to detailed studies on the biochemical peculiarities of the estrogen receptor in pregnant and lactating mammary glands.

2.1.2.1. Physicochemical Characteristics of the Estrogen Receptor in the Mouse Mammary Gland

The equilibrium binding constants of estrogen binding to mouse mammary receptor do not vary significantly during pregnancy and lactation (Auricchio *et al.*, 1976; Muldoon, 1978) but the characteristics of the receptor on sucrose density gradients undergo transformation from a 4 S form in virgin mice to a progressively greater 8 S component during pregnancy so that by the end of pregnancy and during lactation all of the receptor sediments as an 8 S entity (Muldoon, 1978; Muldoon, 1979) (Table 2.10). This transformation of receptor form is not only a biochemical trait but is also potentially of physiological importance since although the equilibrium binding parameters are similar for both forms, the kinetic parameters are different. At 4° C, the 4 S complex from virgin mice forms more rapidly ($k_{+1} = 9.5 \times 10^5 \, \mathrm{M}^{-1} \mathrm{s}^{-1}$) than the 8 S complex from late pregnant mammary gland ($k_{+1} = 1.9 \times 10^5 \, \mathrm{M}^{-1} \mathrm{s}^{-1}$) but the 8 S complex dissociates more slowly ($k_{-1}, 4° \mathrm{C} = 7.2 \times 10^{-6} \mathrm{s}^{-1}$) than the 4 S complex ($k_{-1}, 4° \mathrm{C} = 2.2 \times 10^{-5} \mathrm{s}^{-1}$). The half-life of the 8 S complex is 26.7 h at 4° C compared to 9 h for the 4 S complex (Muldoon, 1978 and 1979). The 8 S receptor is also less specific than the 4 S form for estrogens (Muldoon, 1981). These observations imply that at a time when available hormones are high as is the case at late pregnancy in the mouse, the 8 S receptor would bind and retain estrogens or even slow-acting estrogens over a longer period even when the estrogen levels may fall. In addition, Muldoon (1981) has also shown that chronic estradiol administration to virgin mice will not only increase estrogen receptor levels (2.5-fold above untreated controls) but also lead to an almost complete shift from the 4 S to the 8 S form. Prolactin treatment also resulted in even greater amounts of estrogen receptor (3.4-fold above untreated controls) and the same shift to the 8 S form. In the late pregnant mouse, concomitant administration of prolactin and estradiol resulted in increased binding and retention of estrogen receptor

TABLE 2.10. *Physicochemical Properties of Cytosol Estrogen Receptor in Mammary Glands of the Mouse in Different Physiological States*

	Virgin	Pregnant 16–20 days	Lactating 6–10 days
Number of sites			
fmol/mg protein	33–45	25	53
fmol/mg DNA	177	169	71
fmol/g tissue	733	909	276
fmol/animal	31	110	69
K_d ($\times 10^{-9}$ M), 4° C	0.42–0.44	0.81	0.28–0.54
k_{+1} ($\times 10^5$ M^{-1} sec^{-1}), 4° C	9.5	1.9	
k_{-1} ($\times 10^{-6}$ sec^{-1}), 4° C	22	7.2	
Binding specificity	Estradiol > 5αDHT > testosterone > estrone	Estradiol = estrone > 5αDHT = testosterone	
Sedimentation coefficient	4 S	8 S	8 S

Quoted from Richards *et al.* (1974); Auricchio *et al.* (1976); Hunt and Muldoon (1977); Muldoon (1978; 1981).

in the nucleus, indicating the complementarity of these two hormones in altering the molecular form of the receptor, increasing its concentration and favoring nuclear binding (Muldoon, 1981).

It remains, however, to be remarked that another report has suggested that shifts in sedimentation coefficients of the mouse mammary cytoplasmic estrogen receptor may actually be artefacts of the buffers used in the preparation of the cytosol fractions and of an increased level of endogenous proteases in mammary glands of virgin mice (Gaubert *et al.*, 1982). Although Haslam and co-workers (1984) were not able to demonstrate any differences in receptor activation, Gaubert and co-workers (1986) showed that upon exposure to 0.4 M KCl only 20% of the total estrogen receptor from lactating mammary glands bound to DNA cellulose while 60–80% of the receptor from nulliparous mice could bind to DNA. Furthermore, Shyamala *et al.* (1986) showed that binding of mammary estrogen receptor to mammary chromatin from lactating mice was also impaired compared to chromatin from nulliparous mice.

2.1.2.2. Changes in Estrogen Receptor Levels During
Pregnancy and Lactation in the Mouse

Figure 2.18 indicates the levels of estrogen receptor in mouse mammary glands during pregnancy and lactation. When expressed as receptors per cell (fmol per

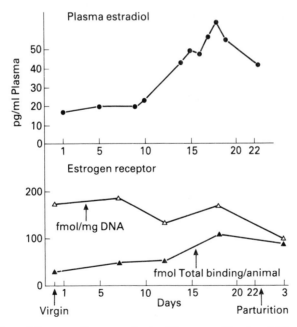

FIG 2.18. Cytosol Estrogen Receptors in the Mammary Gland and Plasma Estradiol Concentrations in the Mouse during Pregnancy and Lactation.
The day of detection of a vaginal plug was designated day 1 of pregnancy. Plasma estradiol data taken from Barkley *et al.* (1977). Cytosol estrogen receptor data adapted from Hunt and Muldoon (1977) and Muldoon (1979) and expressed either as fmol/mg DNA or fmol bound in the combined mammary tissue from one animal.

mg DNA), the numbers are higher during pregnancy and decrease during lactation. More striking is the increase in total receptor per mouse which reaches a maximum at the end of gestation due to the great increase in tissue weight (42.3 mg dry weight/mouse in nonpregnant mice to 121.1 mg dry weight/mouse at 16–19 days of gestation) which, however, does not compensate for the decrease in receptor concentration per cell which occurs during lactation (335.7 mg dry weight/mouse at 15 days post-partum in a lactating mouse) (Hunt and Muldoon, 1977; Muldoon, 1978, 1979; Shyamala and Haslam, 1980). The rise in estrogen receptor levels coincides with rising titers of estradiol (Fig. 2.18) (Barkley *et al.*, 1977) and prolactin (Bast and Melampy, 1972; Murr *et al.*, 1974). Prolactin has been shown to increase estrogen receptor levels in virgin mice (Muldoon, 1981) and in mammary explants (Leung and Sasaki, 1973).

2.1.2.3. Physicochemical Characteristics of Estrogen Receptors in the Rat Mammary Gland

The presence of a specific estrogen binding component has also been demonstrated in the mammary gland of the pregnant and lactating rat whose characteristics are very similar to those of the receptor in the mouse (Table 2.11). The estrogen binding protein of the late pregnant and lactating rat mammary gland sediments at 8.6 S in a low salt sucrose density gradient and at 4–5 S in a high salt gradient (Wittliff *et al.*, 1972; Gardner and Wittliff, 1973a). Mohla and co-workers (1981) observed that between days 14 and 16 of gestation the receptor was in a 4 S form which shifted to the 8 S form by days 2–3 post-partum. However, Gardner and Wittliff (1973a) could only detect binding activity in the 8–9 S region of the gradient in the late pregnant and in the

TABLE 2.11. *Physicochemical Properties of Cytosol Estrogen Receptor in Mammary Glands of the Rat During Pregnancy and Lactation*

	Pregnant (16–20 days)	Lactating (10–21 days)
Number of sites		
fmol/mg protein	4–9	10–50
fmol/mg DNA	–	45–160
fmol/mg tissue	–	200–650
K_d (10^{-9} M), 4° C		0.1–1.0
Binding specificity	Estrogens	Estrogens
		No binding of nonestrogens
Sedimentation coefficient	8–9 S (late pregnant) 4 S (mid-pregnant)	8.6 S (low salt) 4.5 S (high salt)
Proteolysis	–	Destroyed
Thermal stability	–	Labile at 25° C

Quoted from Gardner and Wittliff (1973a); Hsueh *et al.* (1973); Leung *et al.* (1976); Mohla *et al.* (1981); Yu and Leung (1982).

virgin mammary glands which is in contrast to the shift observed in the mouse. During lactation, estradiol binds with high affinity in the cytosol with no significant difference between early and late lactation (Mohla *et al.*, 1981). Receptors acquire higher affinity for nuclear binding sites by either *in vivo* or *in vitro* exposure to estradiol during pregnancy and lactation (Gardner and Wittliff, 1973a; Hsueh *et al.*, 1973).

2.1.2.4. Variations in Rat Mammary Gland Estrogen Receptors During Pregnancy and Lactation

Observations in the literature are contradictory as to how the concentrations of mammary gland estrogen receptors vary during pregnancy and lactation in the rat. Yu and Leung (1982) found receptor levels of approximately 10 fmol/mg protein between days 16 and 20 of gestation which declined abruptly on day 21 of gestation and only began to rise 6 h after delivery and increased to the predelivery level by 18 h. Bohnet and co-workers (1977) reported that there is a sudden dramatic increase from 4 fmol/mg protein during pregnancy to 20 fmol/mg protein in the lactating mammary gland within two days of parturition followed by only a slight decline until day 15. Other groups (Hsueh *et al.*, 1973; Leung *et al.*, 1976; Mohla *et al.*, 1981) have observed a gradual increase in receptor concentrations between days 14–16 of gestation and day 20 of lactation regardless of whether the values are calculated on the basis of protein, DNA or wet weight of the tissue. By days 1 to 3 after the termination of lactation, receptor concentrations have already declined to prelactation levels (Leung *et al.*, 1976). In contrast to the rat, it should be recalled that in the lactating mammary gland of the mouse, estrogen receptor concentrations decrease progressively during lactation.

Estrogen administration for three days does not cause any significant change in the levels of estrogen or progesterone receptors in the lactating mammary gland of the rat although both receptors increase approximately three-fold in uteri from the same animals, suggesting estrogen refractoriness in the mammary gland (Mohla *et al.*, 1981). However, the activity of RNA polymerases I and II are significantly increased by estradiol treatment (Mohla *et al.*, 1981).

The administration of ovine prolactin within 8 h post-partum has no significant effect on estrogen binding in the lactating mammary gland and although bromocriptin suppression of prolactin secretion decreases the number of prolactin binding sites, it does not affect the estrogen binding sites (Bohnet *et al.*, 1977).

In summary, receptors which bind estrogens with high affinity and great specificity tend to be relatively abundant during lactation in both the mouse and rat mammary gland, although the concentrations are much less than in the uterus of the same animal. A conformational change in receptor form results in a shift in sedimentation coefficient from the 4 S to the 8 S form during gestation which alters the kinetics of formation of the estrogen-receptor complex to a more slowly dissociating form. In the lactating mammary gland receptor activation is impaired. Receptor is capable of binding in the nucleus when challenged with estradiol but in the untreated, intact lactating animal, very little receptor is already bound in the nucleus, probably due to a low level of estrogen in the blood (Hsueh *et al.*, 1973). Estrogen receptor concentrations may be increased by prolactin, at least in the pregnant animal, but during lactation, the mammary gland is relatively refractory to estrogen stimulation. It has been suggested that this is due to the differentiation of the gland itself during lactation into a secretory organ.

2.1.2.5. Estrogen Responses in Mammary Glands

The estrogen sensitivity of normal mammary tissue becomes altered by the physiological state of the gland itself since the mammary glands of lactating mice are not responsive to estradiol (Haslam and Shyamala, 1979a; Shyamala and Ferenczy, 1982). Haslam and co-workers (1984) showed that although the lactating mouse mammary gland is biochemically potentially competent to respond to estradiol, it is remarkably estrogen-insensitive. Estradiol does not stimulate progesterone receptor (Haslam and Shyamala, 1981), glucose metabolism or DNA synthesis (Shyamala and Ferenczy, 1982) although the basal levels of the latter two parameters were already high (but not influenced by ovariectomy of lactators). The nonresponsiveness of lactating mammary glands could be associated with the modifications that have been observed in the estrogen receptor, but the relationship is still not clear. It should be noted that administration of estradiol to lactating mice does lead to accumulation of estrogen receptor in the nucleus (Shyamala and Nandi, 1972). (For a review of these aspects of estrogen responsiveness in the mammary gland see Shyamala, 1985.)

The regulation of the progesterone receptor by estrogens in the mammary gland is related to the differentiation of the gland since progesterone is important for alveolar growth during pregnancy (Topper and Freeman, 1980). During lactation, the function of the mammary gland is deviated from growth to milk production so that elevated progesterone receptor concentrations would not be an advantage. This response to estrogen seems to be associated with the process of differentiation.

Other studies showing that estrogen-induced DNA synthesis is initiated earlier in the mammary fat pad (adipose and connective tissue) than the epithelium have led to the conclusion that the apparent estrogen insensitivity of the lactating mammary gland also lies in the morphology of the lactating tissue itself (large number of secretory epithelial cells) and not to the hormonal environment (Shyamala and Haslam, 1980; Shyamala and Ferenczy, 1982, 1984). *In vitro* experiments using cultures of mammary epithelial cells have shown that the epithelial cells are estrogen responsive only in the presence of fibroblasts or factors from the fibroblasts, indicating that epithelial–stromal interactions can determine and modulate epithelial cell responses to estrogen (Haslam, 1986). Moreover, the refractoriness of lactating mammary cells may also depend on their sensitivity to other hormones such as insulin (Oka *et al.*, 1974) and prolactin (Bolander and Topper, 1981) since growth and differentiation of mammary glands are under multihormonal control (Topper and Freeman, 1980).

2.2. Other Mammals

Studies in other mammalian species help to elucidate the role of receptors in the process of implantation and the maintenance of gestation.

2.2.1. RABBITS

2.2.1.1. Uterus

In the rabbit, ovarian estradiol does not appear to be required for initiation of implantation (Chambon, 1949) so that it is possible that the hormonal stimulus derives from the implanting blastocyst since estrogen synthesis by the 6-day rabbit blastocyst has been demonstrated (Seamark and Lutwak-Mann, 1972; Dickmann *et al.*, 1975; Dey *et al.*, 1976).

The cytosol fraction of oviducts and uteri of pregnant rabbits contain a putative estrogen receptor with an affinity of $0.88-1.17 \times 10^{-10}$ M (K_d at 30° C) for estradiol and sedimenting at 8 S in a low salt sucrose density gradient (Muechler *et al.*, 1974). At 3 h post-coitum (p.c.), the receptor concentrations in both the oviduct and uterus were found to be only slightly lower than levels at estrus, which corresponds to a period of high ovarian secretion of estradiol and progesterone (Hilliard and Eaton, 1971). The concentrations are higher in the uterus than in the oviduct (281 fmol/mg protein in the uterus vs 148 fmol/mg protein in the oviduct). A significant decrease occurs in both tissues (155 fmol/mg protein and 128 fmol/mg protein) at 12 h p.c. when ovulation occurs and ovarian steroid secretions decline. Receptor levels increase 72 h p.c., when fertilized ova are migrating from the oviduct into the uterus but do not attain the concentrations found at estrus. Six days p.c., receptor concentrations in both tissues decline. At this time the blastocyst implants and ovarian steroid production is high. The study indicates that the variations in ovarian secretion of both estradiol and progesterone influence receptor concentrations in both the oviduct and the uterus.

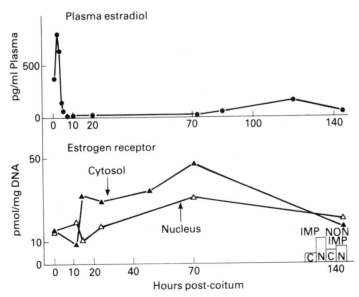

Fig 2.19. Cytosol and Nuclear Estrogen Receptors in the Oviduct and the Uterus and Plasma Estradiol Concentrations in the Rabbit during Early Pregnancy.
Estradiol concentrations in ovarian venous plasma taken from Hilliard and Eaton (1971). Cytosol and nuclear estrogen receptors were measured in the oviduct by Puri and Roy (1981a) and in the implantation (IMP) and nonimplantation (NONIMP) segments of the uterus (columns indicated at 140 h p.c.) by Puri and Roy (1981b).

Estrogen receptor concentrations in specific segments of the rabbit oviduct have also been studied in more detail since in this case estrogen binding in the nucleus was also measured (Puri and Roy, 1981a). In fact, receptor concentrations varied throughout all segments of the oviduct with a similar pattern. At 12 h p.c., nuclear binding through the whole oviduct increases while cytosol binding decreases (note that Muechler *et al.*, 1974 also observed a significant decline in cytosol receptor). At 14 h p.c., when ova are in the ampulla, nuclear receptor decreases and cytosol receptor increases. At 24 h p.c., when ova are in the ampullary-isthmic junction, nuclear and cytosol receptor concentrations increase and remain elevated to 72 h. At 6 days p.c., nuclear receptor is high while cytosol receptor decreases, particularly in the implantation segments (12 pmol/mg DNA vs 7.8 in the interembryonic segment) (Puri and Roy, 1981b). Lescoat *et al.* (1985) also observed a decrease in cytosol receptor in the implantation area as

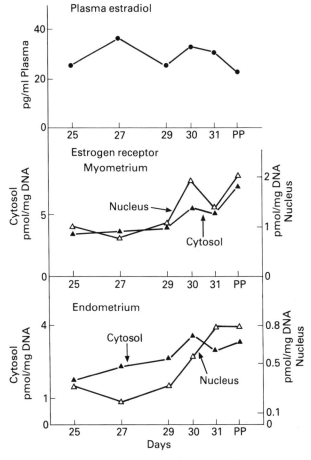

FIG 2.20. Cytosol and Nuclear Estrogen Receptors in the Myometrium and the Endometrium and Plasma Estradiol Concentrations of Rabbits during Late Pregnancy and within 0–10 h Post-partum (PP).

Quoted from Quirk and Currie (1984).

compared to the nonimplantation area. These observations, which resemble those of Logeat *et al.* (1980) in the implanting rat uterus, again tantilizingly suggest a hormonal stimulus from the implanting blastocyst. One report has also suggested the presence of specific estradiol binding proteins in the cytosol fraction of the blastocyst itself (Bhatt and Bullock, 1974). A summary of the observations in the rabbit oviduct and uterus around the time of implantation is presented in Fig. 2.19.

In the rabbit, endometrial and myometrial estrogen receptors rise as the ratio of plasma estradiol to progesterone increases at the end of pregnancy (Quirk and Currie, 1984). Figure 2.20 shows that the cytosolic and nuclear estrogen receptor concentrations in the myometrium and endometrium do not change between days 25 and 29 of gestation but as circulating concentrations of progesterone begin to decline between days 29 and 30, estrogen receptor concentrations in both tissues increase and remain elevated even post-partum. The concentrations of receptors in the myometrium are twice those in the endometrium. Although the plasma concentrations of estradiol do not change during the period, the decrease in plasma progesterone may be the cause of the increase in estrogen receptor.

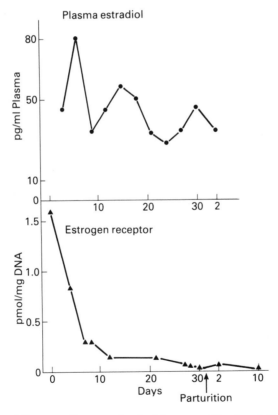

FIG 2.21. Cytosol Estrogen Receptors in the Mammary Gland and Plasma Estradiol Values in the Rabbit during Pregnancy and Lactation.
The day of mating was considered day 0 of pregnancy. Plasma estradiol values taken from Challis *et al.* (1973) and cytosol estrogen receptor data from Kelly *et al.* (1983).

2.2.1.2. Mammary Gland

Estrogen receptors have been found in the mammary glands of virgin rabbits on the day of mating, with significantly higher quantities being present in those females which had accepted the male than in those which had not mated (Kelly *et al.*, 1983). The average concentration of ^{3}H-R2858 (Moxestrol) binding in the cytosol fraction is 36.5 ± 14.0 (SE) fmol/mg protein in the mated females on day 0 of pregnancy with a K_d of $0.23 \pm 0.07 \times 10^{-9}$ M (at 23° C). The receptor is specific for natural and synthetic estrogens and sediments at 8–9 S in a low salt sucrose density gradient. During pregnancy, receptor concentrations decline and remain low during lactation. In contrast, it can be recalled that during the same period the rabbit uterus contains a much higher concentration of estrogen receptor; cytosol receptors rise during the first three days after mating before declining but at day 6 p.c. the level attained is approximately the same as at the time of mating (day 0). As seen in Fig. 2.21, the cytosol receptor concentration decrease occurs during the pre-implantation period when plasma estradiol concentrations tend to rise. Since nuclear receptor concentrations were not measured, it is possible that the binding in the nucleus could account for the loss in more loosely bound receptors found in the cytosol fraction.

2.2.2. HAMSTERS

In the hamster serum estradiol and progesterone increase gradually during pregnancy and both hormones decline abruptly before term on day 16. The estradiol-to-progesterone ratio does not change. Myometrial estrogen receptors (cytosol and nuclear) remain low and constant until day 16 of pregnancy when there is a distinct increase before parturition (Leavitt, 1985). Figure 2.22 illustrates the variations in estrogen receptor concentrations during pregnancy and during the estrous cycle. Although not evident from Fig. 2.22 because different units have been used to express receptor concentrations, estrogen receptor levels in myometrial cytosol and nuclei are lower during gestation as compared with uterine receptor levels during the estrogen-dominated phase of the hamster estrous cycle but tend to approach the pro-estrous values at term. At pro-estrus, myometrial receptor levels (pmol/mg DNA) are: 2.02 ± 0.08 (SE) for cytosol receptor and 1.66 ± 0.06 for nuclear receptor (Leavitt, 1985). The results indicate that estrogen receptor levels are suppressed by progesterone throughout pregnancy and recover when serum progesterone declines at term.

The effect of ovarian steroid hormones on the level of estrogen receptor sites already occupied by endogenous estrogens was also studied by Leavitt and Okulicz (1985). In the pseudopregnant females (induced by sterile mating and ovariectomy) the endometrium was traumatized to induce decidualization, and serum hormone levels were maintained by progesterone and estradiol implants. During the estrous cycle occupied estrogen receptor in the nucleus reaches a value of 1.54 ± 0.18 (SE) pmol/mg DNA at estrus and in the cytosol fraction 0.78 ± 0.11 pmol/mg DNA. The appearance of receptor in both fractions parallels the increase in serum estradiol during the follicular phase. Rising titers of progesterone down-regulates the occupied receptors in the nucleus. Progesterone withdrawal in the presence of increasing serum estradiol concentrations leads to a re-establishment of the distribution of occupied receptor between

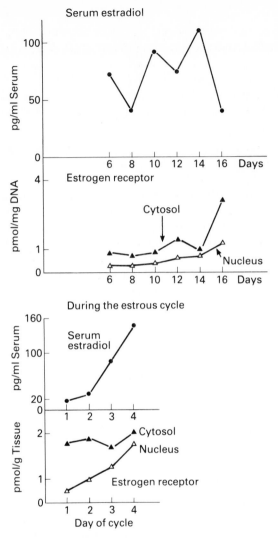

FIG 2.22. Estrogen Receptor Concentrations in the Myometrium or Whole Uterus and Serum Estradiol Concentrations during Pregnancy and the Estrous Cycle in the Hamster.

Day 1 of pregnancy was the day immediately after mating (day 4 of the cycle). Parturition occurred in the morning of day 16. Receptor values in the myometrium during pregnancy taken from Leavitt (1985) and in the whole uterus during the estrous cycle from Evans *et al.* (1980). Serum estradiol values taken from Leavitt (1985) and Saidapur and Greenwald (1978).

nucleus and cytosol. The same pattern of occupied estrogen receptor was observed during progesterone withdrawal in pseudopregnancy where steady-state levels of serum estradiol were maintained. This study also shows the importance of circulating progesterone levels on the regulation of estrogen receptor concentrations under physiological conditions.

2.2.3. CATS

In the pregnant cat, nuclear estrogen receptor concentrations vary closely with the systemic levels of estradiol and progesterone (West *et al.*, 1977). In both the oviduct and the uterus, nuclear receptor levels are maximal at estrus and between day 2–4 p.c. (3–4 pmol/mg DNA as compared to 0.5–1 pmol/mg DNA at anestrus) when estradiol concentrations are highest (16–18 vs 9 pg/ml at anestrus), declining between days 8 to 40 p.c. to 1.5–2 pmol/mg DNA when the circulating progesterone concentration has risen from 0.9 ng/ml at anestrus to 12 ng/ml.

2.2.4. PIGS

The pregnant pig endometrium possesses binding sites with high affinity (7.3 ± 0.6 (SE) $\times 10^{-10}$ M, K_d at 30° C) and specificity for estradiol (Deaver and Guthrie, 1980). In both the pregnant and the nonpregnant (nonbred) pigs, endometrial cytoplasmic estrogen receptors are maximal (1–1.5 pmol/mg DNA) during the mid-luteal phase in the pig (days 8–12 after the onset of estrus) which would seem to contradict observations in other animal species in which estrogen receptor concentrations decline during the progesterone-dominated phase. However, in the pig the presence of endometrial estrogen receptors may be a prerequisite for the process by which the blastocyst could block the luteolytic effect of the uterus and favor the maintenance of pregnancy. In the pig, on days 10 and 12, blastocysts must be present in both uterine horns to prevent luteolysis (Dhindsa and Dziuk, 1968) and estrogen secretion by blastocysts may mediate maternal recognition of pregnancy (Heap *et al.*, 1975; Bazer and Thatcher, 1977). It is interesting to note that changes in estrogen receptor levels in the ampullar and isthmic segments of the pig oviduct precede those occurring in the uterus during the estrous cycle. Maximal concentrations of cytosol and nuclear receptors were observed in the ampulla at estrus parallel to the pro-estrus rise in plasma estradiol (Stanchev *et al.*, 1985).

2.2.5. COWS

High affinity binding sites for estradiol could also be demonstrated in the cytosol fraction of the endometrium of pregnant cows (dissociation constant in the range of 10^{-10} M) (Senior, 1975; Henricks and Harris, 1978) and in nuclei (Erdos and Friès, 1979). The concentration of estrogen binding sites per cell in endometria from cows between days 15 and 35 of gestation is about 7000 sites/cell, which is similar to that observed during the luteal phase of the estrous cycle (Senior, 1975) as compared to a mean concentration of 48 000 sites/cell found during the follicular phase. Receptor concentrations in individual animals do not vary with estradiol concentrations measured in the cytosol (12–143 pg/g wet weight). No significant difference was observed in binding between the two uterine horns so that whatever influence the blastocyst may have on the uterus is not a marked generalized effect on receptor binding, although the implantation sites were not specifically examined.

The results of Henricks and Harris (1978) are very similar, indicating that the binding affinity and concentrations of estrogen binding sites at days 2–3 or at days 13–14 of pregnancy are not significantly different from those of cycling animals at the same stage after estrus. Mean receptor concentrations are 1975 fmol/mg DNA at days 2–3 and 1062 fmol/mg DNA at days 13–14 with a K_d of 1.2×10^{-10} M. Estradiol concentrations are higher in the cytosol of 2–3-day pregnant animals (33.8 pg/g) than in the 13–14-day pregnant animals (10.7 pg/g).

2.2.6. BRUSH-TAIL POSSUMS (*TRICHOSURUS VULPECULA*)

A marsupial has also been studied because of certain characteristics (Curlewis and Stone, 1986). The female brush-tail possum is monovular with an oestrous cycle length of 24–26 days. Gestation length is 17–18 days. Serum estradiol concentrations are high during estrus and low from days 5 to 13, while progesterone concentrations increase rapidly between days 7 and 13. Peripheral estradiol and progesterone concentrations are not altered by pregnancy. In marsupials, the left and right uteri are separate so that during pregnancy, changes in receptor concentration can be studied in the ipsilateral and contralateral uterus to the ovary with the corpus luteum. The concentration of estrogen receptors in pooled right and left uteri from cycling adult possums reaches 11.5 ± 0.65 (SE) pmol/mg DNA at day 5 of the estrous cycle and declines to 2.6 ± 0.21 at day 13. The levels of estrogen receptor on day 13 in the ipsilateral and contralateral uteri of the pregnant possum are similar (2.32 and 2.65, respectively) despite the increase in weight and DNA content of the ipsilateral uterus (Curlewis and Stone, 1986). These variations seem to follow the serum estradiol and progesterone levels.

2.3. Humans

2.3.1. UTERUS

Estrogen receptor binding has been measured in human endometrium during pregnancy in both the cytosol fraction and the nucleus using methods which take into account the presence of receptor sites occupied by endogenous hormone and also plasma binding proteins in the endometrial homogenate (Kreitmann and Bayard, 1979). Previous reports were incomplete due to the inadequate techniques available at the time (Limpaphayom *et al.*, 1971; Trams *et al.*, 1973; Haukkamaa, 1974). Table 2.12 compares the concentrations of cytosol and nuclear estrogen receptors during early pregnancy (8–10 weeks) and at term (38–40 weeks) with those of the late proliferative and late secretory phases of the menstrual cycle. Despite the limited number of samples assayed (seven to thirteen), no differences were found during pregnancy whose values were comparable to those of the late secretory phase of the menstrual cycle and much less than the late proliferative phase. From 60–67% of the total estrogen receptor binding sites are in the nuclei during pregnancy and in the late secretory phase.

In another study, Padayachi and co-workers (1987) measured cytoplasmic and nuclear estrogen receptors in decidua of ectopic pregnancy (6–8 weeks gestation) and therapeutic abortions (8–16 weeks). The concentrations in the decidua are lower than in the endometrium of the luteal phase studied at the same time. In contrast to the study by Kreitmann and Bayard (1979), this group was not able to detect estrogen receptors in full-term pregnant tissue obtained during elective or emergency Cesarean section, irrespective of whether the patients were in labor or not. It was concluded from

TABLE 2.12. *Estrogen Receptors (Cytosol + Nuclear) in the Human Endometrium During Pregnancy and the Normal Menstrual Cycle*

	pmol/mg DNA	Sites/cell
Gestation		
8–10 weeks	0.33 ± 0.17	1314 ± 672
38–40 weeks		
Cesarean section	0.41 ± 0.16	1627 ± 622
Spontaneous delivery	0.61 ± 0.43	2413 ± 1715
Menstrual cycle		
Late proliferative	1.93 ± 1.51	7732 ± 6040
Late secretory	0.65 ± 0.47	2592 ± 1868

Means ± SD
Quoted from Bayard *et al.* (1978); Kreitmann and Bayard (1979).

this study that estrogen receptors decrease with advancing pregnancy. Khan-Dawood and Dawood (1984) were able to show that estrogen receptors were present in decidua in term pregnancies with a ratio of cytosol to nuclear receptors of 3:1.

The human myometrium has been investigated for estrogen receptor binding during pregnancy using exchange assays for cytosol and nuclear binding by Giannopoulos and co-workers (1980). Table 2.13 demonstrates that the total concentrations of cytosol and nuclear estrogen receptors in the myometrium at term are similar to the values reported for the endometrium and are five times less than the levels during the menstrual cycle. However, all receptors were found to be located in the nucleus during pregnancy or during labor while most (72–76%) were found in the cytosol during the menstrual cycle. The levels of nuclear receptors at term and during the proliferative phase are similar. Khan-Dawood and Dawood (1984) found similar results in eight women who underwent elective Cesarean section at term. The myometrium contained nuclear

TABLE 2.13. *Estrogen Receptors in the Human Myometrium in Pregnancy at Term and During the Menstrual Cycle*

	Cytosol	Nuclear
	pmol/mg DNA	
Gestation		
38–42 weeks		
Cesarean section	not detected	0.31 ± 0.12
Spontaneous delivery	not detected	0.17 ± 0.01
Menstrual cycle		
Proliferative phase	1.11 ± 0.17	0.44 ± 0.07
Secretory phase	1.18 ± 0.18	0.38 ± 0.05

Means ± SE
Quoted from Giannopoulos *et al.* (1980).

estrogen receptor but no measurable cytosol receptors, in contrast to the decidual tissues studied at the same time which had more cytosol than nuclear receptors. It can be seen in Table 2.13 that the total receptors in the myometrium do not appear to vary during the menstrual cycle as they do in the endometrium. The group of Padayachi and co-workers (1987) was not able to detect estrogen receptors in the myometrium at full term.

2.4. Primates

The quantity of nuclear and cytosolic estrogen receptors in endometria during early gestation compared with the secretory phase of the normal ovulatory cycle of the rhesus monkey (*Macaca mulatta*) has been studied recently by Ghosh and Sengupta (1988). As seen in Table 2.14, estrogen receptor concentrations remain stable on days 2–6 of gestation, but in the secretory phase, the receptor levels decline significantly in the cytosol fraction. From day 4, both cytosol and nuclear receptor concentrations are significantly higher in endometria during gestation than those obtained from secretory phase tissues. These changes in concentration are not caused by changes in the apparent equilibrium dissociation constants (K_d) (3.1×10^{-10} M on days 5 and 6 of gestation and 2.9×10^{-10} M during the mid-luteal phase) (Ghosh and Sengupta, 1988).

TABLE 2.14. *Estrogen Receptors in Rhesus Monkey Endometrium during the Pre-implantation Stages of Gestation and the Secretory Phase of the Normal Menstrual Cycle*

Days	Cytosol	Nuclear
	pmol/mg DNA	
Gestation		
2	1.67 ± 0.14	0.63 ± 0.06
3	1.50 ± 0.14	0.66 ± 0.05
4	1.40 ± 0.04	0.58 ± 0.05
5	1.41 ± 0.08	0.56 ± 0.04
6	1.57 ± 0.12	0.61 ± 0.05
Postovulation		
2	1.60 ± 0.06	0.54 ± 0.05
3	1.46 ± 0.09	0.44 ± 0.05
4	1.22 ± 0.05	0.37 ± 0.04
5	1.28 ± 0.03	0.42 ± 0.04
6	1.20 ± 0.03	0.39 ± 0.07

Means $\pm$ SE
Day of ovulation for non-fertile females = 24 h after the peak of serum estradiol. Day of gestation = 24 h after the peak of serum estradiol for females mated during days 8–16 of their cycles.
Quoted from Ghosh and Sengupta (1988).

Nuclear estrogen receptors have been measured in the monkey endometrium around the time of implantation which occurs around day 24 of the fertile menstrual cycle in these primates (9–10 days after fertilization). Kreitmann-Gimbal and co-workers (1981) report that the endometrial nucleus possesses receptor binding sites with high affinity and specificity for estrone, separate from the estradiol binding sites. The K_d of the nuclear binding of estrone is 5×10^{-10} M which is in the range of values found for cytosol binding of estradiol. In the fertile menstrual cycle, on day 24 the ratio of nuclear estrone receptor to nuclear estradiol receptor shifts to as much as 2.5 (from < 1 during the proliferative phase) which coincides with the late secretory phase increase in serum progesterone. The ratio could be mimicked by either chorionic gonadotrophic stimulation of progesterone secretion by the corpus luteum or by treatment with progesterone (Kreitmann-Gimbal *et al.*, 1981). The physiological significance of specific estrone binding sites in the nucleus of the monkey endometrium has not yet been explained (Kreitmann-Gimbal *et al.*, 1981).

3. In the Placenta

3.1. Rats

3.1.1. CHARACTERISTICS AND ONTOGENY OF A PLACENTAL ESTROGEN RECEPTOR

Receptor-like macromolecules have been characterized in the rat placental trophoblast, yet the role of estrogen receptors in placental function remains to be elucidated.

Specific estradiol binding was measured in the cytosol fraction and in nuclei of the basal zone trophoblast of the rat placenta (McCormack and Glasser, 1976). Table 2.15 shows the physicochemical characteristics of this putative receptor from mid-gestation placentae. The values are similar to those reported for estrogen receptors from the uterus except for the sedimentation coefficient of 4 S for the cytosol macromolecule. The placental receptor has a high affinity for estradiol ($K_d = 1.65 \times 10^{-10}$ M) and is

TABLE 2.15. *Physicochemical Properties of Cytosol and Nuclear Estrogen Receptors in Rat Placental Trophoblast (Day 11 of Pregnancy)*

	Cytosol	Nucleus
Number of sites sites/cell	12 000	21 000
K_d ($\times 10^{-9}$ M), 4° C	0.17	0.19
k_{+1} ($\times 10^6$ M^{-1} sec^{-1}), 20° C	1.17	–
k_{-1} ($\times 10^{-4}$ sec^{-1}), 20° C	1.28	–
Binding specificity	DES = 17β-estradiol > estriol, estrone, 17α-estradiol	
Sedimentation coefficient	4 S	5 S

Quoted from McCormack and Glasser (1976).

specific for estrogens. The number of binding sites per cell in the day-11 trophoblast (12 000 sites/cell) is in the range of concentrations found in the rat uterus. Although the basal zone trophoblast has areas of syncytial character along with cytotrophoblast which is not syncytial, receptor was never found in the labyrinthine zone.

The number of binding sites in the cytosol fraction of the basal zone decreases from approximately 5 pmol/mg DNA (30 000 sites/cell) on day 9 of pregnancy to 0.2 pmol/mg DNA (1000 sites/cell) on day 15, with no change in the apparent binding affinity (Fig. 2.23) (McCormack and Glasser, 1978). From day 16 until delivery, estrogen receptor concentrations remain undetectable in both the cytosol fraction and the nucleus. On the other hand, the plasma estrogen levels tend to increase during this time (Fig. 2.23) (de Lauzon *et al.*, 1974). On day 11 the trophoblast contains about five times more receptor than the decidua. Removal of the fetus on or before day 12 of gestation arrests the development of the labyrinthine zone and produces a relative shift in placental type to a preponderance of trophoblast giant cells, but fetectomy on day 12 does not affect the ontogeny of the estrogen receptor in the placenta suggesting that these receptors disappear at a predetermined rate and not because of an increase or loss of a particular cell population. However, administration of progesterone or progesterone plus estrogen to intact pregnant rats provokes a significant loss of nuclear estrogen receptor although it has no effect on cytosol receptor (McCormack and Glasser, 1978). Since progesterone secretion by trophoblast giant cells is maximal on day 12 of pregnancy in the rat placenta (Marcal *et al.*, 1975), it is suggested that this

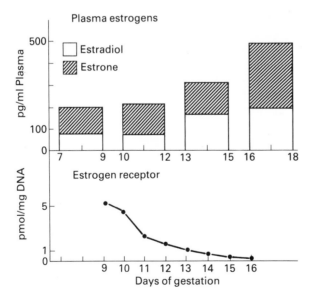

FIG 2.23. Comparison of Cytosol and Nuclear Estrogen Receptors in the Rat Placenta and Plasma Estrogen Concentrations during Gestation.
Plasma estradiol and estrone concentrations are quoted from de Lauzon *et al.* (1974). (The values are the means of pools indicated by the width of the columns whose heights represent the sum of the estradiol plus estrone concentrations.) Estrogen receptor concentrations (cytosol + nuclear) are quoted from McCormack and Glasser (1978).

local secretion of progesterone acting with estrogen from the ovary regulates the concentrations of estrogen receptors in the developing placenta.

3.1.2. RESPONSE TO EXOGENOUS ESTROGEN

When pregnant rats are treated with estradiol between days 10 and 12 of gestation, progesterone receptor concentrations are increased by 200% of the saline-injected control value (Ogle, 1980). This activity of estradiol can be antagonized by subsequent treatment with progesterone (Ogle, 1980). It is clear that exogenous estrogen treatment can elicit a response in the placenta, but the actual receptor-mediated role of estrogens in the placenta remains to be elucidated.

3.2. Humans

An estradiol-binding protein with characteristics similar to those found in the rat placenta has been described in the human term placenta (Younes et al., 1981; Kneussl et al., 1982). Khan-Dawood and Dawood (1984) were also able to confirm these observations but the study by Padayachi and co-workers (1987) showed no detectable cytosolic or nuclear estrogen receptors in any of the term pregnancy tissues studied (placenta, decidua, myometrium, amnion or chorion). Table 2.16 shows that the binding of estradiol is of high affinity ($K_d = 7.35 \times 10^{-9}$ M) and specificity with a sedimentation coefficient of 4–4.5 S as in the rat placenta. Using the technique of autoradiography, estrogen binding was found to be localized in the syncytiotrophoblast and continuous layer of the cytotrophoblast in early placental villi (Fujimori and Yamada, 1977). The syncytiotrophoblast is the site of biosynthesis of progesterone and estrogen during primate pregnancy. Since the human placenta produces large amounts of estrogens by aromatization of C_{19} precursors, the receptor-like binding in the placenta may play a role in controlling the action of these estrogens on such parameters as fetal and placental growth rate.

TABLE 2.16. *Physicochemical Properties of the Cytosol Estrogen Receptor in Human Term Placenta*

Number of sites	
fmol/mg protein	55 ± 18 (SD)
K_d ($\times 10^{-9}$ M), 4° C	7.4 ± 1.1
Binding specificity	Estradiol = DES > estrone
	No binding of nonestrogens
Sedimentation coefficient	4–4.5 S

Quoted from Younes *et al.* (1981).

B. PROGESTERONE RECEPTORS

The specific binding of progesterone to macromolecules in a target organ like the uterus of mammalian and avian species has been known for some time (Sherman et al., 1970; Corvol et al., 1972; Feil et al., 1972). Progesterone by itself does not produce the secretory uterine epithelium characteristic of the second half of the menstrual cycle; previous exposure to an estrogen is required for the expression of the progesterone effect. In fact, estrogen priming significantly stimulates the synthesis of the progesterone receptor (Sherman *et al.*, 1970; Corvol *et al.*, 1972). Progesterone is also a well known estrogen antagonist, and this action of progesterone involves both progesterone and estrogen receptors (for a review, see Clark and Peck, 1979). Thus, the activity of progesterone depends on an interplay between estrogens and progestins (see *Hormones and the Fetus*, Vol. 1, Chapter 1). It is evident that this progestin–estrogen interaction is important during the implantation phase of pregnancy which may depend on elevated estrogen and estrogen receptor levels at the implantation site and the maintenance of pregnancy which depends on progesterone.

The placenta and the fetus are also potential sites of progestin action which may be part of the maintenance of pregnancy or the onset of parturition and the normal development of the reproductive organs during the prenatal stage. The presence of progesterone receptors in the maternal as well as in the fetal compartments and in the placenta lend credence to the possible action of progesterone at all three levels.

1. In the Fetal Compartment

1.1. Guinea-pigs

1.1.1. Uterus, vagina and ovary

1.1.1.1. Physicochemical Characteristics of the Progesterone Receptor

The presence of progesterone receptors in the uterus of the guinea-pig fetus was first demonstrated by measurement of specific binding of ^{3}H-progesterone as well as the synthetic progestin ^{3}H-R5020 in the cytosol fraction (Pasqualini and Nguyen, 1979a). Receptor binding is readily detectable in untreated fetuses and is increased seven- to ten-fold in estrogen-primed fetuses (Pasqualini and Nguyen, 1980).

Complementary studies using the technique of autoradiography confirmed the retention of ^{3}H-progesterone by the fetal uteri and suggested a selective retention of the radioactivity by cells of the uterine stroma and muscle of estrogen-primed fetuses (Tardy and Pasqualini, 1980).

Table 2.17 shows some characteristics of the specific binding of ^{3}H-R5020 in fetal uterine cytosol which are similar to those for the progesterone receptor identified in the adult guinea-pig (Corvol *et al.*, 1972).

Since the guinea-pig is a species that possesses a plasma protein that has a high binding affinity for progesterone (progesterone binding globulin or PBG) (see Chapter 1) during gestation in both the maternal and the fetal compartments (Diamond *et al.*, 1969; Millet and Pasqualini, 1978; Perrot and Milgrom, 1978), it is necessary to distinguish this form of binding from the putative progesterone receptor binding found in the cytosol fraction of the fetal uterus. The principal characteristic used to distinguish the two types of binding is the fact that, although progesterone binds to both proteins,

TABLE 2.17. *Physicochemical Characteristics of the Cytosol Progesterone Receptor (Specific Binding of ^{3}H-R5020) in the Fetal Guinea-pig Uterus, Vagina and Ovary (55–65 Days of Gestation)*

	Uterus	Vagina	Ovary
Number of sites			
pmol/mg DNA	2.2 ± 0.5 (SD)	1.7 ± 0.7	–
fmol/mg protein	136 ± 35	116	72 ± 12
pmol/g tissue	13	4	–
pmol/organ	1.1	0.3	–
sites/cell	~1300	~1000	–
K_d (×10^{-9} M), 4° C	0.7 ± 0.3	0.4	0.6 ± 0.2
Binding specificity	R5020 = progesterone > 5α-dihydroprogesterone. No binding of cortisol, 20α-dihydroprogesterone, estrogens or testosterone	R5020 = progesterone = 5α-dihydroprogesterone. No binding of cortisol	R5020 = progesterone > 5α-dihydroprogesterone. No binding of cortisol
Sedimentation coefficient	6–7 S and 4 S in low salt	–	–
Isoelectric point	5–5.5	–	–
Thermal stability	Labile at 37° C	–	Labile at 37° C

Quoted from Pasqualini and Nguyen (1980); Nguyen *et al.* (1986).

the synthetic progestin R5020 does not bind specifically to PBG. Table 2.18 shows further differences between the binding of progesterone to cytosol receptor and to PBG. The differences clearly indicate that the specific binding of ^{3}H-R5020 measured in fetal guinea-pig uterine cytosol represents receptor binding and not binding to PBG.

Estrogen treatment of the maternal guinea-pigs leads to a seven- to ten-fold increase in the progesterone receptor, in the fetal guinea-pig uteri, which has the same characteristics as the receptor binding found in untreated fetuses (Pasqualini and Nguyen, 1979a,b; 1980). The estrogen-stimulated progesterone receptors show increased

TABLE 2.18. *Comparison of the Physicochemical Properties of the Specific Binding of ^{3}H-Progesterone in Fetal Uterine Cytosol and Plasma of the Guinea-pig*

	Uterus	Plasma
K_d (×10^{-9} M), 4° C	3.3 ± 1.2 (SD)	0.88 ± 0.35 (SD)
Binding specificity	Natural and synthetic progestins	No specific binding of R5020
Sedimentation coefficient (S)	6.7 S and 4 S	4.6 S
Isoelectric point (pI)	5–5.5	<3
Thermal stability	Labile at 37° C	Thermoresistant

Quoted from Millet and Pasqualini (1978); Pasqualini and Nguyen (1980).

retention in the nucleus when exposed to progesterone either *in vivo* or *in vitro* (Sumida *et al.*, 1982). Nuclear retention of the progesterone–receptor complex *in vitro* is temperature-dependent and specific for receptor bound to progestins.

Progesterone receptors are synthesized by explants of fetal uterine tissue in organ culture (Sumida *et al.*, 1983). Synthesis is independent of the addition of estradiol to the organ culture medium and is down-regulated by progestins. On the other hand, progesterone receptors are induced by estradiol in cells of the fetal uterus grown as monolayers in medium containing steroid-poor fetal calf serum (Sumida *et al.*, 1988).

1.1.1.2. Ontogeny of the Progesterone Receptor in the Uterus

Estrogen receptors are already detectable in the cytosol fraction of the fetal uterus at about mid-gestation (34–35 days) (see Section 1.1.1.3.) which is just after the time of differentiation of the uterus. In contrast, progesterone receptors only appear around day 50 of gestation and continue to rise until after birth (Fig. 2.24) (Pasqualini *et al.*, 1976c; Sumida *et al.*, 1980). The temporal relationship between the appearance of the estrogen and the progesterone receptors suggests that the progesterone receptor is induced in the fetal guinea-pig uterus by endogenous estrogens through the estrogen receptor system.

1.1.1.3. Action of Progesterone in the Fetal Uterus

In the adult mammalian uterus, progesterone acts on the estrogen-primed uterus as an endogenous antagonist of estrogen action (Lerner, 1964). In the immature rat, progesterone has been shown to antagonize the uterotrophic effect of estradiol probably by inhibiting the new synthesis of estrogen receptor and decreasing the concentration of its own receptor (Hsueh *et al.*, 1976; Walters and Clark, 1979).

In the fetal guinea-pig uterus, the action of progesterone could be demonstrated by its capacity to modulate estrogen responses. When administered to estradiol-primed fetuses, progesterone inhibits the uterotrophic effect of estradiol (Fig. 2.25) (Sumida *et al.*, 1981). Progesterone appears to act by reducing the retention of the estrogen

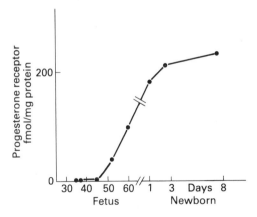

FIG 2.24. Ontogeny of Cytosol Progesterone Receptors in the Guinea-pig Uterus. Data adapted from Pasqualini *et al.* (1980b).

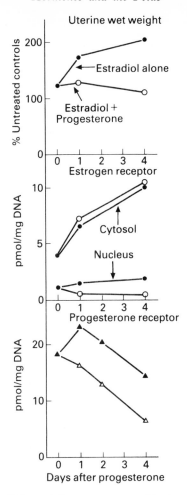

FIG 2.25. Antagonistic Effect of Progesterone on Uterine Wet Weight, Estrogen Receptors and Progesterone Receptors in the Estradiol-treated Fetal Guinea-pig uterus.

Fetuses were treated with estradiol one day before the administration of progesterone. The ● = effects of estradiol treatment alone; ○ = antagonistic effects of subsequent treatment with progesterone. Adapted from Sumida *et al.* (1981).

receptor in the nucleus but has no effect on the amount of estrogen receptor found in the cytosol fraction of the fetal uterus (Fig. 2.25). The reduction in estrogen receptors found in the nuclear fraction has also been consistently found in immature and adult animals (West *et al.*, 1978; Okulicz *et al.*, 1981). In contrast, in the neonatal guinea-pig uterus (Gulino and Pasqualini, 1983; Pasqualini *et al.*, 1983b, 1984) as well as in the immature rat (Clark *et al.*, 1977a) progesterone blocks the synthesis of new estrogen receptor which is required for replenishment of cytosol receptor concentrations.

Progesterone also causes a decline in the concentrations of the progesterone receptor (Fig. 2.25) (Sumida *et al.*, 1981). Since the progesterone receptor is induced by estrogens, the effect of progesterone on its own receptor could also be through its suppression of nuclear estrogen receptors.

In the fetal guinea-pig uterus, the acetylation of nuclear histones is stimulated by estrogens and progesterone antagonizes the estradiol-stimulated acetylation of histones (Pasqualini *et al.*, 1983a).

In conclusion, the fetal uterus can respond to exogenously administered progesterone when the uterus has previously been primed with estrogen. The action of progesterone can be perceived by the antagonism of estrogen responses. The mechanism of action of progesterone involves both the progesterone and the estrogen receptor systems. A change occurs between the pre- and post-natal periods since, in the fetus, exposure to progesterone leads to a rapid clearance of estrogen receptor from the nucleus while in the newborn or immature animal, progesterone also inhibits new estrogen receptor replenishment.

1.1.1.4. Progesterone Receptors in the Fetal Vagina

The fetal vagina shows specific, high affinity binding of the synthetic progestin R5020 (see Table 2.17). The concentrations are similar to those found in the fetal uterus at the same stage of development. The administration of estradiol to the pregnant guinea-pig also increases the concentrations of progesterone receptor in the fetal vagina similar to that seen in the fetal uterus (Nguyen *et al.*, 1986).

1.1.1.5. Progesterone Receptors in the Fetal Ovary

Progesterone receptors have also been found in the fetal guinea-pig ovary (see Table 2.17). The dissociation constant for the binding of ^{3}H-R5020 in ovarian cytosol is 0.6 ± 0.2 (SD) $\times 10^{-9}$ M and the concentration at 55 to 65 days of gestation is 72 ± 12 (SD) fmol/mg protein, somewhat less than in the uterus at the same age (136 ± 35 fmol/mg protein). The characteristics of the ovarian progesterone receptor are similar in all respects to those found in the fetal uterus (Pasqualini and Nguyen, 1980). Like the uterine receptor, ovarian progesterone receptor concentrations increase seven times in estradiol-treated fetuses (498 ± 171 (SD) fmol/mg protein). The finding that significant levels of progesterone receptors are present in the fetal ovary suggests that this receptor may be involved in fetal ovary maturation.

In contrast, although other fetal tissues such as the lungs, kidney, brain, heart and the placenta were also studied at the same time for possible progesterone receptor binding, no other tissues other than the uterus, vagina and ovary showed specific binding of progestins. Moreover, no significant induction by estradiol was observed (Pasqualini and Nguyen, 1980).

1.2. Rabbits

1.2.1. LUNG

1.2.1.1. Physicochemical Characteristics of the Progesterone Receptor

Fetal rabbit lung contains binding sites with high affinity and low capacity for progestins (Table 2.19) (Giannopoulos *et al.*, 1982). The high affinity binding sites are

TABLE 2.19. *Physicochemical Characteristics of the Progesterone Receptor (Specific Binding of ^{3}H-R5020) in the Cytosol from 29-Day-Old Fetal Rabbit Lung*

Number of sites	31.8 ± 1.6 (SE) fmol/mg protein
K_d (×10^{-9} M), 4°C	0.17 ± 0.02
Binding specificity	Natural and synthetic progestins
	Little binding of corticosterone
	No binding of dexamethasone or
	nonprogestins.
Sedimentation coefficient	7.1 S

Quoted from Giannopoulos *et al.* (1982).

specific for progestins, the glucocorticoids having very little affinity. The sites sediment at 7.1 S in low salt sucrose density gradients. The investigators also remarked the presence of two other types of binding sites in fetal rabbit lung. The second type of binding site is also specific for progestins but has a lower affinity and higher capacity. The third type of binding site binds glucocorticoids and progestins but is distinct from the glucocorticoid receptor.

1.2.1.2. Ontogeny of the Fetal Lung Progesterone Receptor

As seen in Table 2.20, a significant increase in the concentration of progesterone receptors occurs in the fetal lung between day 26 and 29 of gestation in the rabbit although these values are still far below the adult lung levels. The physiological significance of progesterone receptors in fetal lung and their increase at the end of gestation is, of course, not as clear as the role of glucocorticoids in fetal lung development. Giannopoulos and co-workers (1982) themselves point to contradictory results in the literature showing either an inhibitory effect of progesterone administration to fetal rabbits on fetal lung maturation or an acceleration of maturation in human fetal lung in organ culture (Pulkkinen and Kero, 1977; Kero and Pulkkinen, 1979; Mendelson *et al.*, 1979).

TABLE 2.20. *Ontogeny of Progesterone Receptors (Specific Binding of ^{3}H-R5020) in Fetal Rabbit Lung*

	fmol/mg protein	K_d (nM), 4° C
Fetus		
20 days	10	0.08
24 days	16	0.13
26 days	20	0.30
29 days	30	0.13
Adult	143	0.39

Quoted from Giannopoulos *et al.* (1982).

TABLE 2.21. *Specific Progestin (³H-R5020) Binding Sites in the Cytosols of Various Fetal Rabbit Tissues (29 Days)*

	fmol/mg protein	K_d (nM)
Lung	31.8 ± 1.6 (SE)	0.17 ± 0.02
Kidney	9.7 ± 1.6	0.40 ± 0.05
Small intestine	9.8 ± 3.4	0.89 ± 0.27
Brain	5.7 ± 1.5	0.25 ± 0.05
Muscle	5.0 ± 0.3	0.59 ± 0.28
Heart	3.8 ± 0.9	0.94 ± 0.49
Skin	2.4 ± 0.4	0.51 ± 0.11
Liver	2.0 ± 1.1	0.85 ± 0.16

Quoted from Giannopoulos *et al.* (1982)

1.2.2. VARIOUS OTHER TISSUES

In the process of studying the specific progestin binding sites in fetal rabbit lung, a number of tissues of the rabbit fetus were investigated for possible progesterone receptor binding sites (Giannopoulos *et al.*, 1982). Fetuses very late in gestation were studied (day 29 of gestation) which is a time when maternal plasma progesterone and cortisol levels decline in the rabbit (Challis *et al.*, 1973; Mulay *et al.*, 1973). As can be seen on Table 2.21, high affinity binding sites for the synthetic progestin R5020 are found in many fetal tissues, including the kidney and brain but by far the highest concentration is to be found in the fetal lung. The dissociation constants for the binding in the various tissues are similar.

1.3. Rats and Mice

1.3.1. UTERUS AND OVARY

In addition to estrogen receptors, the fetal uterus and ovary of the rat have significant quantities of progesterone receptor as measured by the specific binding of the synthetic progestin R5020 (Nguyen *et al.*, 1988). Table 2.22 shows that both fetal tissues contain progesterone receptors at least from day 18 of gestation. Nevertheless, the ontogeny of this receptor diverges; the fetal uterus shows an abrupt decline in receptors to nondetectable levels in 24-h newborns while the fetal ovary manifests a great increase in progesterone receptors after birth. As a comparison, Table 2.22 also indicates the estrogen receptor concentrations measured at the same time. It can be noted that the concentrations of estrogen receptor evolve in the opposite sense in the fetal uterus. This same study also showed that estradiol treatment of the pregnant rats led to an increase in progesterone receptors in both the fetal uterus and the fetal ovary (Nguyen *et al.*, 1988).

TABLE 2.22. *Progesterone Receptor Concentrations (Specific Binding of ^{3}H-R5020) in the Uterus and Ovary of the Fetal and Neonatal Rat: Comparison with Estrogen Receptors (Specific Binding of ^{3}H-R2858)*

	Uterus		Ovary	
	Progesterone receptor fmol/mg DNA ($\pm$SD)	Estrogen receptor fmol/mg DNA	Progesterone receptor fmol/mg DNA	Estrogen receptor fmol/mg DNA
Fetus, 18 days old	195 ± 37	63 ± 21	90 ± 19	105 ± 36
Fetus, 20 days old	97 ± 17	101 ± 18	132 ± 47	520 ± 73
Newborns, 24 h old	Nondetectable	415 ± 147	260 ± 67	410 ± 192

Quoted from Nguyen *et al.* (1988).

1.3.2. OTHER TISSUES

The distribution of ^{125}I-progestin in estrogen-primed 20-day-old fetuses of the mouse was determined by thaw-mount autoradiography (Shughrue *et al.*, 1988; 1989). Nuclear uptake and retention of radioactivity were observed in certain cells of a number of both reproductive and nonreproductive tissues. The most intense uptake and retention of radioactivity were found in nuclei of cells in the mesenchyme of the oviduct and uterus (Shughrue *et al.*, 1988). Uterine epithelium was not labeled. Nuclear concentration of radioactivity was also observed in the pre-optic area of the brain of male and female fetuses, within certain nuclear groups in the basal hypothalamus, in the central gray of the mid-brain, and in the pituitary (Shughrue *et al.*, 1989). No labeling was detected in the cortex or amygdala. The distribution of radioactive progestin is similar to that previously determined by Stumpf and co-workers (1980) for radioactive estrogen in the fetal mouse, suggesting that estrogens and estrogen receptors are involved in progesterone receptor induction in fetal mouse tissues.

1.4. Interaction of Progestins with Androgen Receptors

The interaction of progestins with androgen receptors is important for the understanding of other actions of progestins. Progestins possess androgenic activity in embryonic tissues; medroxyprogesterone acetate is as potent as testosterone propionate in masculinizing the external genitalia of female rat fetuses (Revesz *et al.*, 1960; Suchowsky and Junkmann, 1961). The binding of progestins to the androgen receptor is probably involved (Bardin *et al.*, 1978).

2. In the Maternal Compartment and During Lactation

2.1. Guinea-pigs

2.1.1. UTERUS

The levels of progesterone receptors depend to a great extent on the plasma estrogen and progesterone concentrations. As seen in Fig. 2.26, animals in early pregnancy (days

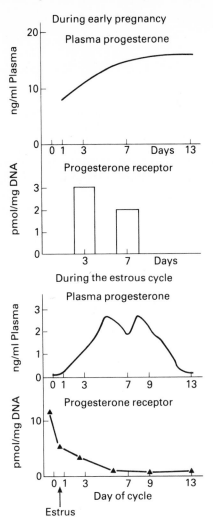

FIG 2.26. Progesterone Receptor Concentrations in the Guinea-pig Uterus during Early Pregnancy and the Estrous Cycle (Comparison with Plasma Progesterone Levels).
Quoted from Challis *et al.* (1971) and Milgrom *et al.* (1972).

3 and 7) do not show any significant difference in progesterone receptor content from nonpregnant animals at the corresponding period of the estrous cycle (Milgrom *et al.*, 1972). The concentrations are very low at the time of implantation (day 7) when circulating plasma progesterone levels are high. This observation probably reflects the down-regulation of the progesterone receptor by progesterone itself. In both the pregnant and non-pregnant uteri, the progesterone receptors sedimented mainly as 4 S binding complexes on low salt sucrose density gradients.

2.2. Rats and Mice

2.2.1. UTERUS

The conditions for interaction between ovum and endometrium which result in successful implantation of the blastocyst and maintenance of pregnancy depend on a series of sequential physicochemical and biological changes which include the development of uterine sensitivity and subsequent receptivity towards the blastocyst. In the rat, the synergistic action of estrogens and progesterone in this process has been well studied. If the rat uterus is progesterone-sensitized, implantation of synchronous blastocysts does not occur as long as progesterone is administered daily although the blastocysts remain viable in the uterus in a state of developmental diapause (delayed implantation) (Psychoyos, 1969; 1973b). However, implantation can be provoked by an injection of estrogen. Progesterone thus plays the predominant role in the maturation of the endometrium to the receptive state. Once gestation has commenced, progesterone is essential for the continuation of pregnancy by the maintenance of uterine quiescence (Davies and Ryan, 1972).

A study by DeHertogh and co-workers (1986) showed that around the time of implantation in the rat, higher concentrations of progesterone receptors can be found at the implantation sites than at the nonimplantation sites of the uterus of the 6-day pregnant rat (Table 2.23), although an earlier study by Logeat and co-workers (1980) had not been able to show this difference. Since the nuclear receptors for estrogens are also higher in the implantation sites, it has been suggested that local estrogenic activity at the implantation sites stimulates the synthesis of progesterone receptors in the close

TABLE 2.23. *Progesterone Receptor Concentrations in the Implantation and Nonimplantation Segments of the Rat Endometrium*

	pmol/mg DNA
6-*day Pregnant*	
Implantation sites	
Cytosol	3.3 ± 1.0
Nuclear	3.0 ± 1.2
Total	6.1 ± 1.9
Nonimplantation sites	
Cytosol	2.0 ± 0.3
Nuclear	1.4 ± 0.7
Total	3.4 ± 0.8

6-day pregnant rats were injected with Evans blue dye to reveal implantation sites. Progesterone receptor = specific binding of ^{3}H-ORG 2058 (16-ethyl-21-hydroxy-19-nor-4-pregnene-3,20-dione). Means $\pm$ SE
Quoted from DeHertogh *et al.* (1986)

TABLE 2.24. *Progesterone Receptor Concentrations in the Endometrium (Deciduoma) and Myometrium of the Rat During Early Pregnancy*

	Endometrium	Myometrium	Reference
Pregnant			
(fmol/mg protein)			
Day 1	–	35	Brodie and Green (1978)
Day 2	–	16	
Day 3	–	8	
Day 5	–	7	
Day 7	–	6	
Pseudopregnant			
(fmol/mg DNA)			
Day 0	3.7	3.7	Martel *et al.* (1984)
Day 1	5.7	5.3	
Day 3	10.5	7.3	
Day 5	11.5	7.1	
Day 7	5.7	5.0	

Day 1 of pregnancy was the day on which sperm was present in the vagina. Pseudopregnancy was provoked by the application of a traumatic decidualizing stimulus.

vicinity of the freshly implanted embryo in the 6-day pregnant rat endometrium (De Hertogh *et al.*, 1986).

During early pregnancy, progesterone receptor concentrations in the myometrium decrease to a low value by days 3–5 (Table 2.24) (Brodie and Green, 1978). Receptors were not measured in the endometrium at this time. On days 9 and 10, these authors report that the endometrium from the implantation sites showed more specific progesterone binding than the myometrium.

In pseudopregnant rats where decidualization is provoked by uterine trauma, progesterone receptor concentrations peak on day 3 after the traumatic stimulus in both the endometrium and the myometrium (Table 2.24) (Martel *et al.*, 1984). Estrogen receptor levels are already high at the time of application of the stimulus and decline by day 7 so that the peak in estrogen receptors precedes the peak in progesterone receptors and probably correlates with a stimulation of the synthesis of progesterone receptors. The development of the decidual reaction is known to be dependent on progesterone (Astwood, 1939; Yochim and DeFeo, 1963) which is consistent with the increase in progesterone receptor during the deciduoma growth phase.

During the course of pregnancy, progesterone receptors in the whole uterus rise until term (Fig. 2.27) (Vu Hai *et al.*, 1978). However, nuclear receptors decrease just before parturition when plasma progesterone also drops. Figure 2.27 also shows the concentration of endogenous progesterone in the uterine tissue during gestation (Wiest, 1970). Cytosol receptors appear to rise as the tissue concentration of progesterone falls.

The pattern of changes that occurs during the estrous cycle is also indicated in Fig. 2.27 to show that cytosol progesterone receptor concentrations are highest during pro-estrus, just before the peak in plasma progesterone. This again shows the downregulation of the progesterone receptor by progesterone itself.

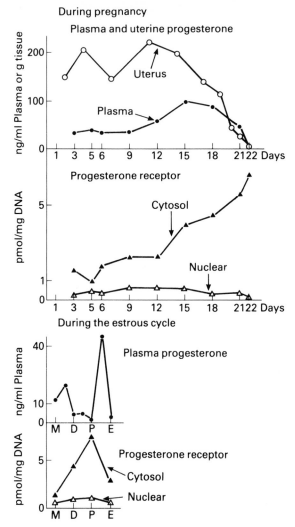

FIG 2.27. Variations in Concentrations of Progesterone Receptors in the Whole
Uterus of the Rat and Endogenous Progesterone during Pregnancy (Comparison
with the Estrous Cycle).

Day 1 of pregnancy was taken as the day of appearance of spermatozoa in the
vagina. Receptor data are taken from Vu Hai *et al.* (1978) and endogenous
progesterone values from Wiest (1970) and Butcher *et al.* (1974). M = metestrus;
D = diestrus; P = proestrus; E = estrus.

Yu and Leung (1982) also observed a rise in cytosol progesterone receptor concentrations in the pregnant rat uterus at the time of parturition with a decline in the two days
following parturition. In their study, the progesterone receptor sedimented as a 4 S
peak in low salt sucrose density gradients which is in contrast to the estrogen receptor
studied at the same time which sedimented in the 8 S region (Yu and Leung, 1982).
When progesterone receptors were measured in the myometrium of the pregnant rat

during gestation, it was also found that the concentrations rose towards parturition and declined thereafter (Alexandrova and Soloff, 1980).

2.2.2. MAMMARY GLAND

The effects of progesterone vary during different stages of mammary gland development. Progesterone cannot by itself support mammary cell proliferation but it acts cooperatively with estrogen during lobuloalveolar development of the mammary gland to sensitize it to mitogenic factors (Lyons *et al.*, 1958; Nandi, 1958; Bresciani, 1965; Freeman and Topper, 1978); progesterone prevents lactogenesis (Kuhn, 1969; Davis *et al.*, 1972; Denamur and DeLouis, 1972; Rosen *et al.*, 1978).

Specific binding of ^{3}H-R5020 could be demonstrated in the cytosols of mammary glands of virgin and pregnant (12–14 days) mice (BALB/c strain) (Haslam and Shyamala, 1979b). However, binding at mid-pregnancy was 3.5 times lower than in virgin mice. By day 1 of lactation binding decreased by 10-fold and was totally undetectable during established lactation (days 2–15 post-partum). On the other hand, Muldoon (1981) found progesterone receptor levels to be higher in mouse mammary tissue (C3H+ strain) in late pregnancy compared to levels in virgin animals (26 vs 3 fmol/mg DNA). Shyamala and McBlain (1979) and Yu and Leung (1982) were not able to detect any significant quantities of progesterone receptors in the late pregnant to the lactating period. Estradiol has very little effect on progesterone receptor binding in late pregnant or lactating mice (Haslam and Shyamala, 1979a; Muldoon, 1981). It appears that low levels of progesterone receptor are negatively correlated with lobulo-alveolar differentiation and the lactational state of the mammary gland. This is corroborated by the observation that in normal, virgin mammary glands, most of the progesterone receptor is present in the glandular epithelium and only progesterone receptor present in the epithelial tissue undergoes modulation in concentration as a function of the developmental state of the mammary gland. The lack of detectable progesterone receptor in lactating mammary glands is most likely the result of the dilution of progesterone receptor present in adipose and connective tissues by the large number of secretory epithelial cells which do not contain progesterone receptor. Whatever progesterone receptor is present in these populations of cells is not inducible by estrogen (Haslam and Shyamala, 1981).

Similar to the situation in the mouse mammary gland, progesterone receptors in the rat show a remarkable decrease with the onset of lactation (15.7 ± 1.4 (SE) fmol/mg protein during pregnancy (14–16 days) to 7.1 ± 2.8 at early lactation (2–3 days post-partum)). By mid and late lactation progesterone receptors are practically undetectable (Mohla *et al.*, 1981; Quirk *et al.*, 1984).

2.2.3. THYMUS

Cytosol and nuclear progesterone receptors have been reported to be present in the thymus of pregnant and pseudopregnant rats (Pearce and Funder, 1986). Binding of R5020 in the thymus is lower in the 12-day pregnant rat than during estrous but slightly higher than during the nonestrous phase of the cycle. The receptor levels in the thymus (40–140 fmol/mg protein) are an order of magnitude lower than in the uterus (350–1300 fmol/mg protein). Thymic receptors are inducible by estrogen and decreased by progesterone as in the uterus. Pearce and Funder (1986) suggest that the existence of progesterone receptors in the thymus indicates the possibility of direct effects of progesterone on the thymus during pregnancy which may be related to thymus-related immunosuppression during pregnancy (Finn *et al.*, 1972; Miller *et al.*, 1973; Carter, 1976; Le Hoang *et al.*, 1981a,b).

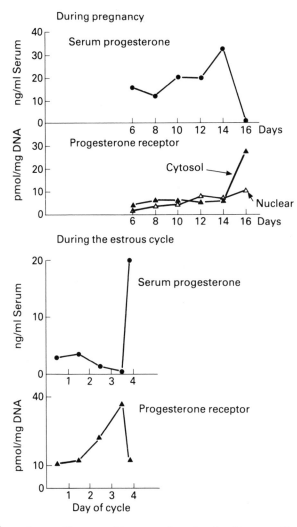

FIG 2.28. Progesterone Receptor Concentrations in the Hamster Uterus or My-ometrium during Pregnancy and the Estrous Cycle (Comparison with Serum Progesterone Concentrations).
Day 1 of pregnancy was the day immediately after mating (day 4 of the cycle). Parturition occurred in the morning of day 16. Progesterone receptor concentrations were measured in the myometrium during pregnancy (Leavitt, 1985) and in the whole uterus during the estrous cycle (Leavitt *et al.* 1974). Serum progesterone values were determined concomitantly.

2.3. Hamsters

2.3.1. UTERUS

The golden hamster has been used as a model system to study variations in estrogen and progesterone receptors with fluctuations in endogenous hormones during the estrous cycle because of its regular 4-day cycle and the predictability of events occurring during the cycle. It has thus also been used to study the regulation of progesterone receptors during pregnancy (Leavitt, 1985). Figure 2.28 shows that progesterone receptor concentrations in the myometrium are low during pregnancy when compared to the levels seen during the estrous cycle which are also indicated in the figure. The progesterone receptor levels rise when serum progesterone declines at term. The serum estradiol and progesterone-myometrial progesterone receptor relationship observed during pregnancy indicate not only that the progesterone receptor is down-regulated by progesterone itself but also that receptor recovery during progesterone withdrawal occurs whether estrogen levels are sustained or not (Leavitt, 1985).

2.4. Rabbits

2.4.1. UTERUS

2.4.1.1. Progesterone Receptors During Pregnancy

In the rabbit, progesterone withdrawal at the end of pregnancy is associated with events leading to parturition (Schofield, 1957; 1960; Csapo and Takeda, 1965; Fuchs, 1978). In 1974, Davies and co-workers determined progesterone receptor concentrations in the myometrium of the pregnant rabbit and related this to progesterone concentrations in the myometrium and plasma. Their findings identified a specific, high affinity ^{3}H-progesterone binding component in the cytosol fraction of the myometrium sedimenting in the 4 S region of low salt sucrose density gradients. The K_a (association constant) of this binding in pregnant rabbits is 1.64 ± 0.06 (SE) $\times 10^9 \, \mathrm{M}^{-1}$. The concentration of progesterone receptor sites in the myometrial cytosol decreases in the first three days post-coitum to 1.35 ± 0.09 (SE) pmol/mg protein as compared to 4.5 ± 0.5 (SE) pmol/mg protein in nonpregnant rabbits. As seen in Fig. 2.29, there is a further drop after mid-pregnancy followed by an increase by day 30. The increase occurs when plasma and myometrial progesterone decreases toward the end of gestation. As seen in the previous sections, a similar relationship was also observed in the pregnant rat and hamster.

Quirk and Currie (1984) confirmed the pattern of change in progesterone receptors in the uterus of the rabbit at the end of gestation by using the synthetic progestin R5020 as specific ligand and measuring receptor levels in both the myometrium and endometrium. Their findings confirmed the increase at the end of gestation of both endometrial and myometrial receptors in both the cytosol and nuclear fractions concomitant with the decrease in plasma progesterone. The K_d (dissociation constant) values for R5020 binding in the cytosol of the myometrium and endometrium of rabbits from days 25–31 of gestation are 2.37 ± 0.22 (SE) and $2.65 \pm 0.28 \times 10^{-10}$ M, respectively.

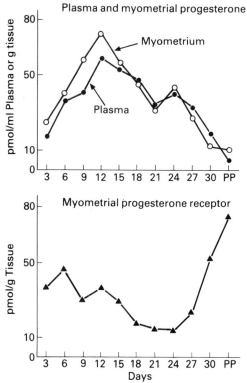

FIG 2.29. Concentration of Progesterone Receptor Sites in the Myometrium and Concentrations of Progesterone in Myometrium and Plasma during Gestation in the Rabbit.

Adapted from Davies *et al.* (1974) PP = post-partum.

Despite the recurring pattern of progesterone receptor increase at the end of gestation concomitant with a decrease in circulating endogenous progesterone, it is still not clear how changes in progesterone receptors affect the onset of labor, especially in a species like the rabbit that shows such profound changes in uterine function in response to progesterone withdrawal.

2.4.1.2. Uteroglobin: A Progesterone-stimulated Protein

Uteroglobin (see also Chapter 1, Section 1.6.) was first discovered because it is a major protein secreted into rabbit uterine fluid around the time of implantation (Krishnan and Daniel, 1967; Beier, 1968). Uteroglobin secretion was found to be stimulated by progesterone (Beier, 1968; Arthur and Daniel, 1972).

Uteroglobin begins to accumulate in uterine secretions on day 3 of pregnancy, reaches a peak on days 4–6 and then becomes virtually undetectable by day 9 (Beier, 1976). Both progesterone and estradiol can stimulate uteroglobin synthesis, but sequential estrogen and progesterone treatment is synergistic, indicating that uteroglobin gene expression in the rabbit endometrium is probably under dual hormonal control (Bullock, 1980).

The function of uteroglobin during the implantation period has not been demonstrated (Bhatt and Bullock, 1978). Among its many properties, uteroglobin binds progesterone so that it has been proposed to be an intraluminal progesterone carrier (Bochskanl and Kirchner, 1981; Bochskanl *et al.*, 1984). Uteroglobin also has anti-inflammatory/immunosuppressive properties and has been suggested to be a mediator of the pregnancy-related immunosuppressive action thought to be exerted by progesterone (Siiteri *et al.*, 1977; Mukherjee *et al.*, 1980). Uteroglobin has been found to be a phospholipase A_2 inhibitor, suggesting that its primary function is immunomodulatory (Miele *et al.*, 1987).

2.4.2. MAMMARY GLAND

In contrast to the uterus, progesterone receptors (specific binding of ^{3}H-R5020) of the cytosol fraction of the rabbit mammary gland are high in virgin mammary glands (364 ± 102 (SE) fmol/mg protein) and decline during the first week of pregnancy (43.4 ± 1.8 fmol/mg protein), but they remain low even at the end of gestation and during lactation (Kelly *et al.*, 1983).

2.5. Humans

The level of progesterone in the plasma and uterine tissue of pregnant rats and rabbits decrease prior to parturition. Such a decline has not been seen in women (Tulchinsky *et al.*, 1972). It has been suggested that the concentration of progesterone receptors in the uterus may be more important than changes in blood progesterone levels in the initiation of labor in women (Giannopoulos and Tulchinsky, 1979). Several studies have been carried out to measure progesterone receptors in either the endometrium or the myometrium of first trimester or term pregnancies. Although conflicting results have been reported, Table 2.25 gives an indication of some of the positive results and compares them to the pattern seen during the menstrual cycle. In the study of Giannopoulos and Tulchinsky (1979), progesterone receptor concentrations in myometria obtained at term were considerably lower than the levels in either the proliferative or secretory phase of the cycle. The dissociation constants of the binding of R5020 in myometria of pregnant and nonpregnant women are similar (1.9 ± 0.2 (SE) and $1.3 \pm 0.2 \times 10^{-9}$ M, respectively). These results were confirmed by Khan-Dawood and Dawood in 1984 (2.9 pmol/mg DNA in the myometrium in term pregnancy). It can be remarked that the highest level of receptor observed in the myometrium or endometrium during the menstrual cycle is in the proliferative phase and not in the progesterone-dominated secretory phase (MacLaughlin and Richardson, 1976; Bayard *et al.*, 1978; Giannopoulos and Tulchinsky, 1979). In the endometrium, receptor concentrations are significantly higher at term than in the first trimester of pregnancy; the highest concentration reached is comparable to that observed in the pre-ovulatory period of the menstrual cycle (Kreitmann and Bayard, 1979). Since plasma progesterone concentrations are high at term (about 200 ng/ml), it would appear that the myometrium is responding to the increased peripheral progesterone concentration by a down-regulation of the progesterone receptor similar to what is observed during the cycle while the endometrium is responding to the higher concentrations of estrogens (principally estriol). In contrast to these observations, Haukkamaa (1974) and

TABLE 2.25. *Progesterone Receptor Concentrations in Human Endometrium My-ometrium and Fallopian Tubes During Pregnancy and the Menstrual Cycle*

	Endometrium pmol/mg DNA	Myometrium pmol/mg DNA	Fallopian tube fmol/mg protein
Pregnancy			
8–10 weeks	1.31 ± 0.19 (SD)		170 ± 70 (SE)
38–40 weeks	2.77 ± 2.04	2.0 ± 0.2 (SE)	
Menstrual cycle			
Early proliferative	1.52 ± 0.74		400 ± 200
Late proliferative	3.01 ± 1.69	25.3 ± 2.8	1910 ± 490
Early secretory	1.90 ± 1.42		340 ± 130
Late secretory	0.89 ± 0.82	11.0 ± 1.9	160 ± 40

Binding in the endometrium and Fallopian tubes was measured with ^{3}H-proges-terone and in the myometrium with ^{3}H-R5020.
Quoted from Bayard *et al.* (1978); Giannopoulos and Tulchinsky (1979); Kreit-mann and Bayard (1979); Verhage *et al.* (1980).

Padayachi and co-workers (1987) were not able to detect any specific binding of progestins in myometria at term.

A specific progesterone receptor was also found in the human Fallopian tube (Verhage *et al.*, 1980) (Table 2.25). The binding affinity is 6×10^{-9} M (K_d) and the binding complexes sediment in the 7–8 S region of low salt sucrose density gradients. Receptor concentrations in early pregnancy and the late secretory phase of menstrual cycle are comparable, probably due to the elevated levels of circulating progesterone.

2.6. Other Mammals

2.6.1. Cows

Specific, high affinity binding of ^{3}H-R5020 has been detected in mammary tissue of prepartum, nonlactating and post-partum, lactating cows (Capuco *et al.*, 1982). In this species, progesterone concentrations are elevated throughout pregnancy and decline at parturition when copious secretion of milk begins. Progesterone receptor concentrations are higher in cytosol from pregnant than post-partum, lactating cows (179 ± 53 (SE) vs 41 ± 15 fmol/mg protein, respectively). The mean dissociation constant is 1.9 ± 0.3 (SE) $\times 10^{-9}$ M in pregnant cow mammary tissue.

2.6.2. Brush-tail Possums (*Trichosurus vulpecula*)

In the brush-tail possum (*Trichosurus vulpecula*), histological studies of the uterus have shown that maximum metabolic activity in the pregnant and nonpregnant cycle occurs between day 8 and 13 of the reproductive cycle (Shorey and Hughes, 1973). Cytosol progesterone receptor concentrations are highest at day 0 (estrus) and decline to a mini-mum at day 13 when the uterus is progesterone-dominated (Curlewis and Stone, 1986).

3. In the Placenta

3.1. Rats

Progesterone is required in numerous processes involved in the maintenance of pregnancy among which are the preparation of the endometrium for implantation and the proliferation of trophoblastic tissue. In the placenta, it is possible that progesterone interacts with a specific trophoblastic receptor and that the resulting progesterone receptor complex plays an essential regulatory role in maintaining pregnancy. The binding of porgesterone to placental receptors has been most extensively studied in the rat.

Specific binding of ^{3}H-progesterone was measured in placenta from rats on day 12 of pregnancy (Ogle, 1980). Binding in these placental cytosols was found to be stabilized by glycerol and molybdate (Ogle, 1983a) and was shown to require sulfhydryl groups for binding (Ogle, 1980). Binding is of high affinity with a K_d of 3.4 ± 0.3 (SE) $\times 10^{-9}$ M and a mean concentration of 250 ± 40 fmol/mg protein. The physico-chemical characteristics of the rat placental progesterone receptor are summarized in Table 2.26. The receptor concentration is similar to that found in deciduomata cytosol between days 3–5 of pseudopregnancy (Armstrong *et al.*, 1977) and the apparent K_d is similar to that reported for the rat uterus (Walters and Clark, 1977).

During gestation, the affinity of placental cytosol progesterone receptor for progesterone decreases between day 9 and 19 of pregnancy in the rat from 1.5 ± 0.2 nM to 4.8 ± 0.5 nM (K_d) (Ogle, 1983b). A low molecular weight inhibitor which decreases the affinity of progesterone for its receptor has been described in the placenta (Ogle, 1981; Ogle and Mills, 1983; Ogle, 1987). The potency of the inhibitor substance remains constant from days 9 to 14 but disappears by day 19 (Ogle, 1983b). Although the inhibitor decreases the association rate of progesterone with the placental receptor three- to four-fold, it does not alter the availability of binding sites (Ogle, 1981) so that

TABLE 2.26. *Physicochemical Characteristics of the Progesterone Receptor in Placental Cytosol on Day 12 of Gestation in the Rat*

Number of sites	
fmol/mg protein	250 ± 40 (SEM)
fmol/placenta	$11\,300 \pm 1\,800$
$K_d \times 10^{-9}$ M (4° C)	3.4 ± 0.3
Association rate constant	
k_{+1} (10^4 M^{-1} sec^{-1})	1.28 ± 0.22
Dissociation rate constant	
k_{-1} (10^{-5} sec^{-1})	3.20 ± 0.61
Sedimentation coefficient	7.9 S in low salt with glycerol and molybdate
Specificity	Progesterone > DOC > Corticosterone 5α-DHP > 20α-OHP > 5α-DHP. No binding of cortisol.
Thermal stability	Labile at 30° C

Quoted from Ogle (1980; 1981); Ogle and Beyer (1982).

the number of binding sites increases from 60 fmol/placenta on day 9 to 100 on day 19. The nuclear binding sites increase three-fold during the same time period (Ogle, 1983b).

The progesterone receptor in the placenta appears to differ from that of the reproductive organs since progesterone regulates its own receptor by rapid and reversible nuclear processing mechanisms with no depletion of cytosolic receptor (Ogle, 1986). This would allow the placenta to be responsive to the hormone throughout pregnancy.

3.2. Humans

Cytosols from term placental tissue were tested for their ability to bind the synthetic progestin R5020. High affinity binding sites having a K_d of 8.13 ± 1.07 (SD) $\times 10^{-9}$ M and a number of binding sites of 35 ± 10 fmol/mg protein were found (Younes *et al.*, 1981). Binding is specific for the synthetic and natural progestins. Corticosterone and dexamethasone are not able to compete for the binding sites. The receptor binding is thermolabile, in contrast to the thermostability of corticosteroid binding globulin (CBG).

3.3. Other Mammals

Progesterone receptors have also been reported in the placenta of rabbits and hamsters. In the rabbit, cytosol receptors were found only in the maternal, not the fetal, part of the placenta (Guerne and Stutinsky, 1978). The apparent association constant varied from 3.04×10^8 M^{-1} on day 10 of gestation to 0.70×10^8 M^{-1} on day 30. The number of binding sites is maximal from day 10 to 16 of gestation ($361-401$ fmol/mg protein) and decreases rapidly thereafter to 114 fmol/mg protein on day 27. Deoxycorticosterone competes significantly with progesterone for the binding sites.

Progesterone receptors were also found in the utero-placental unit (implantation site with surrounding uterine decidual tissue plus placenta) of the hamster on day 6 of pregnancy (Luzzani and Soffientini, 1980). Leavitt and Reuss (1975) found progesterone receptors in decidual tissue.

C. ANDROGEN RECEPTORS

1. In the Fetal Compartment

Androgens secreted by the fetal testes of the male embryo determine the expression of the male phenotype in mammals (Jost, 1961; 1985). The two androgens involved, testosterone and its 5α-reduced metabolite dihydrotestosterone, have been shown to have different sites of action. Dihydrotestosterone is formed from testosterone in the urogenital sinus (anlage of the prostate) and urogenital tubercle (anlage of the external genitalia), before the onset of male phenotypic differentiation and dihydrotestosterone is required for appropriate male differentiation (see Volume 1, Chapter 2). In contrast, the Wolffian ducts (anlage of the epididymis, vas deferens and seminal vesicles) cannot convert testosterone to dihydrotestosterone until after male differentiation of the ducts is far advanced so that virilization of the Wolffian ducts appears to require testosterone (Wilson and Lasnitzki, 1971; Wilson and Siiteri, 1973). Besides their requirement for differentiation of the male organs, androgen secretion during a critical period either before or after birth (depending on the animal species) is a determining factor in the sexual differentiation and maturation of the brain (McEwen, 1983). Although the two androgens act in different tissues, they both bind to the same androgen receptor protein.

1.1. Rabbits

1.1.1. REPRODUCTIVE TRACTS

In 1973, Wilson demonstrated the specific uptake of ^{3}H-testosterone by the Müllerian and Wolffian ducts (not separated), mesonephros, and undifferentiated gonads of 17–21-day-old rabbit fetuses, the critical period of male differentiation of the sex organs of the rabbit. On the other hand, the uptake of ^{3}H-dihydrotestosterone was found to be very low in the ducts. However, ^{3}H-dihydrotestosterone is present in significant quantities in the urogenital sinus and urogenital tubercle. The results suggest that testosterone is the predominant androgen elaborated and retained by the fetal rabbit gonad at the time of differentiation of the male phenotype and gonads and that within the developing urogenital sinus and urogenital tubercle testosterone is reduced to dihydrotestosterone, which is probably the effective intracellular androgen for the masculinization of these structures.

More recently, George and Noble (1984) were able to show that in the urogenital sinus and tubercle from rabbit fetuses from days 18 to 21, dihydrotestosterone had a several-fold higher apparent binding affinity ($K_d = 1.1$ nM) than testosterone ($K_d = 8.5$ nM) and a higher concentration of binding sites. Some characteristics of ^{3}H-dihydrotestosterone binding in urogenital tracts are listed on Table 2.27; the binding characteristics are similar to those of the adult prostate. No significant

TABLE 2.27. *Physicochemical Characteristics of Androgen Receptors in Urogenital Tracts and Lungs of Rabbit Fetuses*

	Urogenital tracts[a] (18–29 days)	Lungs[b] (26–29 days)
Number of sites fmol/mg protein	13–39	6–17
K_d ($\times 10^{-9}$ M), 4° C	0.1–1.9	0.13–0.31
Binding specificity	5α-DHT > testosterone No binding of estradiol, progesterone or cortisol	R1881 > 5α-DHT > testosterone > progesterone
Sedimentation coefficient (S)	8–9 S in low salt	9.2 S in low salt 4.6 S in high salt

[a]Specific binding of ^{3}H-dihydrotestosterone (DHT); [b]Specific binding of ^{3}H-R1881
Quoted from Giannopoulos and Smith (1982); George and Noble (1984).

differences between male and female fetal urogenital tissues and no increase with fetal age throughout the critical period were observed. This group was, however, unable to demonstrate specific binding of either testosterone or dihydrotestosterone in Wolffian ducts although Wilson (1973) had observed the specific uptake of ^{3}H-testosterone in this tissue. From these studies, it was not possible to provide the molecular basis for the different effects of these two androgens in different target tissues.

Other factors must also come into play to confer the difference in sites of action of testosterone and dihydrotestosterone. One of these is probably the actual *in situ* concentration of the respective androgen. The embryonic rabbit testes synthesize and secrete testosterone from the onset of genital tract differentiation (Veyssière *et al.*, 1976). From there, circulating testosterone can then reach the urogenital sinus and urogenital tubercle where it has been shown to be converted to dihydrotestosterone (Wilson and Lasnitzki, 1971; Wilson and Siiteri, 1973). The quantity of testosterone in the fetal rabbit testis increases from a low value on day 18 (166 pg/2 testes) to 2830 pg/2 testes on day 20 (Veyssière *et al.*, 1979). Testicular dihydrotestosterone is detectable only from day 20 and the quantities are very small compared to testosterone. Plasma testosterone is higher in male fetuses (38–66 pg/ml) than in female fetuses from day 19 on, and is always much higher than dihydrotestosterone (see Volume 1, Chapter 2).

1.1.2. LUNG

Specific, high affinity binding of a synthetic androgen ^{3}H-R1881 (17β-hydroxy-17α-methyl-estra-4,9,11-trien-3-one) was identified in the lungs of male and female rabbit fetuses from as early as the day 26 of gestation (Giannopoulos and Smith, 1982). As seen in Table 2.27, the characteristics of androgen binding in fetal lungs are very similar to those of the urogenital tracts. The concentration of binding sites significantly increases with age from 3.6 fmol/mg protein in the 26-day-old fetus to 5.0 fmol/mg protein on days 28–29 of fetal age and 12 fmol/mg protein in the adult. Binding affinity is high, in the range of 0.2 nM (K_d). No significant sex difference in number of binding sites or in binding affinity was observed.

The presence of androgen receptors in fetal lungs may have implications in lung terminal differentiation and fatal respiratory distress syndrome of the newborn (RDS). It has been reported that RDS is observed more frequently in males than in females (Farrell and Wood, 1976; Miller and Futrakul, 1968). RDS is caused by deficient synthesis or secretion of pulmonary surfactant (Farrell and Avery, 1975). Studies have shown that surfactant phospholipid indices of fetal lung maturity are more favorable in female fetuses than males (Torday *et al.*, 1981; Nielsen and Torday, 1981) although no sex differences in glucocorticoid receptors and glucocorticoid responses were observed that could explain the difference in lung maturity (see Section 1.1.1.2 of Part D in this chapter, p. 149). It has been suggested that high concentrations of circulating androgen metabolites could directly inhibit surfactant phospholipid synthesis via a receptor-mediated mechanism (Nielsen *et al.*, 1981). Nielsen (1985) reported that surfactant production is 28% higher in the lungs of female fetal mice than of normal male fetuses but surfactant production in the lungs of fetuses of the testicular feminization mouse (Tfm mouse) is similar to that of the normal females. Tfm mice lack androgen receptors in all tissues (Verhoeven and Wilson, 1976). The presence of higher circulating androgen levels in the male and androgen receptors in the fetal lung (Veyssière *et al.*,

1976) could be the reason for the delay in fetal lung maturation in the male. Although no sex differences were observed in fetal lung androgen receptors towards the end of gestation (Giannopoulos and Smith, 1982), studies would have to be performed at an earlier point in gestation at the period of a maximum sex difference in circulating androgens. No sex-related differences were observed in other hormone receptors such as the glucocorticoid and the progesterone receptors and in the circulating plasma concentrations of their respective hormones (Giannopoulos and Smith, 1982).

1.2. Rats and Mice

1.2.1. REPRODUCTIVE TRACTS

In 14.5–15-day-old rat fetuses, high affinity, specific binding sites for ^{3}H-testosterone can be isolated from mesonephros, genital ducts, urogenital sinus and urogenital tubercle (Table 2.28) (Gupta and Bloch, 1976). Androgen receptors are not detectable in muscle, lung, heart, intestine, stomach and liver by the methods used. ^{3}H-testosterone binding was found to increase with fetal age (between 14.5 and 20.5 days) in Wolffian ducts. There is no difference in binding capacity between male and female genital ducts in the 14.5-day-old embryo, but by days 20.5 specific binding is five times higher in the male ducts. During this period in the rat fetus, the Wolffian ducts (present in both sexes) differentiate through the influence of androgens secreted from the fetal testes. The administration of dihydrotestosterone to pregnant rats causes virilization of the urogenital tract of female fetuses (Schultz and Wilson, 1974).

Recent data have shown that in the rat fetus the plasma levels of testosterone are higher in the males while dihydrotestosterone is similar in male and female fetuses (Habert and Picon, 1984). In the fetal testes, the testosterone content is measurable from 15.5 days and increases to a maximum on day 18.5 (about 2 ng/testis), suggesting that target organs situated close to the testes such as the Wolffian ducts may receive a constant testosterone supply even by diffusion (Habert and Picon, 1984). On the other hand, intratesticular concentrations of dihydrotestosterone are minute so that dihydrotestosterone in the urogenital sinus and urogenital tubercle is formed from the conversion of testosterone *in situ* as has been demonstrated (Wilson and Lasnitzki, 1971). The formation of dihydrotestosterone is already high in the urogenital sinus and

TABLE 2.28. *Physicochemical Characteristics of Androgen Receptors in Genital Tracts of Fetal Rats (14.5–15 Days)*

Number of sites	
fmol/mg protein	16
K_d ($\times 10^{-9}$ M), 4° C	2
Binding specificity	Testosterone > 5α-DHT
	No binding of estradiol or progesterone
Proteolysis	Destroyed

The data represent the specific binding of ^{3}H-testosterone.
Quoted from Gupta and Bloch (1976).

tubercle at day 15 (Wilson and Lasnitzki, 1971) when putative androgen receptors can be detected (Gupta and Bloch, 1976).

From an autoradiographic study, it is possible to localize androgen binding sites within the urogenital sinus of the fetal rat. At day 14 of fetal age neither male nor female sinuses show labeling with tritiated androgens except after a prolonged exposure period when the mesenchyme showed weak nuclear labeling (Takeda *et al.*, 1985). On days 16.5 and 18.5, heavy nuclear labeling becomes apparent in the mesenchyme while the epithelium remains unlabeled. There are no sex differences and no difference between the localization of ^{3}H-testosterone and ^{3}H-dihydrotestosterone at all fetal ages. On day 20.5 the uptake of androgens by the mesenchyme surrounding the ventral epithelium of the female sinuses is greatly reduced. These observations suggest that androgens act at the level of the mesenchyme of the fetal urogenital sinus to affect prostatic morphogenesis (Takeda *et al.*, 1985). From studies using a 5α-reductase inhibitor, it was shown that treatment from days 14–22 of gestation to inhibit dihydrotestosterone formation, impaired development of the prostate and virilization of the external genitalia in male offspring, indicating that dihydrotestosterone is the active androgen responsible for prostate morphogenesis (George and Peterson, 1988).

Development of prostate-like acini in a variety of embryonic, neonatal and adult epithelia can be induced by recombination experiments that associate these tissues with urogenital sinus mesenchyme in intact, male hosts (Cunha and Lung, 1978; Cunha *et al.*, 1980a,b). Once the epithelium develops into a prostate-like, glandular epithelium, ^{3}H-dihydrotestosterone is then found in the nucleus of the epithelium (Cunha *et al.*, 1980c). The induction of androgen-binding sites in epithelium where they are previously absent seems to indicate the important role played by the target mesenchyme in directing epithelium development and steroid sensitivity (Cunha *et al.*, 1980c).

1.2.2. MAMMARY GLAND

In the embryonic mouse, fetal testicular androgens cause fetal male mammary gland primordia to either undergo atrophy or lose their connection with the ectoderm (Raynaud and Frilley, 1949). However, androgen sensitivity is a peculiarity of the mammary glands of Muridae and is not common to all mammals (Raynaud and Delost, 1977). The mesenchyme is the target for androgen action (Kratochwil and Schwartz, 1976; Drews and Drews, 1977; Dürnberger and Kratochwil, 1980) and it becomes sensitive to testosterone on embryonic day 14 (Kratochwil, 1977).

Using autoradiographic techniques, Heuberger and co-workers (1982) demonstrated that ^{3}H-testosterone or [^{3}H]dihydrotestosterone is localized in the 14-day-old mouse embryo mammary gland in a distinct population of mesenchymal cells surrounding the glandular epithelium. Mammary epithelium, epidermis or the more distant mesenchyme are not labeled. Mesenchymal cell retention of ^{3}H-testosterone could even be detected in the 12.5-day-old embryo. These results could be duplicated in mesenchyme–epithelium recombination studies *in vitro* (Heuberger *et al.*, 1982), but it seems that a stimulus from the epithelium is still required. The total amount of radioactive testosterone bound by the recombinants is 11 times greater than the radioactivity bound by mesenchyme not associated with epithelium (Heuberger *et al.*, 1982) suggesting that embryonic mouse mammary epithelium sends a signal that triggers the formation of androgen-binding sites in adjacent mesenchyme and androgen responsiveness.

The ontogeny of high-affinity, androgen-binding sites in the embryonic mouse mammary gland has been studied by Wasner and co-workers (1983) from the initial formation of the primordial, epithelial bud (day 12) through the androgen-responsive stage (day 14) until term (day 19). Specific ^{3}H-testosterone binding is first detectable in the 12-day-old embryos, increases about 20-fold by day 14 ($\sim$30 000 sites per cell) and persists until birth. These results confirm the autoradiographic data previously obtained (Heuberger *et al.*, 1982).

Regression of the nipple anlage in the male rat fetus is also under androgenic control. Nipple formation can be arrested in female fetuses treated with testosterone, dihydrotestosterone or 5α-androstane-3α,17β-diol at a critical period (Goldman *et al.*, 1976) and treatment of male fetuses with the anti-androgen cyproterone acetate leads to development of nipple and mammary gland tissue (Neumann and Elger, 1966). A recent study has shown that inhibition of 5α-reductase activity and dihydrotestosterone formation from days 12–21 of gestation inhibits nipple regression in male rat fetuses so that dihydrotestosterone is implicated not only in the masculinization of the external genitalia but also in the inhibition of nipple development in the male rat fetus (Imperato-McGinley *et al.*, 1986). It is interesting to note that in this study, the mammary gland also developed in both the males and the females; males treated with the 5α-reductase inhibitor also showed evidence of feminization of the external genitalia (Imperato-McGinley *et al.*, 1986).

1.2.3. BRAIN

Specific androgen receptors are present in brains of fetal rats and mice (Vito *et al.*, 1979; Lieberburg *et al.*, 1980; Vito and Fox, 1982). Like the estrogen receptor, androgen receptor can be detected as early as seven days before birth and both receptors are more abundant in the hypothalamus–pre-optic area. In both rats and mice, the concentration of estrogen receptors is higher than that of the androgen receptors. The ontogeny of the two receptor systems differ considerably: estrogen receptor concentrations increase or are already high during the last week of gestation, but androgen receptors increase in a gradual fashion postnatally (Lieberburg *et al.*, 1980; Vito and Fox, 1982). These observations suggest that besides the estrogen receptors, androgen receptors could also be involved in some aspects of masculinization and defeminization of sexually dimorphic behaviors.

1.3. Humans

1.3.1. FETAL AMNION

High affinity, specific androgen binding sites are found in human fetal membranes from normal term pregnancies (DeCicco Nardone *et al.*, 1984). ^{3}H-R1881 has a binding affinity of 1.03 ± 0.7 (SD) nM (K_d, 4° C) with a mean concentration of 20.2 ± 10.4 (SD) fmol/mg protein; R1881 and dihydrotestosterone have higher affinity than testosterone. In contrast, McCormick and co-workers (1981) reported no significant specific binding of ^{3}H-R1881 in the fetal membranes although they were able to study the placental androgen receptor.

1.3.2. SEX SKIN FIBROBLASTS

Sex skin fibroblasts from external genitalia of human fetuses in the week 8 of intra-uterine life contain ^{3}H-dihydrotestosterone binding sites (Sultan *et al.*, 1980). Binding capacity is four times higher in genital skin fibroblasts than nongenital skin (474 vs 124 fmol/mg DNA).

1.4. Primates (**Macaca fascicularis**)

1.4.1. SEX SKIN FIBROBLASTS

Androgen receptors are found in skin fibroblasts from the external genitalia of 100-day-old male and female fetal monkeys (*Macaca fascicularis*) (Sultan *et al.*, 1981). In these primates, differentiation of the external genitalia occurs between days 57 and 75 of gestation. No significant difference in binding was observed between male and female fetuses. The number of binding sites of ^{3}H-dihydrotestosterone is between 500 and 800 fmol/mg DNA, and the binding affinity is 0.3 to 0.4 nM (K_d at 37° C). Since the number of androgen receptors is similar in males and females, it seems that the concentration of hormone in the tissue rather than receptors would be the decisive factor in masculinization of the genitalia.

1.4.2. BRAIN AND PITUITARY

Fetal rhesus monkey brains contain specific androgen receptor binding sites in the cytosol fraction (Pomerantz *et al.*, 1985; Handa *et al.*, 1988). The apparent dissociation constant (K_d) of the binding of ^{3}H-R1881 (methyltrienolone) is 1.6×10^{-10} M in the hypothalamus of 150-day-old female fetuses (Handa *et al.*, 1988). In the hypothalamus–pre-optic area, androgen receptor concentrations increase steadily from 1.3 fmol/ mg protein at 50 days of fetal age to 6.2 fmol/mg protein at 150 days (Handa *et al.*, 1988). No sex differences were observed.

Like the estrogen receptors, the concentration of androgen receptors is higher in the anterior pituitary than in the hypothalamus–pre-optic area/amygdala and cerebral cortex (Pomerantz *et al.*, 1985). In the anterior pituitary, the concentration of androgen receptors is lower than that of estrogen receptors (6 vs 10 fmol/mg protein). They are approximately the same in the hypothalamus (0.8 fmol/mg protein) and, in the cerebral cortex, androgen binding is greater (0.2 vs 0.1 fmol/mg protein). In rodents, the concentration of estrogen receptors is higher than that of androgen receptors in the hypothalamus (Vito and Fox, 1982).

Sholl and Pomerantz (1986) have characterized androgen receptor binding sites in the cerebral cortex of fetal female rhesus monkeys (125–135 days of fetal age). The dissociation constant (K_d) of the binding of tritiated R1881 (methyltrienolone) to cytosol receptors is 2.5×10^{-10} M and binding capacity is 5.5 fmol/mg protein. The presence of androgen receptors in female fetal primate brain could confer sensitivity to abnormal androgen levels.

The presence of androgen receptors in fetal reproductive tracts, lungs and mammary glands coincides with the onset of reproductive tract differentiation, lung differentiation and male mammary gland regression. At this developmental period, no significant sex differences in the receptors were observed, suggesting that androgen receptor protein synthesis is not a genotypic mechanism. However, the further synthesis appears to be sex-linked, possibly related to testosterone biosynthesis and secretion by the fetal testes. The *in situ* conversion of testosterone to dihydrotestosterone is also important in determining the specificity of the site of action of testosterone and dihydrotestosterone.

2. In the Placenta

2.1. Humans

The human placenta contains high affinity, specific binding sites for androgens at various gestational periods ranging from 16 weeks to term (Table 2.29) (Barile *et al.*, 1979; McCormick *et al.*, 1981; Younes *et al.*, 1982). This binding could be distinguished from binding to SHBG (sex hormone binding globulin) by the use of the synthetic androgen [3H]-R1881 and by the lack of competitive binding inhibition by estradiol (see Chapter 1). [3H]-R1881 has a binding affinity of 3.8 nM (K_d at 4° C) in term placental cytosol; similar binding affinitites were also found at 16 weeks and between 33 and 37 weeks. McCormick and co-workers (1981) found no significant difference in the concentration of receptor with length of gestation, but Younes and co-workers (1982) reported an approximate three-fold increase in binding sites in term placentas as compared to placentas from 20–34 weeks of gestation. More receptor was found in term placentas corresponding to male children than female (McCormick *et al.*, 1981). At the present time, except for the possible function of androgen receptors in permitting anabolic effects of testosterone, the function of androgen receptors in the placenta is unknown.

TABLE 2.29. *Physicochemical Characteristics of Androgen Receptors in Human Term Placenta*

Number of sites	
fmol/mg protein	1.4–15
fmol/mg DNA	20–340
fmol/g tissue	~1200
K_d ($\times 10^{-9}$ M), 4° C	1.3–27
Binding specificity	R1881 > 5α-DHT > testosterone
	Little or no binding of estradiol
	or progesterone
Sedimentation	
coefficient (S)	4–5 S in low and high salt
Thermal stability	Labile at 45° C

The data represent the specific binding of [3H]-R1881 (McCormick *et al.*, 1981; Younes *et al.*, 1982) or [3H]-testosterone (Barile *et al.*, 1979).

D. GLUCOCORTICOID RECEPTORS

1. In the Fetal Compartment

Glucocorticoids are crucial for the development of certain fetal tissues and trigger specific developmental events in a number of fetal organs (Liggins, 1976). The mechanism of action of glucocorticoids in fetal lung has been particularly well studied because they are involved in the maturation of the fetal lung (Giannopoulos, 1980). To function adequately, the lung must contain alveoli of appropriate quantity and structure and adequate amount of surfactant. Pulmonary surfactant is required to reduce surface tension at the alveolar air–tissue interface and to prevent alveolar collapse at low lung volumes (Goerke, 1974). A deficiency in surfactant is considered to be the primary cause of respratory distress syndrome in the premature newborn, a major cause of death in human infants (Avery and Mead, 1959). In 1969, Liggins observed that following infusion of dexamethasone into sheep fetuses, lambs born prematurely showed precocious lung maturation. At this time, Liggins already suggested that the glucocorticoid had accelerated the appearance of surfactant in fetal lungs, 'possibly as a result of premature activity of enzymes involved in a biosynthetic pathway'. Since then, numerous studies have been carried out to elucidate the effect of glucocorticoids, including work on the ontogeny of fetal glucocorticoid receptors in the lung as well as in other tissues.

Other fetal organs such as the liver, intestine, kidney and thymus are also responsive to glucocorticoids, but acquisition of sensitivity differs in each tissue.

1.1. Rabbits

Some of the first studies on glucocorticoid binding in the fetal rabbit included measurements of receptor concentrations in numerous fetal tissues since glucocorticoids have multiple functions. Table 2.30 shows that some specific, high affinity binding of a

TABLE 2.30. *^{3}H-Dexamethasone Binding in Various Tissues of the Fetal Rabbit at the End of Gestation*

Tissue	fmol/mg protein[a]	pmol/mg DNA[a]	K_d nM $(4° C)$[b]
Lung	510	1.62	2.7
Kidney	460	1.83	3.1
Thymus	220	0.35	4.6
Skin	230	1.25	2.5
Muscle	210	0.95	2.6
Small intestine	170	0.80	8.0
Liver	170	0.49	5.0
Heart	190	0.69	6.3
Brain	80	0.41	5.7
Fetal placenta	250	1.78	3.7

[a]Quoted from Giannopoulos *et al.* (1974); [b]Quoted from Ballard *et al.* (1974).

synthetic glucocorticoid, ^{3}H-dexamethasone, could be found in a whole range of tissues studied. The lung clearly contains a higher concentration of binding sites, but the other fetal tissues also contain substantial amounts, including the fetal placenta. The higher level of binding activity in lung tissue may reflect a potentially greater responsiveness of fetal lung compared with other fetal tissues.

1.1.1. LUNG

1.1.1.1. Ontogeny of Glucocorticoid Receptors

Fetal rabbit lung contains high affinity binding sites for glucocorticoids which have often been studied using the synthetic glucocorticoid ^{3}H-dexamethasone because of its particularly high affinity for the glucocorticoid receptor and low affinity for corticosteroid binding globulin (CBG). Table 2.31 indicates the physicochemical characteristics of the glucocorticoid receptor found in the cytosols of fetal rabbit lungs at the end of gestation. One notable particularity is the higher affinity of the receptor for cortisol than for corticosterone. This receptor also binds progestins and androgens but with lesser affinity. The rabbit is a cortisol-secreting species and this is reflected in the specificity of its glucocorticoid receptor. Receptor binding can be distinguished from binding to CBG by the high affinity for ^{3}H-dexamethasone, by the sedimentation coefficient of 7 S in low salt sucrose density gradients and by the thermolability of the receptor.

Receptor binding could be detected in rabbit fetal lung in 18-day-old fetuses (380 fmol/mg protein) (Ballard and Ballard, 1972). During fetal development, very little or no difference could be found in receptor concentrations between days 18 and 29 when binding was expressed per mg cytosol protein (Ballard and Ballard, 1972; Giannopoulos, 1974b), but receptor concentrations gradually increased when expressed

TABLE 2.31. *Physicochemical Characteristics of Cytosol Glucocorticoid Receptor in Fetal Rabbit Lung (27–30 Days of Gestation)*

Number of sites	
fmol/mg protein	430–520
pmol/mg DNA	1.6–2.2
pmol/g tissue	18
sites/cell	7000–12 000
K_d ($\times 10^{-9}$ M) 4° C	2.7
Binding specificity	Cortisol > corticosterone > progestins > androgens
Sedimentation coefficient	7 S in low salt
	4 S in high salt
Proteolysis	Destroyed
Thermostability	Labile at 37° C

The values represent the specific binding of ^{3}H-dexamethasone.
Quoted from Ballard and Ballard (1972); Giannopoulos (1973, 1974a, 1976); Giannopoulos and Keichline (1981); Ballard *et al.* (1984a).

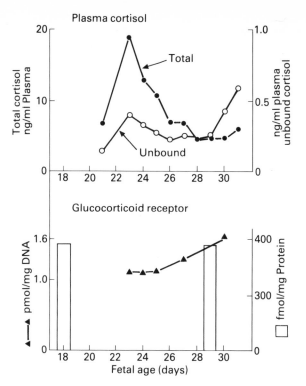

FIG 2.30. Ontogeny of Cytosol Glucocorticoid Receptors in Fetal Rabbit Lung and
Plasma Cortisol Concentrations.
Quoted from Ballard *et al.* (1984a) and Hümmelink and Ballard (1986).

per mg DNA (Ballard *et al.*, 1984a) (Fig. 2.30). Receptors are, thus, present early in
fetal lung development so they are probably not the limiting step in the development
of glucocorticoid sensitivity.

In order to determine whether a relationship exists between fetal plasma glucocorticoid concentrations and receptor concentrations, the evolution of these values during
fetal development is also shown in Fig. 2.30. Some groups have reported an increase in
unbound plasma cortisol only at the end of gestation (Mulay *et al.*, 1973) while others
have observed a peak on day 25 (Barr *et al.*, 1980). Hümmelink and Ballard (1986)
found that total cortisol (bound and unbound) rose to a peak on day 23 of gestation in
fetal plasma, but unbound cortisol plateaued between days 23 and 29 as seen in Fig.
2.30. The presence of receptors as early as day 18 and the subsequent increase with
advancing fetal development do not coincide with changes in the plasma concentrations
of unbound cortisol.

Glucocorticoid metabolism could also be an important regulatory factor in lung
development. Cortisone, a biologically inactive corticoid with little affinity for the fetal
lung glucocorticoid receptor, is, nevertheless, the prevailing glucocorticoid circulating in
unbound (bioavailable) form (Barr *et al.*, 1980). Cortisone is converted to cortisol in
fetal rabbit lung but this capacity develops with age (Giannopoulos, 1974b; Torday *et
al.*, 1976). No 11β-hydroxysteroid dehydrogenase activity was observed on day 21 but

it appeared on day 23. A significant increase in activity could be seen between days 23 and 29 (Torday *et al.*, 1976). This coincides with the peak in unbound cortisol in fetal plasma and would favor the appearance of the physiological effects of cortisol on fetal lung maturation observed shortly thereafter.

1.1.1.2. Fetal Lung Development and Ontogeny of Glucocorticoid Receptors

The physiological importance of the relationship between receptors and endogenous active glucocorticoids in fetal lung maturation may be more apparent if they can be temporally associated with key events in lung development. Differentiation of alveoli is characterized by increasing formation of type II cells, which occur at the junction of branching alveoli and which are the sites of synthesis of surfactant. Type II cells can be recognized by osmiophilic lamellar bodies that are probably the sites of surfactant production and storage. Lamellar bodies appear in type II cells on days 24–25 (Kikkawa *et al.*, 1971).

Surface-active phospholipids are present in whole lung homogenates on days 21–23 of gestation (Gluck *et al.*, 1967a,b; Gluck *et al.*, 1970) but can be detected in the alveolar washes only several days later (days 26–27) (Rooney *et al.*, 1976; Torday and Nielsen, 1981). Synthesis and storage of surfactant thus occurs before its secretion. A good temporal correlation can be seen between intracellular storage of surfactant and increasing numbers of lamellar bodies in fetal lung as gestation progresses.

From Table 2.32, it can be seen that the onset of lung maturation occurs around day 23 of gestation in the rabbit, but development culminates toward the end of gestation. The surfactant content of lung tissue increases by about 70% between days 27 and 31 and, more significantly, the amount of surfactant in lung washes increases 10-fold. The most dramatic rise occurs on day 31 (Rooney *et al.*, 1976). Decapitation of the fetal rabbit delays morphological development of the fetal lung and leads to decreased levels

TABLE 2.32. *Time course of Events in Fetal Lung Maturation in the Rabbit*

	Days of Gestation	Reference
Cytodifferentiation		
Appearance of lamellar bodies	24–25	Kikkawa *et al.*, 1971
Accumulation of lamellar bodies	27	Wang *et al.*, 1971
Surfactant		
Detectable in whole lung homogenates	21–23	Gluck *et al.*, 1967a,b; Gluck *et al.*, 1970
Increases in lung tissue	26–31	Gluck *et al.*, 1970 Rooney *et al.*, 1976
Increases in alveolar washes	27–31	Torday and Nielsen, 1981; Rooney *et al.*, 1976
Rate of synthesis increases	28	Gross *et al.*, 1983

of surfactant in lung extracts probably due to the diminution of hormones in the fetal compartment (Blackburn *et al.*, 1972).

A specific protein that is associated with surfactant glycerophospholipids as well as the mRNA of this protein increases as a function of gestational age in rabbit fetal lung (Mendelson *et al.*, 1986; Boggaram *et al.*, 1988). This 28–36 kDa glycoprotein (SP-A, SP 28–36) is found in the cytoplasm of type II pneumonocytes but not in fibroblasts (Liley *et al.*, 1987). SP-A mRNA is undetectable in rabbit fetal lung tissue until day 26 of gestation, and the steady-state levels then increase to a maximum on day 31 of gestation (Boggaram *et al.*, 1988). The rates of transcription of SP-A mRNA also increase during fetal lung development (Boggaram and Mendelson, 1988).

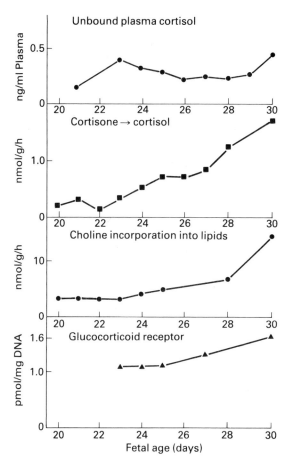

Fig 2.31. Comparison of Unbound Plasma Cortisol Levels, Rates of Conversion of Cortisone to Cortisol, Surfactant Formation and Glucocorticoid Receptor Concentrations in the Fetal Lung of the Rabbit during Development.
Unbound cortisol levels in fetal plasma adapted from Hümmelink and Ballard (1986). The rates of conversion of ^{14}C-cortisone into ^{14}C-cortisol and incorporation of ^{14}C-choline into total lipids by fetal lung tissue taken from Nicholas *et al.* (1978). Glucocorticoid receptor concentrations in the cytosol and nuclear fractions of fetal lung taken from Ballard *et al.* (1984a).

A close correlation has been observed between the ability of fetal lung tissue to reduce cortisone to cortisol and the rate of *de novo* synthesis of choline-containing lipids (Fig. 2.31) (Nicholas *et al.*, 1978). Pulmonary surfactant is composed largely of phospholipid, the major component of which is phosphatidylcholine. As seen in Fig. 2.31, the conversion of cortisone to cortisol by fetal lung tissue increases during fetal development (Giannopoulos, 1974b; Torday *et al.*, 1976) and leads to increased levels of cortisol actually retained in the lung tissue probably because of the presence of receptors (Nicholas *et al.*, 1978).

Ballard and co-workers (1984a) reported a close correlation between glucocorticoid receptor concentrations found in a series of 27-day-old fetal lungs and the rate of choline incorporation into phosphatidylcholine by explants of fetal lung in organ culture. However, glucocorticoid receptors are present long before the increase in surfactant formation. The abrupt rise in plasma cortisol on day 23 and the increasing capacity of fetal lung tissue to convert cortisone to cortisol may be the principal factors in the timing of lung maturation while receptor concentrations may play a permissive role (Fig. 2.31). Another possibility is that since concentrations of receptors and the endogenous active glucocorticoid are maximal well before the acquisition of glucocorticoid sensitivity, both factors may be permissive, priming the lung for stimulation by other hormones such as thyroid hormones (Smith and Sabry, 1983; Ballard *et al.*, 1984b) or prolactin (Hamosh and Hamosh, 1977).

It has been reported that male and female fetuses differ in pulmonary development and glucocorticoid responsiveness (Kotas and Avery, 1980; Nielsen and Torday, 1981). In the human, male newborns have a higher incidence of respiratory distress syndrome and, in some studies, are less responsive to prenatal glucocorticoid treatment for prevention of this disease (Farrell and Wood, 1976; Ballard *et al.*, 1980a). In fetal rabbits, it has been reported that males are less responsive to corticosteroid treatment than females (Kotas and Avery, 1980). Nielsen and Torday (1981) observed significantly higher amounts of surfactant in lung lavage in female fetuses at 26 and 28 days as compared to males. No differences were detected on days 24 or days 30. On the other hand, when the rate of choline incorporation into phosphatidylcholine was studied *in vitro*, no difference between sexes was found from days 24 to 28 of gestation (Gross *et al.*, 1983). Also, there was no male–female difference when a glucocorticoid was injected to the mother on day 25 and the rate of choline incorporation was examined in fetal lungs on day 26 (Gross *et al.*, 1983). Finally, no sex differences in receptor binding were found in lungs of 27-day-old rabbit fetuses (Ballard *et al.*, 1984a).

1.1.1.3. Ontogeny of Responsiveness to Exogenous Glucocorticoids

Cortisol accelerates maturation of the fetal lung when injected into rabbit fetuses as early as the day 19 of gestation (Kikkawa *et al.*, 1971). Injection of glucocorticoids into fetal animals increases the number of lamellar bodies in type II alveolar epithelial cells (Kikkawa *et al.*, 1971) and the amount of lung tissue surfactant at least from day 23 (Farrell and Zachman, 1973). Administration of glucocorticoid to rabbit fetuses on day 25 of gestation results in 70% more surfactant in lung lavage than in the untreated littermates (Rooney *et al.*, 1979a). It appears that fetal lung tissue is capable of responding to exogenous glucocorticoids before surfactant appears in the alveolar lining during normal development because glucocorticoid receptors are already present as early as day 18 of gestation. Exogenously administered glucocorticoids stimulate the activities of several enzymes involved in surfactant production (Rooney, 1979).

In 1973, Farrell and Zachman were able to demonstrate that treatment of rabbit fetuses with a single dose of glucocorticoid (9α-fluoroprednisolone acetate) on days 23–24 days of gestation leads to a 40% increase in surfactant in fetal lungs three days later (Fig. 2.32). In these same animals, incorporation of ^{14}C-choline into lecithin increases by 50% in lung slices of glucocorticoid-treated animals. This stimulation cannot be blocked by prior treatment of the fetuses with actinomycin D but cyclohex-imide abolishes the glucocorticoid effects (Farrell and Zachman, 1973), suggesting that increased lecithin production requires protein synthesis.

In vitro studies using organ culture of fetal lung tissue explants and fetal lung cells in monolayer cultures have confirmed the activity of glucocorticoids in the fetal rabbit lung. The ability of glucocorticoids to stimulate choline incorporation into phos-phatidylcholine when compared with untreated lung tissue of the same age was found

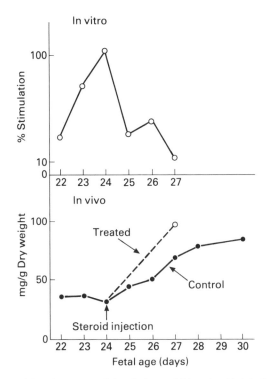

FIG 2.32. Effect of Fetal Age on Stimulation of Phosphatidylcholine Synthesis by Glucocorticoids in Fetal Rabbit Lung *in vivo* and *in vitro*.

In vitro: explants of fetal rabbit lung were cultured for two days with and without 100 nM dexamethasone and the rate of incorporation of ^{3}H-choline into phos-phatidylcholine was measured; *In vivo*: fetuses received one injection of 9α-fluoroprednisolone acetate at 24 days of gestation, and the surfactant content of lung tissue was measured. Quoted from Farrell (1977) with the permission of the Journal of Steroid Biochemistry.

to be greatest on days 23–24 of gestation (Fig. 2.32) (Gross *et al.*, 1983). In mixed fetal lung cell cultures, ^{3}H-choline incorporation into phosphatidylcholine could be increased two-fold by glucocorticoids in a dose-dependent manner (Torday *et al.*, 1975). This effect was specifically obtained with glucocorticoids in both cell and organ cultures (Torday *et al.*, 1975; Gross *et al.*, 1983). Table 2.33 shows the close correlation between the effects of various steroids on choline incorporation into phosphatidylcholine and their relative capacities to bind to receptors in the nucleus (Gross *et al.*, 1983). Furthermore, the dose-response curves of ^{3}H-dexamethasone bound in the nucleus and the stimulation of choline incorporation into phosphatidylcholine are superimposable (Gross *et al.*, 1983).

In the fetal lung explants, cortisol increases the levels and rates of transcription of the mRNA corresponding to the 28–36 kDa surfactant protein (SP-A) in incubations lasting more than 24 h (Boggaram and Mendelson, 1988). The increases in the rates of transcription of SP-A mRNA during development of rabbit fetal lung and the stimulating effect of cortisol *in vitro* are similar to the changes in the steady-state levels of SP-A mRNA, suggesting that regulation of SP-A mRNA occurs primarily at the transcriptional level (Boggaram and Mendelson, 1988).

The overall result of glucocorticoid treatment in the fetal lung is an acceleration of maturation, and the net biochemical effect is an enhanced capacity of the lung to produce surfactant at an earlier time in gestation than would normally occur. The activities of enzymes involved in phospholipid biosynthesis increase during normal development, and these same enzyme activities can be stimulated by hormones. At the time when the fetal lung is responsive to exogenously administered glucocorticoids, glucocorticoid receptors are already relatively high.

TABLE 2.33. *Effects of Various Steroids on the Rate of Incorporation of Choline into Phosphatidylcholine and on the Binding of ^{3}H-Dexamethasone to the Glucocorticoid Receptor in Fetal Rabbit Lung in Organ Culture*

Steroid	Choline incorporation %	^{3}H-Dexamethasone binding %
Dexamethasone	100	100
Cortisol	96	71
Cortisone	92	47
Corticosterone	43	22
Dehydrocorticosterone	27	13
Progesterone	0	2
17α-Hydroxyprogesterone	0	0
17β-Estradiol	0	0
Testosterone	0	0

Choline incorporation into phosphatidylcholine and the competition for nuclear binding sites of ^{3}H-dexamethasone are expressed as the percentage of the effect of dexamethasone (assigned the value of 100%)

Adapted from Gross *et al.* (1983).

1.1.2. INTESTINE

In the rabbit, intestinal enzymes such as alkaline phosphatase and lactase appear only towards the end of gestation (Moog, 1953; Sterk and Kretchmer, 1964). Glucocorticoids may play a role in the development of these enzyme systems in the fetal intestine since the decapitation *in utero* of fetal rabbits abolishes the increase in alkaline phosphatase, and the administration of ACTH to these fetuses increases the enzyme activity to normal levels (Bearn, 1973).

1.1.2.1. Ontogeny of Glucocorticoid Receptors in the Fetal Small Intestine

The characteristics of glucocorticoid receptors present in the small intestine of the rabbit fetus are shown in Table 2.34 (Lee *et al.*, 1976). Binding is specific for natural and synthetic glucocorticoids; cortisol has a slightly higher affinity than corticosterone for the receptor. As seen in Fig. 2.33, cytosol and nuclear binding sites for ^{3}H-dexamethasone are already detectable as early as 21 days of gestation (Lee *et al.*, 1976). The concentrations rise to a peak at 26 days and decline thereafter. The peak in binding occurs three days after the peak in unbound plasma cortisol (Hümmelink and Ballard, 1986).

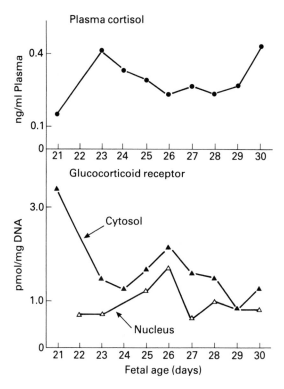

FIG 2.33. Ontogeny of Cytosol Glucocorticoid Receptors in the Small Intestine of the Rabbit Fetus and Fetal Plasma Cortisol Concentrations.
Glucocorticoid receptor values adapted from Lee *et al.* (1976) and Lee and Solomon (1978). Plasma cortisol data taken from Hümmelink and Ballard (1986).

TABLE 2.34. *Physicochemical Characteristics of Cytosol Glucocorticoid Receptors in Fetal Rabbit Small Intestine (27–29 Days of Gestation)*

Number of sites	200–250 fmol/mg protein
	1.4–1.6 pmol/mg DNA
	10–12 pmol/g tissue
	3–6 pmol/intestine
K_d ($\times 10^{-9}$ M), 4°C	1.7–4.4
Binding specificity	Cortisol > corticosterone
Sedimentation coefficient	7 S and 4 S in low salt
	4 S in high salt
Proteolysis	Destroyed
Thermal stability	Labile at 37° C

Binding was determined using ^{3}H-dexamethasone
Quoted from Lee *et al.* (1976); Solomon and Lee, 1977.

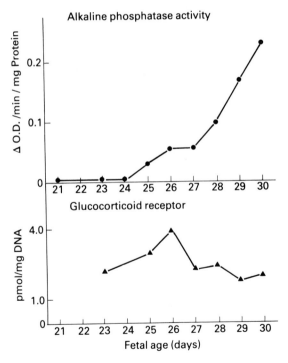

FIG 2.34. Development of Alkaline Phosphatase Activity and Glucocorticoid Receptors in the Fetal Rabbit Small Intestine.
Alkaline phosphatase activities taken from Lee *et al.* (1976). The glucocorticoid receptor concentrations are the sum of cytosol and nuclear receptor values reported by Lee *et al.* (1976) and Lee and Solomon (1978).

1.1.2.2. Development of Alkaline Phosphatase Activity and Glucocorticoid Receptors

Alkaline phosphatase activity develops in the small intestine with fetal age and continues to increase after birth. Activity of this enzyme is absent prior to day 25 of gestation and increases rapidly thereafter (Fig. 2.34) (Lee *et al.*, 1976). Glucocorticoid receptors are already present in high concentrations before the appearance of alkaline phosphatase activity and do not parallel the increase, suggesting that the availability of a sufficient level of receptors allows the increase in enzymes such as alkaline phosphatase but a continuing increase in activity does not depend on a parallel increase in binding.

1.1.3. LIVER

The first evidence for the role of fetal endocrine function in the biochemical differentiation of fetal liver was obtained by Jost and co-workers (Jost and Hatey, 1949; Jost and Jacquot, 1955, 1958). They showed that decapitation of fetal rabbits prevents the accumulation of liver glycogen and that the administration of glucocorticoids restores this capacity in fetuses.

1.1.3.1. Ontogeny of Glucocorticoid Receptors in Fetal Liver

Specific binding of the synthetic glucocorticoids dexamethasone and triamcinolone acetonide has been observed in fetal liver with concentrations of approximately 150 fmol/mg protein or 0.5 pmol/mg DNA in the cytosol at the end of gestation and an affinity of $1-7 \times 10^{-9}$ M (K_d at 4° C) (Ballard and Ballard, 1972; Giannopoulos *et al.*, 1974; Bourbon *et al.*, 1979). During fetal development, binding was found as early as day 22 of gestation (91 fmol/mg protein); no difference was observed on either day 24 (98 fmol/mg protein) or on day 29 (104 fmol/mg protein) (Bourbon *et al.*, 1979).

Livers from fetuses decapitated on day 22 and studied on day 29 exhibited lower concentrations of glucocorticoid receptor (78 fmol/mg protein) than control litter mates (104 fmol/mg protein) (Bourbon *et al.*, 1979).

1.1.3.2. Development of Glucocorticoid Responses

Rapid accumulation of glycogen occurs after day 25 in the liver of the rabbit fetus. No storage of glycogen occurs in fetuses decapitated before day 25, and glucocorticoids alone cannot compensate for the absence of the pituitary (Jost and Hatey, 1949; Jost and Jacquot 1955, 1958). Since the concentration of glucocorticoid receptors is constant in the fetal liver before and after the onset of glycogen storage and the effect of fetal decapitation, they do not appear to be the limiting factor preventing glycogen storage before day 26. The difference in binding between decapitated and control fetuses is also not sufficient to explain the lack of effects of glucocorticoids on glycogen storage in fetuses decapitated before day 26.

1.1.4. KIDNEY

Fetal kidney contains ^{3}H-dexamethasone binding sites with high affinity for both natural and synthetic glucocorticoids but not for other steroids except for progesterone (Table 2.35) (Giannopoulos *et al.*, 1974).

TABLE 2.35. *Physicochemical Properties of Glucocorticoid Receptors in the Cytosol of Fetal Rabbit Kidney (28–30 Days of Gestation)*

Number of sites	240–260 fmol/mg protein
	~2 pmol/mg DNA
K_d ($\times 10^{-9}$ M), 4° C	3.1
Binding specificity	Cortisol > corticosterone
	> progesterone
Sedimentation coefficient	7–8 S, 4 S in low salt

Glucocorticoid binding was measured using ^{3}H-dexamethasone

Quoted from Giannopoulos *et al.* (1974).

1.2. Rats

The rat has been most often used as an animal model for the study of the action of glucocorticoids on the developing liver. Glucocorticoids are important in the maturation of rat liver during the end of gestation and act on both the hepatocyte and hemopoietic cell populations of the fetal liver (Jacquot, 1959; Jost, 1966a; Jost and Picon, 1970; Jacquot *et al.*, 1973).

1.2.1. Lung

1.2.1.1. Physicochemical Properties of the Fetal Glucocorticoid Receptor

At the end of fetal development, fetal rat lung contains binding sites with high affinity for natural and synthetic glucocorticoids (Table 2.36). The characteristics are very similar to those of the receptor from the lungs of fetal rabbits except for the higher

TABLE 2.36. *Physicochemical Characteristics of Cytosol Glucocorticoid Receptors in Fetal Rat Lung (19–22 Days)*

Number of sites	210–220 fmol/mg protein
	0.68–0.72 pmol/mg DNA
	~8000 sites/cell
K_d ($\times 10^{-9}$ M), 4° C	4.7
Binding specificity	Corticosterone > cortisol
	> progestins
Sedimentation coefficient	7 S

The values represent the specific binding of ^{3}H-dexamethasone

Quoted from Giannopoulos (1975a); Ballard *et al.* (1978); Giannopoulos and Keichline (1981); Mulay *et al.* (1982).

affinity for corticosterone than cortisol. Corticosterone is the biologically potent gluco-corticoid in the rat.

1.2.1.2. Ontogeny of Glucocorticoid Receptors

Glucocorticoid receptors could be found in fetal rat lungs from the earliest period studied, 16 days (Fig. 2.35) (Ballard *et al.*, 1984a; Brönnegard and Okret, 1988). The receptor concentration then doubles by 20 days of fetal age and remains at a plateau until birth (Ballard *et al.*, 1984a). No differences in ligand affinity for the receptor were observed (Brönnegard and Okret, 1988). Fetal plasma corticosteroid concentration also rises towards the end of gestation. Total (bound and unbound) corticosteroids peak on day 20, but the unbound fraction continues to increase sharply due to the decrease in CBG concentrations (Fig. 2.35) (Martin *et al.*, 1977). Fetal plasma corticosterone concentrations (bound and unbound) show the same temporal profile as that of total corticosteroids (Dupouy *et al.*, 1975).

Receptor binding has also been determined in the alveolar type II cells of fetal rat lung which is the site of surfactant synthesis. Specific binding of ^{3}H-dexamethasone is

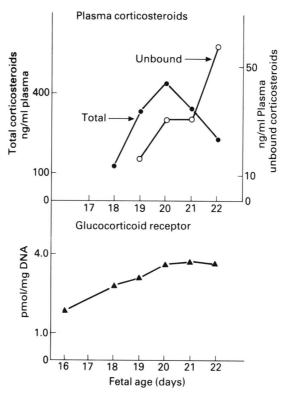

FIG 2.35. Ontogeny of Glucorticoid Receptors in the Fetal Rat Lung (Comparison with Plasma Corticosteroid Concentrations).
Glucocorticoid receptors (^{3}H-dexamethasone binding) were measured by Ballard *et al.* (1984a). Plasma corticosteroid levels were taken from Martin *et al.* (1977).

higher than in whole tissue with a mixed cell population (13 500 sites/cell in type II cells vs 4000–8000 sites/cell in whole tissue), with a slightly lower affinity ($K_d = 10.2 \pm 0.8$ (SE) $\times 10^{-9}$ M at 4° C) (Ballard *et al.*, 1978).

1.2.1.3. Comparison of the Development of Surfactant Formation and Glucocorticoid Receptors

The rise in glucocorticoid receptor concentrations in the fetal lung during development in the rat, the increase in unbound plasma corticosteroids and the abrupt increase in surfactant content of the lung appear to be more closely associated in the rat than in the rabbit. Figure 2.36 shows that the rate of phosphatidylcholine formation form choline begins to rise significantly after day 20 (Farrell *et al.*, 1974), at a time when

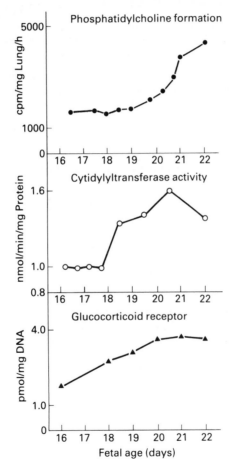

FIG 2.36. Development of Surfactant Formation and Glucocorticoid Receptors in Fetal Rat Lung.
Phosphatidylcholine formation and the specific activity of cytidylyltransferase adapted from Farrell (1977). Receptor measurements representing the binding of ^{3}H-dexamethasone in whole lung tissue adapted from Ballard *et al.* (1984a).

receptor concentrations have reached a maximum. The phosphatidylcholine content of whole lung tissue follows a very similar curve (Bourbon *et al.*, 1987). The activity of one of the key enzymes in phosphatidylcholine formation increases sharply on day 18.5, before surfactant production appears (Fig. 2.36). Phosphocholine cytidylyltransferase (EC 2.7.7.15) is the enzyme that catalyses the rate-limiting reaction in the formation of phosphatidylcholine. In contrast, in the rabbit, the activity of this enzyme is not closely correlated with surfactant synthesis during fetal lung development (Heath and Jacobson, 1984). In the rat, the major surfactant-associated protein SP-A and its corresponding mRNA are detected in fetal lung at 17 days and increase between days 19 and 22, similar to the increase in the production of surfactant phospholipid (Phelps *et al.*, 1987; Gross *et al.*, 1989).

1.2.1.4. Development of Glucocorticoid Responsiveness

As in the rabbit, fetal lung maturation can be accelerated by providing exogenous glucocorticoids. Administration of dexamethasone to pregnant rats on day 18 of gestation increases the phosphatidylcholine content of fetal lung tissue by about 70% on day 19 (Post *et al.*, 1986), but not on days 16 or 17 of gestation (Brönnegard and Okret, 1988). Glucocorticoid receptors are already present on day 16 of gestation and the lack of response to glucocorticoids at this stage cannot be attributed to any physicochemical deficiency in the receptor (Brönnegard and Okret, 1988).

Table 2.37 shows that the glucocorticoid-induced increase in phosphatidylcholine synthesis is accompanied by a stimulation of phosphocholine cytidylyltransferase and lipoprotein lipase activities, the former a key phospholipid synthesizing enzyme and the latter an enzyme which plays an important role in supplying fatty acid precursor for phospholipid synthesis through hydrolysis of circulating triglyceride. At this stage of fetal rat development, glucocorticoid receptors in the lung are rising but phosphatidylcholine formation has not yet matured (see Fig. 2.36). Glucocorticoid treatment has, therefore, provoked a precocious development of surfactant, probably due to the presence of a sufficient quantity of receptors at an early stage in fetal rat lung development.

The surfactant-producing alveolar type II cells have also been shown to respond to glucocorticoid treatment *in vitro* (Sanders *et al.*, 1981; Post *et al.*, 1984a). As seen in Table 2.37, cortisol stimulates the synthesis of phosphatidylcholine and the activity of phosphocholine cytidylyltransferase in type II cells isolated from mixed cell cultures of lungs from fetal rats 19 days of age (Post *et al.*, 1986). Explants of fetal lung in organ culture contain about 3.5 pmol/mg DNA of specific binding sites for ^{3}H-dexamethasone (Ballard *et al.*, 1984a) and the alveolar type II cells themselves have a high concentration of binding sites (Ballard *et al.*, 1978) which could mediate these glucocorticoid responses.

Evidence from a variety of studies has indicated that the glucocorticoid effect on lung maturation depends on intercellular interaction and is not a direct effect on surfactant production by the type II cells (Smith, 1979; Smith and Sabry, 1983; Post *et al.*, 1984a,b; Post and Smith, 1984). Glucocorticoids induce the production of a protein, fibroblast-pneumonocyte factor, in fetal lung fibroblasts that stimulates surfactant formation by fetal alveolar type II cells. Isolated fetal type II cells in primary culture show a two-fold stimulation of cytidylyltransferase activity by fibroblast-pneumonocyte

TABLE 2.37. *Glucocorticoid Responses* In Vivo *and* In Vitro *in Fetal Rat Lung*

	Ratio of treated/control	Reference
In vivo		
Phosphatidylcholine content	1.68	Post *et al.* (1986)
Phosphocholine cytidylyltransferase	1.34	Post *et al.* (1986)
Lipoprotein lipase	2.68	Mostello *et al.* (1981)
Mixed lung cell cultures		
Phosphatidylcholine formation	1.64	Post *et al.* (1986)
Phosphocholine cytidylyltransferase	2.04	Post *et al.* (1986)
Primary culture of Type II cells		
Phosphocholine cytidylyltransferase	2.00	Post *et al.* (1986)

In vivo: Pregnant rats were treated with dexamethasone (0.2 mg/kg) on day 18 except for the studies in lipoprotein lipase where pregnant animals were infused from day 16 with dexamethasone (400 μg/kg/day) and fetuses were sacrificed on day 19. *Mixed lung cell cultures*: Lung cells from fetal rats on day 19 of gestation were incubated with and without cortisol for 20 h. Type II cells were then isolated from the cultures. *Primary culture of Type II cells*: Alveolar Type II cells were isolated from day-19 fetal rat lung and cultured as monolayers. Cells were incubated with either cortisol alone (control) or medium containing fibroblast pneumonocyte factor (treated).

factor compared to cells treated with cortisol (Table 2.37) (Post *et al.*, 1986). The mechanism of action of fibroblast-pneumonocyte factor is not yet known. Besides the alveolar type II cells, lung fibroblastic cells (human) also contain glucocorticoid receptors (Ballard *et al.*, 1978), but a relationship with fibroblast-pneumonocyte factor cannot be concluded especially since isolated alveolar type II cells do respond to glucocorticoid treatment.

1.2.2. LIVER

Glucocorticoids are involved in the maturation of the rat liver, particularly in the development of glycogen accumulation in rat hepatocytes before birth (Jacquot, 1959). Glucocorticoids are necessary for the induction of some enzymes required for glycogen deposition; in the fetus deprived of glucocorticoid the formation of enzymes and glycogen deposition is inhibited (Greengard, 1970).

1.2.2.1. Properties of Fetal Liver Glucocorticoid Receptor

Table 2.38 shows the characteristics of glucocorticoid receptors in the liver of rat fetuses from days 19 to 20 of gestation. The properties of receptors in hepatocytes and hemopoietic cells are also compared since fetal rat liver contains, in addition to hepatocytes, a large population of hemopoietic cells (Oliver *et al.*, 1963; Greengard *et al.*, 1972). Both hepatocytes and hemopoietic cells contain glucocorticoid receptors.

TABLE 2.38. *Comparison of the Physicochemical Properties of the Glucocorticoid Receptor in Liver, Hepatocytes and Hemopoietic Cells of the Fetal Rat (19–20 Days of Gestation)*

	Liver	Hepatocytes	Hemopoietic cells
Number of sites			
fmol/mg protein	110–250	220	–
pmol/mg DNA	0.76	0.3–0.5	–
pmol/g tissue	3.1	–	–
pmol/liver	0.6	–	–
sites/cell	–	$\sim$50 000	$\sim$2000
K_d ($\times 10^{-9}$ M), 4° C	3.6–5.0	$\sim$6	5.4–6.9
Binding specificity	Corticosterone > cortisol	Corticosterone = cortisol > progesterone	Corticosterone $\gg$ progesterone
Sedimentation coefficient	7 S in low salt	–	–
Thermal stability	Labile even at 0° C	–	–

Glucocorticoid receptor was measured using ^{3}H-dexamethasone as ligand.
Quoted from Feldman (1974); Giannopoulos (1975b); Billat *et al.* (1981); Cake *et al.* (1981); Kalimi and Gupta (1982); Mayeux *et al.* (1983); Plas and Duval (1986).

1.2.2.2. Ontogeny of Fetal Liver Glucocorticoid Receptors

Receptors for glucocorticoids have been found in the cytosol fraction of whole livers of rat fetuses from at least 16 days of gestation (Feldman, 1974; Giannopoulos, 1975b). Figure 2.37 shows the quantitative values from day 18 to birth. It can be seen that the concentration declines after day 20, reaching undetectable levels at birth (Giannopoulos, 1975b). Total bound and unbound plasma corticosteroids reach a peak on day 20 of gestation in fetal rat plasma, but the unbound (potentially active) fraction increases to day 22 (Dupouy *et al.*, 1975; Martin *et al.*, 1977). Maximum receptor levels appear to coincide with the peak of total plasma corticosteroids but minimum concentrations correspond to the increase in unbound plasma corticosteroids. Receptor values may be underestimated because the high concentrations of endogenous unbound plasma corticosteroids can interfere with receptor measurements by occupying receptor binding sites so that only available binding sites are measured.

Conflicting results were observed when glucocorticoid receptors were measured in a fetal hepatocyte cell population essentially free of hemopoietic cells (Fig. 2.37). Cake and co-workers (1981) could only detect significant amounts of receptor binding in 19-day-old fetuses while Plas and Duval (1986) found that hepatocytes already contained $\sim$50 000 sites/cell on day 15, and the concentrations remained constant until day 18.

In hemopoietic cells, the concentration of glucocorticoid receptors is already highest on day 13 of gestation, and levels decline thereafter (Fig. 2.37) (Billat *et al.*, 1981).

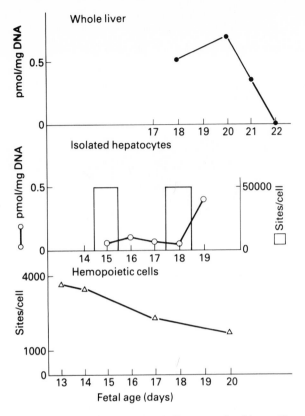

FIG 2.37. Ontogeny of the Glucocorticoid Receptor in Liver, Hepatocytes and
Hemopoietic Cells of the Fetal Rat.
Adapted from Giannopoulos (1975b), Cake *et al.* (1981) and Billat *et al.* (1981).

1.2.2.3. Glucocorticoid Responsiveness of the Fetal Rat Liver in Relation to the Ontogeny of Glucocorticoid Receptors

Glucocorticoids appear to trigger glycogen synthesis in fetal liver since glycogen synthesis and storage in fetal liver accompanies the increase in unbound plasma corticosteroids (Fig. 2.38). The liver is competent to produce glycogen if exposed to glucocorticoid at least from day 17 of gestation, at a time when glucocorticoid receptors are already present in the fetal liver (Fig. 2.38) (Greengard, 1970). Fetal decapitation inhibits the accumulation of some enzymes involved in glycogen formation manifested by the complete inability of glycogen synthesis and storage to proceed normally (Fig. 2.38) (Jacquot and Kretchmer, 1964). Cortisol has been shown to induce glycogen synthesis and storage in fetal hepatocytes on day 15 (Fig. 2.39) (Plas *et al.*, 1973) and induction appears to be correlated with increased receptor concentrations because these cells develop receptors and hormone responsiveness during the course of the culture period (Cake *et al.*, 1980, 1981).

Tyrosine aminotransferase (TAT) is one of a cluster of enzyme activities that first appears at birth when overall liver metabolism is shifted toward gluconeogenesis

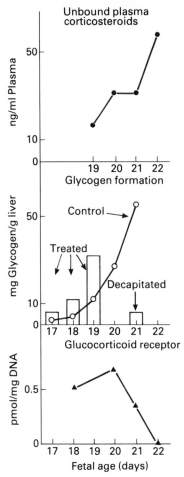

FIG 2.38. Ontogeny of Glycogen Deposition and Glucocorticoid Responsiveness in the Fetal Rat Liver Compared with Glucocorticoid Receptor and Unbound Plasma Corticosteroid Concentrations.
Fetal plasma corticosteroid concentrations taken from Martin *et al.* (1977), glycogen contents from Greengard (1970) and glucocorticoid receptors from Giannopoulos (1975b).

(Greengard, 1971). TAT catalytic activity is virtually absent in fetal rat liver up to day 20 of gestation (Yeoh *et al.*, 1979); detectable amounts have been reported on day 21 (Andersson *et al.*, 1980). In contrast to their observed effect on glycogen deposition, glucocorticoids do not induce TAT in fetal rat liver but do so 24 h after birth (Sereni *et al.*, 1959; Holt and Oliver, 1968). Ruiz-Bravo and Ernest (1985) confirmed that the *in utero* injection of cortisol to 20-day-old rat fetuses fails to induce TAT activity in fetal liver, but cortisol could potentiate the action of cyclic AMP, a known inducer of TAT.

Studies using isolated fetal hepatocytes have shown that hepatocytes isolated from 15-day-old fetal rats are initially unresponsive to glucocorticoids, but TAT activity can be induced if the cells are maintained in culture for three days (Fig. 2.39) (Cake *et al.*,

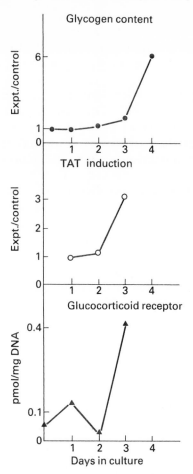

FIG 2.39. Glucocorticoid Responsiveness of Hepatocytes from 15-day-old Rat Fetuses. Comparison with Glucocorticoid Receptor Concentrations.
Hepatocytes from 15-day-old fetal rats were cultured in the presence of a glucocorticoid. TAT = tyrosine aminotransferase activity. The glucocorticoid effect is expressed as the ratio of results from treated cells to untreated cells. Data combined from Plas *et al.* (1973) and Cake *et al.* (1981).

1981). In this report, glucocorticoid receptors were not detectable in 15-day-old fetal hepatocytes before culture, but a significant correlation could be established between the increase in receptors during the culture period and the inducibility of TAT by dexamethasone. Another *in vitro* study using organ culture of fetal liver (19 days of gestation) has also shown that both glycogen content and TAT activity are increased by cortisol *in vitro* (Monder and Coufalik, 1972). In this organ culture study, glycogen synthesis and TAT activity were shown to be independent since the cortisol-provoked increase in TAT activity could be inhibited without any effect on glycogen synthesis and suppression of glycogen synthesis by omission of glucose did not prevent the induction of TAT by cortisol (Monder and Coufalik, 1972).

The inability of exogenous glucocorticoids to induce TAT activity in fetal liver *in vivo* is not due to the absence of receptors, but adequate receptor concentrations alone are clearly insufficient for this particular response. A lack of maturation of a step distal to receptor binding may be involved, or multiple glucocorticoid receptors may exist that require development. Kalimi and Gupta (1982) found differences in physicochemical properties of the receptor during development. Fetal receptors are more unstable even at 0° C (with or without bound ligand). The elution patterns of the receptor proteins from fetal and adult livers on Sephadex G-100 gel and on DEAE-cellulose chromatography are different. At least three weeks of post-natal maturation are necessary to acquire the adult receptor characteristics. These differences might possibly explain the lack of response.

Glucocorticoid responsiveness may also depend on other factors. Physiological concentrations of insulin have been found to prevent glucocorticoid induction of TAT in hepatocytes which are normally responsive (Cake *et al.*, 1981). On the other hand, glucocorticoids can enhance the insulin stimulation of glycogenesis in fetal hepatocytes in a dose-dependent manner (Plas and Duval, 1986).

The hemopoietic cell population of the fetal liver is also sensitive to glucocorticoids; glucocorticoids induce an accelerated maturation and a precocious depletion of the erythroid line from as early as day 14 (Billat *et al.*, 1980). This is consistent with the finding of glucocorticoid receptors in hemopoietic cells of the fetal liver even at an early stage of development (Billat *et al.*, 1981).

1.2.3. BRAIN

Specific binding of tritiated dexamethasone is present in brains of fetal rats from as early as day 17 of fetal age (Kitraki *et al.*, 1984). The concentration of glucocorticoid receptors is similar to that observed in the adult (about 120 fmol/mg protein). The dissociation constant (K_d) of dexamethasone binding $(2 \times 10^{-8}\,\mathrm{M})$ does not vary during the fetal period studied.

Meaney and co-workers (1985) showed high affinity binding of dexamethasone in the limbic area of the fetal rat brain (hippocampus, septum, amygdala, hypothalamus and caudate). Glucocorticoid receptor concentrations were found to be highest on day 16 of fetal age (111 fmol/mg protein). They decline to 65 fmol/mg protein on day 19 and to 61 fmol/mg protein on post-natal day 2 with no variation in binding affinity $(K_d = 4-6 \times 10^{-9}\,\mathrm{M}.$

1.3. Mice

1.3.1. WHOLE EMBRYOS

In order to gain an approach to the time in development when glucocorticoid receptors first appear, Salomon *et al.* (1978) chose to examine mid-gestation mouse embryos. At this stage, mouse embryos are exposed to high circulating concentrations of endogenous corticosteroids in the maternal circulation (Barlow *et al.*, 1974). Two inbred strains of mice (A/J and C57BL/6J) were chosen for this study because of their very different sensitivities to glucocorticoid-induced teratogenesis. The exogenous administration of glucocorticoids to mice of the A/J strain produced cleft palate in 100% of the offspring while only 20–25% of offspring of similarly treated C57BL/6J mice developed cleft palate (Kalter, 1965).

1.3.1.1. Presence of Specific Glucocorticoid Binding Sites

Specific, high affinity binding of ^{3}H-dexamethasone was found in cytosols of both the A/J and C57BL/6J mouse embryos (Salomon *et al.*, 1978). The binding curves showed two components with an apparent K_d (0°C) of 2.2×10^{-8} M for the high affinity binding site and 1.3×10^{-7} M for the low affinity binding site in embryos of both strains of mice. The concentrations of receptor sites are 20 and 60 fmol/mg protein for the high and low affinity sites, respectively. Dexamethasone, triamcinolone acetonide, corticosterone, cortisol and cortisone bind equally well to the receptor; progesterone also shows some binding ability. The specific binding of ^{3}H-dexamethasone is heat-labile while specific ^{3}H-corticosterone binding is unaffected by pre-incubation of cytosols at 45°C indicating that dexamethasone binds to receptor macromolecules in the embryonic cytosols while corticosterone binds preferentially to serum CBG in the cytosols.

In low salt glycerol density gradients, the specifically-bound ^{3}H-dexamethasone sediments in the 7–8 S regions of the gradient while ^{3}H-corticosterone bound to serum components sediments at 4.6 S.

1.3.1.2. Ontogeny of Glucocorticoid Receptors

No specific binding could be detected in cytosols of day 11 embryos of either strain; binding was first detected in day 12 embryos (Salomon *et al.*, 1978). On day 12, A/J embryos contain about twice as many receptor sites as the C57BL/6J embryos, but on days 13 and 14, this difference is not apparent. When expressed on a per embryo basis, the concentration of receptor sites increases in both A/J and C57BL/6J embryos between days 12 and 14 with no significant changes in apparent binding affinity.

The finding of glucocorticoid receptors in early mammalian embryos at a time when most embryonic tissues are just starting organogenesis may indicate a role for glucocorticoids in the initial stages of differentiation. The difference in receptor levels observed between the two strains on day 12 may possibly be related to the enhanced teratogenic sensitivity of the A/J strain since the initial stages in the formation of the secondary palate occur between days 11 and 12 of gestation and maximal sensitivity to glucocorticoids was also observed at this period (Andrew *et al.*, 1972).

1.3.2. Thymus

In contrast to the liver where glucocorticoids have an anabolic effect, the thymus undergoes involution in response to a glucocorticoid load (Litwack and Singer, 1972; Duval *et al.*, 1977). Immediately after delivery, the size of the maternal thymus of the mouse and the number of thymocytes are greatly reduced, probably due to the increase in corticosteroids during this period (Duval *et al.*, 1977).

1.3.2.1. Glucocorticoid Receptors in Fetal Thymocytes

Glucocorticoid receptors have been found to be present in thymocytes of fetal mice on days 18–20 of gestation (Duval *et al.*, 1979). The receptor concentration was calculated to be 11.7 ± 3.9 (SD) $fmol/10^6$ cells; no significant difference was observed with the values in the neonatal or adult periods. The affinities of the binding sites for ^{3}H-dexamethasone are similar in the fetal and maternal thymocytes (K_d at $37°$ C $= 2.71 \pm 0.15$ (SD) $\times 10^{-8}$ M in the fetus and 2.13 ± 2.01 (SD) $\times 10^{-8}$ M in the mother). The receptor has a lower affinity for corticosterone and some affinity for progesterone but no affinity for estradiol or testosterone.

1.3.2.2. Glucocorticoid Responsiveness

The presence of glucocorticoid receptors in fetal thymocytes at the same levels present in the adult thymocytes could indicate that the fetal thymus is responsive to glucocorticoids. This was studied by Duval and co-workers (1979) by measuring the inhibition of ^{3}H-uridine incorporation in fetal thymocytes induced by dexamethasone, a parameter often used to assess glucocorticoid sensitivity. The dexamethasone-induced inhibition of ^{3}H-uridine incorporation was proportionally similar in fetal and adult thymocytes (40%), indicating good responsiveness in the fetus.

1.3.3. KIDNEY

During fetal development in the mouse, glucocorticoid receptor concentrations in fetal kidneys increase in an almost linear fashion with gestational age followed by a sharp increase just after birth (Ellis *et al.*, 1986). On day 13 of fetal age the concentration of receptors in the cytosol fraction is 100 fmol/mg protein and on day 18 the value is 200 fmol/mg protein. The receptor concentration on day 18 is comparable to that found in the fetal rabbit kidney at the end of gestation (Giannopoulos, 1974a). The dissociation constants do not vary significantly with fetal age (K_d, $4°$ C $= 6.5 \pm 2.9$ (SD) nM) (Ellis *et al.*, 1986) and are similar to those observed in adult rat kidneys (Ballard *et al.*, 1974). The role of glucocorticoids in fetal renal development has not yet been elucidated.

1.4. Sheep

1.4.1. LUNG

Glucocorticoid receptors are present in the lungs of fetal sheep (Flint and Burton, 1984). ^{3}H-Dexamethasone binds with high affinity in the cytosol (K_d at $4°$ C $= 0.5–5 \times 10^{-9}$ M) (100–140 days of gestation), and binding is specific for glucocorticoid agonists or antagonists. On DEAE-cellulose ion exchange chromatography, the receptor elutes in the range of 0.15–0.20 M KCl. When minces of fetal lung were incubated with ^{3}H-dexamethasone, the specific binding in the nuclei reached a maximum of 141 fmol/mg DNA after 3 h at $22°$ C (Flint and Burton, 1984).

The concentrations of receptors vary with fetal age. A peak occurs between days 85 and 115 of fetal age (Flint and Burton, 1984). At this time, the receptor concentrations range from 800 to 1600 fmol/mg protein in the cytosol. From days 60 to 80 and from 120 days to term, binding varies from 400 to 500 fmol/mg protein. Total bound and unbound corticosteroid concentrations in the carotid artery of sheep are 10.6 ± 0.5 (SEM) ng/ml between days 95 and 139 of gestation, and there is a very sharp rise on day 140 (Jones *et al.*, 1977). The mid-gestational peak in fetal lung glucocorticoid receptors occurs at a time when fetal plasma corticosteroid levels are low, but the subsequent decline on day 120 does not correspond to the period of drastic change in the total circulating levels of corticosteroids. It is possible that receptor determinations towards term are under-estimated due to the rise in endogenous corticosteroids, but it would be important to know the quantity of unbound, biologically available circulating corticosteroids during the same period. Moreover, fetal hypophysectomy has no effect on glucocorticoid receptor concentrations (Flint and Burton, 1984).

It is interesting to note that a metabolic switch from corticosterone to cortisol also occurs in fetal sheep. In fetuses on days 97–137 of gestation, the cortisol:corticosterone ratio is 1:7 and in fetuses of 140 days and older, this ratio increases significantly to 4:5 (Jones *et al.*, 1977).

Liggins (1969) showed that dexamethasone caused premature delivery when infused into the fetuses at rates of 0.06–4.0 mg/24 h between days 100 and 121 of gestational age. Six of ten lambs born prematurely on days 117–123 showed partial aeration of the lungs, suggesting accelerated appearance of surfactant due to the dexamethasone treatment. Receptor levels in fetal lungs are highest at the time when the treatment was carried out and could have mediated the glucocorticoid responsiveness.

1.4.2. ADRENAL

Glucocorticoids have been shown to modulate ACTH-induced activation of fetal adrenal function (Lye and Challis, 1984; Challis *et al.*, 1985; Darbeida and Durand, 1987). Yang and Challis (1989) have reported the presence of glucocorticoid receptors in the fetal sheep adrenal cortical cells from as early as day 60 of fetal age. Binding increases 20-fold on days 100–110 and decreases by days 125–130. Receptor concentration on day 100 (207 fmol/10^6 cells) is much higher than that of the adult adrenal cortical cells (5 fmol/10^6 cells). Binding of ^{3}H-triamcinolone acetonide is of high affinity (K_d, $37°$ C $= 2$–3 nM), and binding is specific for glucocorticoids. Intrafetal ACTH treatment on days 125–130 has no significant effect on fetal adrenal glucocorticoid receptor concentrations.

1.4.3. BRAIN AND PITUITARY

Brains and pituitaries from mid-gestation (day 70) sheep fetuses contain specific, high affinity, saturable binding of ^{3}H-triamcinolone acetonide (Rose *et al.*, 1985). The concentrations of binding sites are relatively constant during fetal development. Glucocorticoid receptor concentrations are five to seven times higher in the pituitary than in hypothalamus or hippocampus. The dissociation constants (K_d) in cytosols of all three tissues are similar (2×10^{-9} M).

1.5. Humans

The stimulatory effect of glucocorticoids on surfactant synthesis and lung maturation, extensively studied in experimental animals, has been confirmed in the human fetal lung. The therapeutic benefit of glucocorticoids in reducing respiratory distress syndrome in premature human infants is well established. The effects of glucocorticoids in human fetal lung are also probably mediated by receptors which are found in human fetal lung at a very early stage of development.

1.5.1. ONTOGENY OF GLUCOCORTICOID RECEPTORS IN HUMAN FETAL LUNG

Specific binding of glucocorticoids can be detected as early as week 12 of gestation (Ballard and Ballard, 1974). The concentrations range from 110 to 350 fmol/mg protein in the cytosol of 14–25-week-old fetuses. The cytosol receptor binds dexamethasone with high affinity (K_d ($2°$ C) = 8.9×10^{-9} M). The receptor shows higher affinity for synthetic glucocorticoids such as methylprednisolone, dexamethasone, betamethasone and fluorocortisol than for cortisol (Ballard *et al.*, 1975). The affinity of corticosterone is similar to that of cortisol.

1.5.2. BIOLOGICAL EFFECTS OF GLUCOCORTICOIDS

In the human fetus, differentiation of type II cells occurs late in the second trimester. At about week 24 of gestation, organelles resembling lamellar bodies appear in a few epithelial cells and their number and size subsequently increase (Campiche *et al.*, 1963; Hage, 1973). Before week 25 of gestation, the concentration of saturated phosphatidylcholine in the lung is low (Ballard *et al.*, 1986). Surface active phospholipids can be measured in amniotic fluid at about week 30 and they increase until term (King *et al.*, 1975; Shelley *et al.*, 1982; Kuroki *et al.*, 1985).

Glucocorticoids stimulate choline incorporation into phosphatidylcholine in explant organ cultures of human fetal lungs (Ekelund *et al.*, 1975a,b; Mendelson *et al.*, 1981). Half-maximal stimulation of choline incorporation is observed at a concentration of dexamethasone (2.1 nM) compatible with the affinity of dexamethasone for the receptor ($K_d \approx 5$ nM) (Gonzales *et al.*, 1986). In the absence of hormone, the explants from fetal lungs older than 20 weeks of gestation show some spontaneous morphological maturation of the epithelial cells, but dexamethasone treatment greatly increases the number and size of lamellar bodies in epithelial cells (Mendelson *et al.*, 1981; Gonzales *et al.*, 1986). Thyroid hormones also stimulate phosphatidylcholine synthesis *in vitro* and have been shown to act in synergy with dexamethasone probably because they have different biochemical sites of action (Gonzales *et al.*, 1986).

It has also been possible to demonstrate the stimulatory effect of glucocorticoids on the 28–36 kDa protein SP-A associated with pulmonary surfactant (Liley *et al.*, 1987; Ballard, 1989). Its levels are very low or undetectable in lung from 16- to 23-week fetuses and increase concomitantly with surfactant lipid in amniotic fluid about the beginning of the third trimester of pregnancy. Dexamethasone (10^{-8} M) induces SP-A synthesis in explant cultures of 22-week human fetal lung (Liley *et al.*, 1987). However, biphasic effects of glucocorticoids on the accumulation of SP-A mRNA and protein have also been observed. High concentrations of dexamethasone (10^{-7}–10^{-6} M) (Odom *et al.*, 1988) or explant culture periods longer than three days (Ballard, 1989) inhibit the previously induced SP-A protein and mRNA levels. In human fetal lung, glucocorticoids, thus, appear to have dual regulatory effects on SP-A protein and mRNA synthesis (Ballard, 1989). The observation that surfactant lipid and surfactant protein SP-A are regulated by factors in common has led to the proposal that SP-A could serve as another marker of lung maturity (Shelley *et al.*, 1982; Kuroki *et al.*, 1985; Liley *et al.*, 1987).

1.5.3. METABOLISM OF GLUCOCORTICOIDS IN THE HUMAN FETUS

In the maternal compartment, cortisol is the predominant glucocorticoid but in the mid-term fetus the concentration of cortisone is higher than that of cortisol (see Volume I, Chapter 2). Pasqualini and co-workers (1970) demonstrated that in most of the fetal tissues cortisol is converted extensively to cortisone but cortisone is not reduced to cortisol. Cortisone is biologically inactive because it has very little affinity for the fetal and adult glucocorticoid receptor. This means that although glucocorticoid receptors are already present very early in the human fetal lung, the hormonal environment does not favor a biological activity at this time. However, from about week 33 of gestation, there is a switch towards cortisol production (Murphy, 1979). This correlates well with the appearance of surfactant in amniotic fluid so that lung maturation also depends on the decrease in metabolism of biologically active to biologically inactive cortisone at a critical time in fetal lung development.

1.6. An Overview of Glucocorticoid Receptor-mediated Processes in the Fetus

Glucocorticoids are very ubiquitous hormones and act on so many tissues that it is difficult to generalize. Very interesting aspects of the development of glucocorticoid responsiveness in the fetus have been revealed by the studies performed using the fetal lung as a model system. Table 2.39 shows that the concentrations of glucocorticoid receptors in the fetal lung of several mammalian species including the human are at significant levels except for the guinea-pig fetus. The affinity of triamcinolone acetonide for the fetal lung glucocorticoid receptor is highest in the rabbit, lowest in the guinea-pig and intermediate in the rat and human. Since the levels of circulating glucocorticoids at the end of gestation are very high in the guinea-pig (Dalle and Delost, 1976), relatively low in the rabbit (Mulay *et al.*, 1973) and intermediate in the rat (Dupouy *et al.*, 1975), it appears that receptor affinity is reciprocally correlated with endogenous glucocorticoid levels.

The receptors of all species are highly specific for glucocorticoids but their relative affinities vary with the species. Glucocorticoid receptors bind with higher affinity those glucocorticoids that are normally secreted by the given species (Giannopoulos and Keichline, 1981).

Those fetal tissues that have been shown to be targets for glucocorticoid action contain glucocorticoid receptors with similar characteristics but variable concentrations. Glucocorticoid receptors in fetal lung are present well before hormonal effects are observed so that their levels are not limiting factors.

TABLE 2.39. *Glucocorticoid Receptors in Fetal Lungs of Various Species*

Species	³H-Dexamethasone bound fmol/mg protein	Reference
Rabbit (29 days)	380	Ballard and Ballard (1972)
Rat (21 days)	210	Giannopoulos (1974a)
Sheep (120 days–term)	400–500	Flint and Burton (1984)
Human (15–17 weeks)	180	Ballard and Ballard (1974)
Guinea-pig (55–65 days)	10	Giannopoulos (1975a)

The metabolic switch from cortisone to cortisol that has been observed plays an important role in controlling the biological activity of potent glucocorticoids and the timing of their effect. The changes in levels of plasma binding proteins such as corticosteroid binding globulin also serve as regulators of glucocorticoid action.

Fetal lung maturation (as determined by surfactant production) is also influenced by other hormones and factors, such as estrogens (Khosla and Rooney, 1979), thyroid hormones (Farrell and Hamosh, 1978; Rooney *et al.*, 1979b), cAMP (Farrell and Hamosh, 1978), epidermal growth factor (Whitsett *et al.*, 1987), transforming growth factor β (Ballard, 1989). However, only glucocorticoids increase the synthesis of all surfactant constituents.

Glucocorticoids are involved in the maturation and differentiation of many fetal organs and pathologically high levels may lead to fetal abnormalities. Many of these events are probably receptor-mediated; this has been shown by the correlations between either glucocorticoid induction and receptors or the development of receptors, endogenous glucocorticoid levels and maturational events.

2. In the Maternal Compartment and During Lactation

2.1. Mammary Gland

Several peptide and steroid hormones control the development and differentiation of normal mammary glands during pregnancy and lactation, including adrenal steroids that are required for lactogenesis in many species (Denamur, 1971). Glucocorticoids have been found to be important for both the morphological and functional differentiation of the mammary gland (Elias 1957; Mills and Topper, 1970; Oka and Topper, 1971). Both glucocorticoids and prolactin are required for lactogenesis at parturition (Chatterton *et al.*, 1979) and glucocorticoids are essential for the maintenance of secretory function in the mammary gland of the rat (Banerjee and Banerjee, 1971). Mammary glands of pregnant and lactating mice contain glucocorticoid receptors that may mediate the important effects of glucocorticoids on lactogenesis.

Tritiated dexamethasone binds with high affinity in mammary gland cytosols from C3H/He mice from mid-pregnancy to late lactation. From about day 13 to the end of gestation, the average apparent binding affinity (K_d) was found to be approximately 7×10^{-9} M (Lindenbaum and Chatterton, 1981). After parturition, the affinity constants appear to decline with the duration of lactation, but this was found to be an artefact due to the diminished CBG levels and higher unbound levels of corticosterone during lactation.

During pregnancy and lactation, mammary gland glucocorticoid receptors have high affinity for synthetic glucocorticoids such as dexamethasone and triamcinolone acetonide and for corticosterone. Aldosterone and progesterone have affinities one to two orders of magnitude less than that of dexamethasone (Lindenbaum and Chatterton, 1981).

Receptor concentrations increase about four-fold between day 13 of gestation and parturition (from 1 to 4.5 pmol/mg DNA) and remain at this level throughout lactation (Lindenbaum and Chatterton, 1981). It has been suggested that glucocorticoid receptor levels in the rat mammary gland correspond to the alveolar cell content of the gland (Gardner and Wittliff, 1973b), and alveolar cells develop considerably just before parturition (Munford, 1963), similar to the time course of the development of receptors. Receptor concentrations are highest (Shyamala, 1973; Lindenbaum and Chatterton, 1981) when the glandular epithelium predominates in the mammary gland (Topper and Freeman, 1980). The epithelium is the tissue where synthesis of α-lactalbumin, casein and lactose occurs (Banerjee, 1976; Topper and Freeman, 1980).

The presence of glucocorticoid receptors in mammary epithelial cells was confirmed in freshly dissociated epithelial cells from rat mammary glands (Quirk *et al.*, 1982) and in isolated mouse mammary epithelial cells from mid-pregnant mice cultured on floating collagen gels (Schneider and Shyamala, 1985). High affinity, saturable binding of ^{3}H-dexamethasone was observed with a K_d (4° C) of 0.99 ± 0.14 (SEM) $\times 10^{-9}$ M. The concentration of receptors in the cultured cells is similar to that of the whole mammary gland (day 13 of gestation) (1.39 ± 0.08 (SEM) pmol/mg DNA or approximately 5600 binding sites per cell). The specificity of binding is also similar except for aldosterone and progesterone that showed more competitive binding in the isolated epithelial cells than in the whole mammary gland (Schneider and Shyamala, 1985). The receptor concentrations can be maintained at the same levels for at least ten days. However, it was observed that insulin, cortisol and prolactin are required. The effects of prolactin and cortisol in maintaining the glucocorticoid receptor in culture are elicited at doses corresponding to their affinities for their receptors (Schneider and Shyamala, 1985) and other studies have shown that cortisol is required to maintain the prolactin receptors in mammary epithelial cells in culture (Sakai *et al.*, 1979). These observations confirm the multihormonal control of the differentiation of mammary glands in preparation for lactation.

3. In the Placenta

Glucocorticoids induce steroid metabolic enzymes in the sheep placenta that may be involved in the initiation of parturition (Anderson *et al.*, 1975; Steele *et al.*, 1976; Ricketts *et al.*, 1980). However, it is not clear how glucocorticoids intervene directly in placental function. Glucocorticoid receptors that could potentially be involved as

TABLE 2.40. *Glucocorticoid Receptors in the Placenta of Various Species*

Species	Specific binding of ^{3}H-dexamethasone		Reference
	fmol/mg protein	K_d ($\times 10^{-9}$ M)	
Human			
First trimester	9	30	Lageson *et al.* (1983);
Second trimester	259	46	Lopez Bernal *et al.* (1984)
Third trimester	113	36	
Rat (19–22 days)			
Basal zone trophoblast	203	10	Heller *et al.* (1981)
Labyrinthine zone	187	15	
Sheep			
50–89 days	111	–	Flint and Burton (1984)
90–129 days	177	3–7	
Rabbit (16–26 days)			
Fetal placenta	260	4	Ballard and Ballard (1972)
Maternal placenta	0	0	

mediators of glucocorticoid responses are present in the placentae of several animal species.

Table 2.40 compares the concentrations of specific binding sites for ^{3}H-dexamethasone that are found in the human, rat, sheep and rabbit. It is noteworthy that the concentrations of binding sites are similar in all four species. Receptors could not be detected on the maternal side of the rabbit placenta (Ballard and Ballard, 1972), but, on the contrary, human fetal membranes were reported to contain only extremely low amounts of receptor (Lopez Bernal *et al.*, 1982). In contrast, in the rat, no significant difference was found between the basal zone trophoblast and the labyrinthine zone (Heller *et al.*, 1981).

In the sheep and the human, glucocorticoid receptors are present very early. In the human placenta, several reports concur that there is a sharp increase in receptors between the first trimester and the second and third trimesters (Speeg and Harrison, 1979; Giannopoulos *et al.*, 1983; Lageson *et al.*, 1983). In the sheep, a smaller but significant increase was also observed (Flint and Burton, 1984). These increases seem to suggest an increasing responsiveness of the placenta.

E. MINERALOCORTICOID RECEPTORS

The mineralocorticoids are secreted by the zona glomerulosa of the adrenals. Their principal biologic activity is in the retention of sodium and chloride and the excretion of potassium and hydrogen ion by the kidney, intestine and salivary gland (see *Hormones and the Fetus*, Volume I, Chapter 2; Pasqualini and Sumida, 1977a; Crabbé, 1977). Aldosterone is the most potent natural mineralocorticoid but deoxycorticosterone, corticosterone, and 18-hydroxydeoxycorticosterone also affect electrolyte balance. Cortisol, the physiological glucocorticoid in man also has mineralocorticoid activity because of its interaction with mineralocorticoid receptor binding sites.

The production of aldosterone by the human fetus has been established. Bloch and co-workers (1956) showed that aldosterone was synthesized from the ninth week of gestation. Aldosterone could also be formed from progesterone *in vitro* by incubation of fetal adrenals (Longchampt and Axelrod, 1964; Dufau and Villée, 1969). Pasqualini and co-workers (1966) found that corticosterone perfused into the human fetus was converted to aldosterone in the fetal adrenals. The plasma concentrations of aldosterone in the maternal and the fetal compartments increase near term in human pregnancies as well as during gestation in rats and guinea-pigs (see *Hormones and the Fetus*, Volume I, Chapter 3). Specific binding of a mineralocorticoid to macromolecules in a fetal organ (guinea-pig kidney) was first demonstrated by Pasqualini and Sumida in 1971. Aldosterone binding sites have also been characterized in kidneys of pregnant rats (Quirk *et al.*, 1983).

1. In the Fetal Compartment

1.1. Guinea-pigs

A selective retention of radioactivity by the kidney of fetal guinea-pigs was observed after administration of ³H-aldosterone directly to the fetus (Table 2.41) (Pasqualini *et al.*, 1976a): 57% of the radioactivity found in the kidney was in the form of nonmetabolized aldosterone, while the liver and placenta contained mainly the tetrahydrogenated metabolite, tetrahydroaldosterone. Maximum uptake of radioactivity in the kidney was found 60 min after subcutaneous administration of [³H]-aldosterone to the fetus (Pasqualini *et al.*, 1972). These observations confirmed the presence of specific binding sites for aldosterone in fetal guinea-pig kidney.

TABLE 2.41. *Distribution of Radioactivity and Concentration of Nonmetabolized ³H-aldosterone in Fetal Organs and Placenta of the Guinea-pig 20 min after Subcutaneous Administration of ³H-aldosterone to the Fetus*

Tissues	Total dpm / g tissue	dpm nonmetabolized ³H-aldosterone / g tissue
Kidney	87 182	46 153
Lung	74 103	41 468
Liver	392 052	50 967
Brain	40 282	21 064
Intestine	30 873	14 222
Placenta	52 816	2 242

Quoted from Pasqualini *et al.* (1976a).

1.1.1. CHARACTERISTICS OF THE FETAL KIDNEY MINERALOCORTICOID RECEPTOR

Specific binding of ^{3}H-aldosterone was demonstrated in the cytosol and nuclear fractions of the fetal guinea-pig kidney after *in vivo* administration of ^{3}H-aldosterone to the fetus and after *in vitro* incubation of kidney cell suspensions with ^{3}H-aldosterone at 37° C (Pasqualini and Sumida, 1971). Some characteristics of the binding sites in the cytosol fraction are indicated on Table 2.42. Cortisol also binds to ^{3}H-aldosterone binding sites, but with a lower relative affinity than aldosterone (Pasqualini *et al.*, 1974a). It is well known that mineralocorticoids and glucocorticoids share common binding sites with different affinities; Type I sites have a higher affinity for mineralocorticoids and Type II sites have a higher affinity for glucocorticoids (Funder *et al.*, 1973). This reflects the similarities in the structures of their receptors (Evans, 1988) and accounts for some of their shared biological activities.

Estradiol shows very little competition with aldosterone for the fetal kidney mineralocorticoid receptor. The fetal kidney also contains estrogen receptors with characteristics that are different from those of the mineralocorticoid receptors (Pasqualini *et al.*, 1976b; Pasqualini and Sumida, 1977b).

The retention of ^{3}H-aldosterone binding sites in the nucleus is temperature-dependent but a concomitant decrease in cytosol binding is not seen because the amount of ^{3}H-aldosterone strongly associated with the nuclear fractions represents only 12% of the specific binding found in the fetal kidney (Pasqualini *et al.*, 1972; Pasqualini and Sumida, 1977b).

TABLE 2.42. *Physicochemical Characteristics of Cytosol Mineralocorticoid Receptors in Kidneys of Guinea-pig Fetuses (50–55 Days of Gestation)*

Number of sites	
fmol/mg protein	20–30
fmol/mg DNA	160
fmol/g tissue	934
K_d (10^{-9} M), 4° C	4–5
Binding specificity	*d*-aldosterone > cortisol
	Very little binding of estradiol
Sedimentation coefficient (S)	8–9 S in low salt

Quoted from Pasqualini and Sumida (1977a,b).

Purified nuclei of the fetal guinea-pig kidney (30–50 days of fetal age) bind ^{3}H-aldosterone directly (Pasqualini *et al.*, 1974b). This appears to represent unoccupied receptor tightly bound in nuclei because Giry and Delost (1977) reported that fetal plasma aldosterone concentrations are very low or undetectable before day 62. It is therefore difficult to ascribe the presence of aldosterone receptors in purified nuclei to high endogenous concentrations of the hormone in the fetus.

In the cytosol fraction, 22% of the radioactivity bound to macromolecules after incubation of fetal kidney with ^{3}H-aldosterone is in the form of ^{3}H-tetrahydroaldosterone (Pasqualini *et al.*, 1972). Since very little binding was observed when kidneys were incubated directly with ^{3}H-tetrahydroaldosterone, it was concluded that aldosterone is metabolized to tetrahydroaldosterone while bound to its receptor.

In the fetal guinea-pig, the presence of mineralocorticoid receptors in the kidney (Pasqualini *et al.*, 1972) and the rise in adrenal and plasma concentrations of aldosterone at the end of gestation (Giry and Delost, 1977) suggest that aldosterone is biologically active in the fetal kidney.

2. In the Maternal Compartment and During Lactation

2.1. Rats

2.1.1. KIDNEY

In 1973, Abe showed that ^{14}C-aldosterone administered intravenously to pregnant and nonpregnant female rats was taken up and retained by the maternal kidneys as nonmetabolized aldosterone to a much greater extent than the other tissues studied. No difference was observed between the pregnant and nonpregnant rats. In contrast, there were no differences in uptake of ^{14}C-aldosterone among the fetal tissues studied.

Mineralocorticoid receptors have been characterized in the kidneys of adrenalectomized pregnant and lactating rats (Table 2.43) (Quirk *et al.*, 1983). The number of binding sites is similar in kidneys of pregnant and lactating rats but the receptor has a somewhat higher affinity for aldosterone during lactation. The concentration of binding sites is in the range of that found in the fetal guinea-pig kidney (Pasqualini *et al.*, 1972).

The binding sites have higher affinity for deoxycorticosterone than for aldosterone. Deoxycorticosterone is an intermediate in the biosynthesis of corticosterone and aldosterone and is an active mineralocorticoid. It was observed that aldosterone and corticosterone (the natural glucocorticoid in the rat) have almost equivalent affinities in kidneys from lactating rats. By contrast, in renal cytosols from virgin rats, aldosterone has a higher affinity than corticosterone.

TABLE 2.43. *Physicochemical Characteristics of Cytosol Mineralocorticoid Receptors in Kidneys and Mammary Glands of Pregnant and Lactating Rats*

	Kidneys		Mammary glands	
	Pregnant	Lactating	Pregnant	Lactating
Number of sites				
fmol/mg protein	26	19	22	4
K_d (10^{-9} M), 4° C	2.5	0.7	2.8	1.7
Binding specificity	DOC > aldo > B > DM	DOC > aldo = B > DM	DOC > aldo = B > DM	

DOC = deoxycorticosterone; aldo = aldosterone; B = corticosterone; DM = dexamethasone
Quoted from Quirk *et al.* (1983).

2.1.2. MAMMARY GLAND

Glucocorticoid receptors (Type II) have been characterized in the mammary glands of both pregnant and lactating rats (Quirk *et al.*, 1982), and glucocorticoids are known to be important for the functional differentiation of the mammary gland (see Section D.2.1 above). The mammary glands are not considered to be mineralocorticoid target tissues, but Quirk *et al.* (1983) have identified Type I mineralocorticoid binding sites in mammary glands that are clearly distinct from Type II glucocorticoid receptors. They have shown evidence that these sites bind aldosterone and corticosterone equally well. Table 2.43 shows the characteristics of mineralocorticoid receptors in mammary glands of adrenalectomized pregnant and lactating rats. The characteristics are very similar to those of the receptor in kidneys. Nevertheless, in both pregnant and lactating rat mammary glands, (like the kidneys of lactating rats) binding specificity is different from that of the classical Type I mineralocorticoid receptor; both aldosterone and corticosterone have high affinity for the receptor. Thus, depending on the plasma concentrations of unbound corticosterone under certain physiological conditions, these mineralocorticoid binding sites could be occupied either by aldosterone or by corticosterone.

F. THYROID HORMONE RECEPTORS

Thyroid hormones regulate metabolic processes that are important for fetal growth and development (see Volume I, Chapter 3). The fetal thyroid produces fetal thyroxine (T_4) and 3,5,3′-triiodothyronine (T_3) in response to thyrotropin (TSH) stimulus from the fetal anterior pituitary. TSH secretion is controlled by thyrotropin releasing hormone (TRH) from the fetal hypothalamus. The fetal hypothalamo-pituitary-thyroid axis is considered to be independent of the maternal compartment (Thorburn, 1974; Browne and Thorburn, 1989).

Thyroidectomy of ovine fetuses between days 80 and 96 of gestation reduces body weight and long bone growth and maturation (Hopkins and Thorburn, 1972; Thorburn and Hopkins, 1973; Chapman *et al.*, 1974). Tissue growth and myelination of brain tissue are also impaired (Erenberg *et al.*, 1974; Holt *et al.*, 1975). Hopkins and Thorburn (1972) reported that fetuses thyroidectomized around 90 days of gestation failed to breathe on delivery at normal term, but Nathanielsz (1975) observed that fetuses thyroidectomized later in gestation (130 days) showed no respiratory failure. Therefore, the period of development is an important aspect of thyroid hormone action.

Current knowledge about thyroid hormone receptors in the fetus is presented here following the sections concerning the steroid hormone receptors because they belong to the same superfamily of nuclear receptors with similar structure and mode of action. In contrast, other peptide hormone receptors are located in the cell membrane.

1. In the Fetal Compartment

1.1. Rats

1.1.1. BRAIN

Perez-Castillo and co-workers (1985) reported binding of T_3 in nuclei of fetal rat whole brains (Table 2.44). Binding affinity of T_3 is 100 times higher than that of T_4 and 10 000 times that of rT_3. Study of the ontogeny of T_3 receptor concentrations in the fetal rat brain (Fig. 2.40) revealed the presence of receptors on day 14 of fetal age that

TABLE 2.44. *Characteristics of Triiodothyronine (T$_3$) Receptor in Nuclei of Fetal Rat Brain (17 Days of Gestation)*

Number of sites	210 fmol/mg DNA
K_d ($\times 10^{-9}$ M), 22° C	0.12
Binding specificity	T$_3$ > T$_4$ > rT$_3$

T$_3$ = 3,5,3′-triiodothyronine; T$_4$ = thyroxine; rT$_3$ = reverse T$_3$

Quoted from Perez-Castillo *et al.* (1985).

increase abruptly between days 15 and 17 and are then relatively constant until a second significant rise after birth (Perez-Castillo *et al.*, 1985). No changes in binding affinity were observed during this time. By day 17 of fetal age, the fetal rat brain contains a concentration of T$_3$ receptors about 30% of adult levels. This period of development in the fetal rat brain corresponds to the phase of neuroblast proliferation. Both T$_4$ and T$_3$ cross the placenta in significant amounts from at least day 10 of fetal life (Gray and Galton, 1974) and maternal thyroidectomy or iodine deficiency cause a decrease in thyroid hormone concentrations in embryonic tissues (Morreale de Escobar *et al.*, 1985); therefore, the rat fetus develops in the presence of significant amounts of thyroid hormones that might influence fetal development much before fetal thyroid function is established. The measurement of T$_3$ and T$_4$ concentrations in rat embryos revealed that both hormones are already detectable in 9-day-old embryotrophoblasts (three days after uterine implantation) and the concentrations increase considerably after day 17 of fetal age (Fig. 2.40) (Morreale de Escobar, 1985). An immunohistochemical study has demonstrated the localization of T$_4$ and T$_3$ in the fetal rat thyroid on day 17 day of gestation (Kawaoi and Tsuneda, 1985).

Brain cell cultures using dissociated cells from 17-day-old fetal rat cerebral hemispheres have been used to study the cellular distribution of nuclear T$_3$ receptor in fetal neural tissue (Kolodny *et al.*, 1985). High affinity, specific binding of T$_3$ was observed to be limited to neurons; little binding was found in glial cell nuclei. There are approximately 5000 binding sites per neuronal nucleus initially in 17-day-old fetal rat cortex and this number increases to 12 000 sites/neuronal nucleus after seven days in culture (Kolodny *et al.*, 1985).

T$_3$ acts in synergy with cortisol to induce somatotrope differentiation in the fetal pituitary (Hemming *et al.*, 1988). Somatotropes are capable of synthesizing and secreting growth hormone by day 19 of gestation in the rat (Birge *et al.*, 1967; Blazquez *et al.*, 1974; Rieutort, 1974; Strosser and Mialhe, 1975; Chatelain *et al.*, 1979; Frawley *et al.*, 1985). The effect of T$_3$ in synergy with glucocorticoids on growth hormone synthesis is well known (Martial *et al.*, 1977). T$_3$ stimulates the rat growth hormone gene by binding of the T$_3$-receptor complex to T$_3$ response elements in the 5′-flanking region of the gene (Larsen *et al.*, 1986; Flug *et al.*, 1987; Wright *et al.*, 1987). Hypothyroidism or thyroidectomy is paralleled by growth hormone deficiency (Defesi *et al.*, 1979; Coiro *et al.*, 1979; Morreale de Escobar *et al.*, 1985).

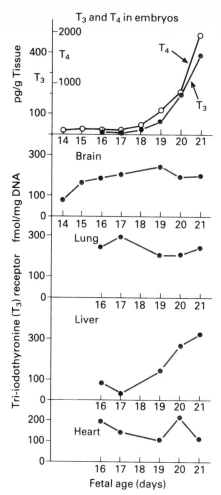

FIG 2.40. Ontogeny of Nuclear Tri-iodothyronine Receptors in Brain, Lung, Liver
and Heart of Fetal Rats.
Quoted from Perez-Castillo *et al.* (1985).

1.1.2. OTHER TISSUES

Fetal rat lung, liver and heart also contain significant amounts of T_3 receptors as seen
in Fig. 2.40. Like the fetal brain, receptor levels in fetal rat lung are fairly constant
during fetal development from day 16 of fetal age and increases post-natally (Perez-
Castillo *et al.*, 1985). In fetal liver, the number of binding sites increases linearly from
day 17 and post-natally. Fetal heart contains lower concentrations of T_3 receptors than
the other fetal tissues studied but the number of binding sites also increase after birth
(Perez-Castillo *et al.*, 1985). The presence of thyroid hormone receptors in various fetal
tissues suggest biological responsiveness to these hormones but direct evidence is not yet
available for all tissues. The fetal lung has received particular attention because of the
synergism between glucocorticoid and thyroid hormone action in fetal lung maturation;
fetal rabbit and human lungs have been studied.

1.2. Rabbits

1.2.1. LUNG

Extensive evidence suggests that both glucocorticoids and thyroid hormones regulate surfactant synthesis in late fetal life. T_4 treatment of fetuses accelerates lung morphologic development (Hitchcock, 1979; Rooney *et al.*, 1976; Wu *et al.*, 1973; Ballard,

TABLE 2.45. *Characteristics of Nuclear Triiodothyronine Receptor in Fetal Rabbit Lung (28 Days of Gestation)*

Number of sites	400–720 fmol/mg DNA
K_d ($\times 10^{-9}$ M), 37° C	0.13–0.5
Binding specificity	$T_3 > T_4 > DIMIT > rT_3$

$T_3 = 3,5,3'$-triiodothyronine; $T_4 =$ thyroxine; DIMIT = 3,5-dimethyl-3'-isopropyl-L-thyronine; $rT_3 =$ reverse T_3
Quoted from Lindenberg *et al.* (1978) and Gonzales and Ballard (1982).

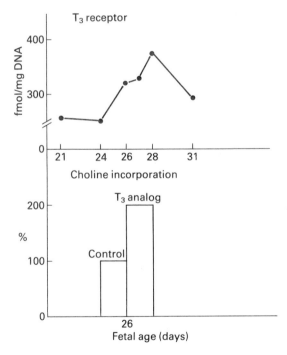

FIG 2.41. Ontogeny of Nuclear Triiodothyronine (T_3) Receptors in Fetal Rabbit Lung and Effect of Triiodothyronine on Choline Incorporation into Surfactant. Nuclear T_3 receptor concentrations adapted from Gonzales and Ballard (1982) and the effect of maternal treatment with a synthetic T_3 analog (DIMIT) on choline incorporation into phosphatidylcholine in fetal lung explant cultures quoted from Ballard *et al.* (1984b).

1982). The effects of thyroid hormone in fetal lung are probably mediated by the presence of nuclear receptors in fetal lung.

Nuclear T_3 receptors are present in fetal rabbit lung (Lindenberg *et al.*, 1978; Gonzales and Ballard, 1982) and the characteristics of specific T_3 binding in lungs at 28 days of fetal age are shown in Table 2.45. The concentration of nuclear binding sites in the fetal lung is approximately twice as high as that of the adult lung which was compared in the same study (Lindenberg *et al.*, 1978). Figure 2.41 indicates that T_3 receptors are present at least from day 21 of fetal age and a maximal value is reached at day 28 (Gonzales and Ballard, 1982).

In order to demonstrate a direct effect of thyroid hormones on fetal rabbit lung, the effects of maternal treatment with 3,5 dimethyl-3'-isopropyl-L-thyronine (DIMIT), a synthetic analog of T_3 that binds poorly to plasma thyroid hormone binding proteins (Ballard *et al.*, 1980b) was studied. As shown in Fig. 2.41, DIMIT increases the incorporation of choline into phosphatidylcholine of fetal lung minces *in vitro* when injected to pregnant rabbits on day 26 of gestation (Ballard *et al.*, 1980b; Ballard *et al.*, 1984b). DIMIT treatment also causes a three-fold increase in saturated phosphatidylcholine content of fetal lung lavage.

Thyroid hormone receptors could mediate direct actions of thyroid hormones on fetal lung maturation and their synergism with glucocorticoids. A relatively close correlation has been found between receptor affinity for T_3 and T_4 and the dose-response curve of stimulation of choline incorporation into phosphatidylcholine in fetal lung explants (Ballard *et al.*, 1984b; Ballard, 1989).

1.3. Sheep

1.3.1. BRAIN

In the sheep, both maternal and fetal thyroid hormones are involved in normal brain maturation. In contrast to the rat, thyroid hormone action matures before birth in the sheep. The length of gestation in the sheep is 150 days and fetal brain growth reaches maximal velocity before birth. From days 40 to 80 of gestation, DNA content is increased due to neuroblast proliferation and from days 95 to 130 glial cell proliferation and myelination occurs (Barlow, 1969).

Triiodothyronine receptors are present in fetal sheep brain from a very early stage of fetal development (Ferreiro *et al.*, 1987; Polk *et al.*, 1989). Table 2.46 indicates that the number of binding sites in fetal sheep on day 100 of gestation is more than twice that found in fetal rat brain (Perez-Castillo *et al.*, 1985). Binding affinity is greater for T_3 than for T_4. Ontogenic studies revealed a marked increase in T_3 receptors between days 50 and 80 of gestation with no significant change thereafter (Fig. 2.42) (Ferreiro *et al.*, 1987; Polk *et al.*, 1989). Total plasma T_4 concentrations increase in the fetal lamb from days 60 to 100 of gestation and decrease between days 135 to 150 (Nathanielsz *et al.*, 1973). As in the rat fetus, the increase in T_3 receptors occurs during the period of neuroblast proliferation (Ferreiro *et al.*, 1987). Fetal plasma T_3 values are 100 times lower than the T_4 concentrations (Chopra *et al.*, 1975). T_3 receptors appear to be present in high concentrations in the fetal sheep brain prior to the maturation of serum T_3 concentrations. Thyroidectomy of fetuses on days 99–107 or 129–132 of fetal age has no effect on the number of T_3 binding sites nor on the binding affinity (Polk *et al.*, 1989).

TABLE 2.46. *Characteristics of Nuclear Triiodothyronine Receptors in Fetal Sheep Brain (100 Days of Gestation)*

Number of sites	400–500 fmol/mg DNA
K_d ($\times 10^{-9}$ M), 22° C	0.1
Binding specificity	T_3 > Triac > T_4

$T_3 = 3,5,3'$-triiodothyronine; Triac = $3,5,3'$-triiodothy-roacetic acid; T_4 = thyroxine

Quoted from Ferreiro *et al.* (1987) and Polk *et al.* (1989).

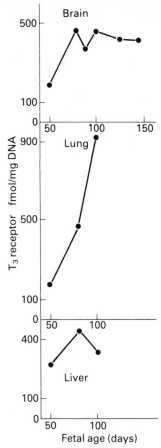

FIG 2.42. Ontogeny of Triiodothyronine Receptors in Brain, Lung and Liver of Fetal Sheep.

Adapted from Ferreiro *et al.* (1987) and Polk *et al.* (1989).

1.3.2. LUNG

The T_3 receptor in fetal sheep lung is similar to that of the fetal rabbit lung (Ferreiro *et al.*, 1987). Moreover, the sedimentation coefficient was determined to be 3.6 S. Figure 2.42 shows that, in contrast to the fetal brain, fetal lung T_3 receptors continue to increase considerably between days 80 and 100 of fetal age.

1.3.3. LIVER

T_3 binding sites are also present in fetal sheep liver at approximately the same concentrations as in fetal brain and lung (Ferreiro *et al.*, 1987). However, receptor affinity is lower in the liver ($K_d = 0.18$ nM) than in fetal brain or lung and in the fetal liver, T_3 and Triac (3,5,3'-triiodothyroacetic acid) have the same affinity for the receptor binding sites. The ontogenic profile of T_3 receptors in fetal liver is similar to that of the fetal brain (Fig. 2.42).

1.4. Humans

1.4.1. BRAIN

Thyroid hormone receptors are present at a very early stage in the human fetal brain (Bernal and Pekonen, 1984). In the nuclear fraction of brains of 16-week-old fetuses, T_3 receptor concentration is 479 fmol/mg DNA. Binding is of high affinity (K_d (22° C) $= 0.5 \times 10^{-10}$ M). Triac (3,5,3'-triiodothyroacetic acid) binds with about ten times the affinity of T_3, and T_4 binds with about ten times less affinity than T_3. Receptor concentrations increase ten times between weeks 10 and 16 of fetal age with no change

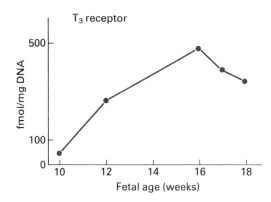

FIG 2.43. Ontogeny of Thyroid Hormone Receptors in Fetal Human Brain. Quoted from Bernal and Pekonen (1984).

TABLE 2.47. *Comparison of Thyroid Hormone Receptor Concentrations in Brain, Lung, Liver and Heart from 16-Week-Old Human Fetuses*

Organ	T_3 Receptor fmol/mg DNA
Brain	479
Lung	544
Liver	352
Heart	201

Quoted from Bernal and Pekonen (1984).

in binding affinity (Fig. 2.43) (Bernal and Pekonen, 1984). In this same study, thyroid hormone receptor binding was also studied in fetal lung, liver and heart. Table 2.47 shows that in the 16-week-old fetus, at the time when receptor concentrations in the brain appear to reach a peak, slightly higher concentrations are found in the fetal lung, and lower concentrations in the fetal liver and heart (Bernal and Pekonen, 1984).

The period of great increase in thyroid hormone receptors in human fetal brain coincides with the development of the fetal thyroid gland (Olin *et al.*, 1970; Fisher and Klein, 1981) and with increased brain growth due to neuroblast multiplication (Dobbing and Sands, 1979). In the human, the appearance of receptor either antedates or is coincident with development of the fetal thyroid.

1.4.2. LUNG

Gonzales and Ballard (1981) have characterized the high affinity binding sites for T_3 found in nuclei of fetal human lung. This group reported a capacity of 420 fmol/ mg DNA for T_3 binding in 16–19-week-old fetal lung and a binding affinity close to that found by Bernal and Pekonen (1984) (K_d, 20° C = 0.35×10^{-10} M) in fetal lung

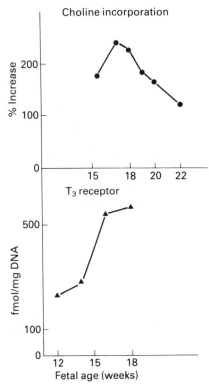

FIG 2.44. Ontogeny of Thyroid Hormone Receptors and the Stimulation of Choline Incorporation into Surfactant by T_3 Plus Dexamethasone in Fetal Human Lung. Choline incorporation into phosphatidylcholine was measured in explant cultures of fetal lung. Quoted from Gonzales and Ballard (1981), Bernal and Pekonen (1984) and Gonzales *et al.* (1986).

and brain. The relative affinities of the thyroid hormones and analogs are similar to those found for nuclei from human brain.

As in the fetal brain, thyroid hormone receptor concentrations increase between weeks 13 and 19 of fetal age (Fig. 2.44) (Gonzales and Ballard, 1981). A study by Gonzales and co-workers (1986) has demonstrated that T_3 alone can increase choline incorporation into phosphatidylcholine by 36% in explant cultures of fetal lungs in weeks 16–25 of gestation, but the synergistic action of T_3 in combination with dexamethasone is dramatic (193% increase). Morphological maturation of the lung epithelium (numerous large lamellar bodies in the apical cytoplasm) was also observed after T_3 plus dexamethasone treatment (Gonzales *et al.*, 1986). Figure 2.44 shows this combined effect of the two hormones on choline incorporation as a function of fetal age in relation to the fetal lung thyroid hormone receptor concentrations. The biological synergistic effect is somewhat greater when T_3 receptors are higher.

The combined biochemical effects of T_3 and dexamethasone and some biochemical differences in their effects indicate that the two hormones act at different biochemical sites (Gonzales *et al.*, 1986). Glucocorticoid treatment of pregnant women reduces the incidence of respiratory distress syndrome in their premature infants, but is not always effective. Intra-amniotic T_4 administration has resulted in reduced incidence of respiratory distress syndrome in premature infants (Mashiach *et al.*, 1979). The synergy between thyroid hormones and glucocorticoid in stimulating surfactant synthesis and lung maturation suggests that combined hormone therapy may be advisable.

G. LUTEINIZING (LH) AND FOLLICLE-STIMULATING (FSH) HORMONE RECEPTORS

1. In the Fetal Compartment

In the adult, the regulation of testicular and ovarian endocrine function by gonadotropic hormones is mediated by specific, high affinity receptors that are located in the plasma membrane of the respective target cells. LH stimulates testosterone synthesis by the fetal testis in several mammalian species (Warren *et al.*, 1975; Veyssière *et al.*, 1977; Huhtaniemi *et al.*, 1977a,b; Brinkmann and van Straalen, 1979), suggesting the presence of functional receptors in the fetal testis. Sexual differentiation in the mammalian fetus depends on the production of androgens by the fetal testis and is, therefore, sensitive to control by the fetal pituitary (Jost, 1966a). On the other hand, the role of FSH in the fetal testis is not yet clear. FSH may be important in regulating Sertoli cell proliferation during the perinatal period (Orth, 1984), a function that seems to be related to the presence of FSH receptors in the fetal testis at this time.

The development of ovarian steroidogenic capacity and responsiveness to gonadotropins varies between species. The human fetal ovary secretes steroids only in the last part of fetal life (Reyes *et al.*, 1973). Other species produce estrogens at early stages of ovarian differentiation (Mauléon *et al.*, 1977; Schemesh, 1980; Sholl and Goy, 1978; Grinsted, 1982; Milewich *et al.*, 1977). The role of gonadotropins in steroid biosynthesis in the ovary is not clear. Gonadotropins stimulate fetal ovarian steroid synthesis in the fetal mouse (Terada *et al.*, 1984), calf (Schemesh, 1980) and pig (Raeside, 1983) but not in the rabbit (George and Wilson, 1979) and the rat (Weniger *et al.*, 1985). Fewer studies have been carried out on gonadotropin receptors in the fetal ovary than in the fetal testis.

1.1. Rats

For binding studies on the gonadal receptors for LH, labeled human chorionic gonadotropin (hCG) has been more frequently employed than labeled LH because hCG is more readily available in highly purified form and is a more stable ligand when labeled with radioactive iodine. The biological properties of hCG and LH are very similar, and the two glycoprotein hormones bind to the same receptor sites in the testis and ovary.

1.1.1. PHYSICOCHEMICAL CHARACTERISTICS OF LH RECEPTORS IN FETAL TESTIS

Gangnerau and co-workers (1982) reported the presence of LH/hCG binding sites in fetal rat testis homogenates that showed the high affinity, limited capacity and specificity characteristic of hormone receptors (Table 2.48). The characteristics are similar to those of LH receptors in adult testis of the rat (Dufau and Catt, 1978).

TABLE 2.48. *Physicochemical Characteristics of LH/hCG Receptor in Fetal Rat Testis (18–20 Days of Gestation)*

Number of sites	7–8 fmol/mg protein
	0.6–1.4 fmol/testis
K_d ($\times 10^{-10}$ M), 22° C and 37° C	0.4–1.2
Binding specificity	hCG > LH
	No binding of FSH

Quoted from Gangnerau *et al.* (1982) and Warren *et al.* (1984).

1.1.2. ONTOGENY OF LH RECEPTORS AND STIMULATION OF TESTOSTERONE BIOSYNTHESIS IN FETAL TESTIS

At 14 days of fetal age, specific binding of ^{125}I-hCG is not significantly different from the nonsaturable binding in the presence of a 1000-fold excess of nonradioactive hCG or from the nonspecific binding present in muscle, ovaries or spleens at any age of gestation (Gangnerau *et al.*, 1982; Warren *et al.*, 1984). By day 15, a significant quantity of ^{125}I-hCG binding can first be detected and the concentration of receptors then begins to rise, reaching a peak on day 21 (Fig. 2.45).

It is interesting to note that binding of hCG is not detectable in fetal rat ovaries, in contrast to the fetal testis (Siebers *et al.*, 1977b; Warren *et al.*, 1984). The fetal rat ovary becomes responsive to gonadotropic stimulation only after the first week of life (Funkenstein *et al.*, 1980).

The endogenous testosterone content and testosterone secretion by fetal testis explants in organ culture also increase sharply by day 18 of fetal age (Fig. 2.45). It is possible that an increase in circulating LH in the fetus could be responsible for the stimulation of androgen production by the fetal testis, but the rise in fetal plasma LH occurs after the increase in androgen content and secretion (Fig. 2.45). Habert and Picon (1982) (bioassay of LH) and Slob and co-workers (1980) (radioimmunoassay of LH) both reported similar changes in fetal plasma LH concentrations and both observed lower

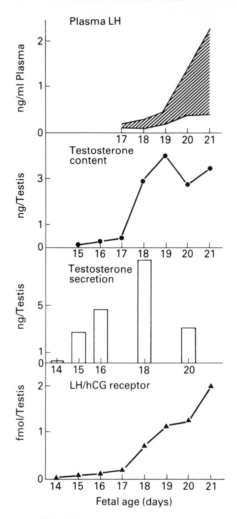

FIG 2.45. Ontogeny of LH/hCG Receptors and Testosterone Production in Fetal
Rat Testis (Comparison with LH Concentrations in Fetal Plasma).
LH receptors measured by binding of ^{125}I-hCG in fetal testis homogenates
(Gangnerau *et al.*, 1982; Warren *et al.*, 1984). Testosterone content represents the
endogenous steroid measured by radioimmunoassay (Warren *et al.*, 1984). Testosterone secretion into culture medium determined in fetal testis explant cultures over
a 3 h period (Gangnerau *et al.*, 1982). Plasma LH-like activity (the range of extreme
values is shown) measured by a bioassay (Habert and Picon, 1982).

values in males than in females, but Chowdhury and Steinberger (1976) (radioimmunoassay) found that LH concentrations decreased with fetal age and that values
were higher in males than in females.

Treatment of fetal testis with LH or hCG both *in vitro* and *in vivo* stimulates
testosterone and cAMP production and LH receptors (Warren *et al.*, 1975, 1982, 1987;
Feldman and Bloch, 1978; Gangnerau *et al.*, 1982). The responses are first observed on
day 15 of fetal age, concomitant with the appearance of LH receptors. The increase in

LH receptors could allow the fetal testis to concentrate LH in the cell despite the low circulating levels of LH.

These observations are in distinct contrast to the response of the adult testis where the ability of Leydig cells to respond to sustained gonadotropic stimulation with increased androgen production is limited by the development of a refractory state associated with down-regulation of LH receptors (Hsueh *et al.*, 1976a). The ability of the fetal Leydig cell to respond to sustained concentrations of gonadotropin without being desensitized would contribute to the maintenance of elevated androgen production during early development.

The inability of the fetal Leydig cell to be desensitized by endogenous gonadotropin appears to be due to low aromatase activity, undetectable estradiol production and lack of increase in estrogen receptor content of fetal testis (Tsai-Morris *et al.*, 1986; 1988). In the adult testis, the estrogen-mediated steroidogenic lesion at the site of conversion of progesterone to androgen leads to a decrease in testosterone response to hCG (Nozu *et al.*, 1981). This regulatory mechanism can be induced in fetal Leydig cells by exogenous estradiol treatment (Tsai-Morris *et al.*, 1986).

1.1.3. BINDING OF FSH IN THE FETAL RAT TESTIS

High affinity binding of ^{125}I-FSH can also be demonstrated in fetal rat testis (Warren *et al.*, 1984; Tsutsui and Kawashima, 1987). The number of binding sites on days 19 and 20 of gestation was found to be $2-7$ fmol/testis. Warren and co-workers (1984) reported that the dissociation constant ($K_d = 1.1 \times 10^{-9}$ M) of FSH for its receptor in fetal testis was similar to that of FSH in adult rat testis (Dufau and Catt, 1978), but Tsutsui and Kawashima (1987) found that the K_d (0.4×10^{-9} M) in the testis of 17.5- and 19.5-day-old fetuses was significantly greater than that of rats on day 50 of post-natal age ($K_d = 0.18 \times 10^{-9}$ M) determined in the same study. The binding affinity of FSH for its receptor is approximately 10% that of LH for its receptor in fetal testis (Warren *et al.*, 1984). LH does not compete with FSH for FSH receptor binding sites.

Like the LH receptors, FSH receptor concentrations of the fetal testis increase with fetal age. However, FSH receptor concentrations become significantly different from nonspecific binding levels only from day 17 of fetal age and a sharp rise is observed on day 20 (Warren *et al.*, 1984). In the fetal rat, Sertoli cells are present at this stage of development (Magre and Jost, 1980) and days 20 and 21 of fetal age correspond to the time of maximal Sertoli cell proliferation (Orth, 1982). Immunoreactive FSH concentrations in fetal rat plasma were reported to decline between days 16 and 20 of fetal age (Chowdhury and Steinberger, 1976), but other data are lacking.

Orth (1984) demonstrated that FSH could be involved in the control of Sertoli cell proliferation in fetal rat testis. On day 18 of fetal age, just before the onset of maximal Sertoli cell proliferation, fetal decapitation or treatment with antiserum to FSH led to reductions in the percentages of Sertoli cells preparing to divide on day 19, suggesting that FSH from the fetal pituitary stimulates Sertoli cell proliferation in fetal testis. Orth (1984) also showed that FSH or cAMP could increase the labeling of Sertoli cell nuclei with ^{3}H-thymidine in explants of fetal testis in organ culture. The close temporal correlation between increasing numbers of FSH-binding sites in the fetal testis and enhanced proliferation of Sertoli cells suggest that FSH regulates Sertoli cell division at a critical period in the establishment of an adequate Sertoli cell population.

1.2. Rabbits

1.2.1. LH/HCG BINDING IN RABBIT FETAL TESTIS

In rabbits, the onset of fetal testicular synthesis and secretion of testosterone occurs between days 18 and 19 of fetal age, just prior to the male phenotypic differentiation of the genital tract (days 20 to 25) (Catt *et al.*, 1975). A concomitant appearance of LH/hCG receptors in the fetal rabbit testis can be observed (Catt *et al.*, 1975), but testicular synthesis and production of testosterone are not stimulated by exogenous LH until day 20 of fetal age (George *et al.*, 1978; Veyssière *et al.*, 1980).

Radio-iodinated hCG binds with high affinity in fetal rabbit testis; binding affinity is similar between days 18 and 29 of fetal age ($K_d = 0.4 \times 10^{-10}$ M) and is of the same order of magnitude as that found in adult rabbit testis (Catt *et al.*, 1975). Receptor concentrations are between 6 and 10 fmol/testis or 5 to 10 fmol/mg gonad weight. No significant amounts of LH/hCG receptors were found in fetal ovaries.

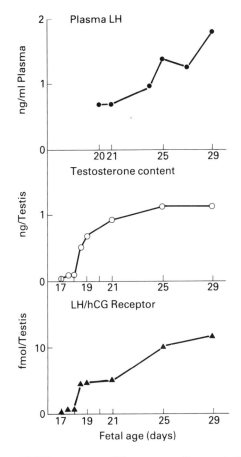

FIG 2.46. Ontogeny of LH Receptors and Testosterone Content in Fetal Rabbit Testis. LH receptor binding data and testosterone contents in fetal testis quoted from Catt *et al.*, (1975). Fetal plasma LH concentrations taken from Veyssière *et al.* (1982).

1.2.2. ONTOGENY OF LH RECEPTORS AND RESPONSIVENESS
IN FETAL TESTIS

Binding of labeled hCG is low on days 17 and 18 but binding increases within the subsequent 12-h period (Fig. 2.46) (Catt *et al.*, 1975). Immunoreactive LH could only be detected in fetal plasma from day 20 (Veyssière *et al.*, 1982). The pattern of testosterone content in the fetal testis is parallel with the profile of LH receptor concentration (Fig. 2.46) and also corresponds to the development of 3β-hydroxy-steroid dehydrogenase activity (Milewich *et al.*, 1977). This temporal sequence is correlated with the histological appearance of the differentiated Leydig cell (Catt *et al.*, 1975). On day 17, the testicular interstitium consists of undifferentiated mesenchymal cells occupying narrow spaces between seminiferous cords. On day 19, larger cells appear between the seminiferous cords with increased cytoplasm containing accumulations of smooth endoplasmic reticulum. By day 21, the interstitium contains numerous

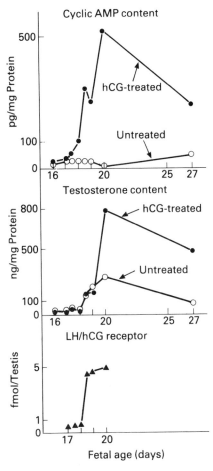

FIG 2.47. Development of Responsiveness to hCG in Fetal Rabbit Testis. Quoted from Catt *et al.* (1975) and George *et al.* (1978).

cells that resemble adult Leydig cells with large quantities of cytoplasm exclusively occupied by smooth endoplasmic reticulum.

To study the development of responsiveness to LH, fetal testes from days 16 to 20 of gestation were incubated with hCG (George *et al.*, 1978). An increase in cyclic AMP formation in response to hCG stimulation was first observed in testes from 18-day-old fetuses, but testosterone content was poorly responsive to hCG until after day 19 of fetal age (Fig. 2.47).

In fetal rabbit testis, testicular testosterone synthesis begins between days 18 to 19 of fetal age at a time when testosterone synthesis is resistant to stimulation by hCG and could, therefore, be pituitary-independent. During this narrow time period, LH/hCG receptors increase strikingly and hCG is capable of stimulating cyclic AMP contents of the fetal testis. From day 20, testosterone biosynthesis becomes greatly responsive to hCG so that receptors appear to be coupled functionally to the testosterone biosynthetic pathway with a delay of one to two days. In contrast, the capacity of the testis to produce testosterone and the response to LH and LH receptors seem to appear simultaneously in fetal testes of rats.

1.3. Humans

In the male human fetus, testosterone levels in the plasma attain peak values around week 15–16 of fetal age (Reyes *et al.*, 1974). This transient increase in testosterone production is necessary for the differentiation and growth of male genitalia (Jost, 1961). The levels of hCG in maternal and fetal plasma also reach peak levels during this period (Clements *et al.*, 1976), suggesting that hCG stimulates fetal testicular steroidogenesis during this critical period of fetal development. hCG binding and stimulation of testosterone biosynthesis by hCG have been demonstrated in testis of human fetuses.

1.3.1. BINDING OF hCG AND BIOLOGICAL RESPONSES TO hCG IN THE HUMAN FETAL TESTIS

Huhtaniemi and co-workers (1977a) reported a single class of binding sites with high affinity and low capacity for ^{125}I-hCG in testicular homogenates of human fetuses (13.5–19.5 cm crown–rump length) at 14–20 weeks of gestational age. The dissociation constant was found to be in the order of 10^{-10} M and the binding capacity, in this study, varied between 25.6 to 42.2 pg/mg wet weight of tissue. In testes from fetuses ranging in age from 10–24 weeks, the dissociation constants range from 0.4–5.5 $\times$ 10^{-10} M (Molsberry *et al.*, 1982). No specific binding could be demonstrated in the ovaries, adrenals, kidneys and livers of human fetuses (Huhtaniemi *et al.*, 1977a).

Between weeks 12 and 24 of fetal age, hCG binding capacity rises and falls, as seen in Fig. 2.48. A sharp increase occurs at week 15 with a decline after week 17 (Molsberry *et al.*, 1982). Human fetal plasma levels of hCG peak between 10 and 14 weeks; in the male fetus, plasma LH levels average 5.1 ng/ml between weeks 12 and 20 of fetal age but the number of samples was too limited to determine a developmental pattern (Reyes *et al.*, 1974; Clements *et al.*, 1976). The increase in testicular content of testosterone (peaking at 13.5 weeks) seems to be concomitant with the peak in fetal plasma levels of hCG that precedes the increases in hCG binding capacity and plasma levels of testosterone (peaking at 15–16 weeks) (Reyes *et al.*, 1974; Tapanainen *et al.*,

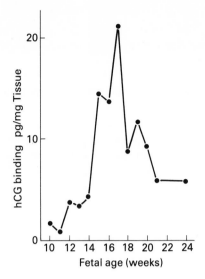

FIG 2.48. Developmental Changes in Concentrations of hCG Binding Sites in Human Fetal Testis.

Adapted from Molsberry *et al.*, 1982.

1981). Physiological concentrations of hCG have been shown to stimulate testosterone biosynthesis in human fetal testes *in vitro* (Huhtaniemi *et al.*, 1977a), suggesting that hCG, and not LH, promotes testosterone production in fetal testis.

The number of Leydig cells in the fetal testis also parallels the concentrations of hCG in fetal serum (Leinonen and Jaffe, 1985). hCG was also reported to increase thymidine incorporation into DNA in cultured human fetal cells (Leinonen and Jaffe, 1985).

Leinonen and Jaffe (1985) found that hCG can repeatedly stimulate testosterone production by the fetal testes, indicating that the human fetal testes (like the rat fetal testes) escapes gonadotropic desensitization that is characteristic of the adult testis.

1.3.2. FSH RECEPTORS IN HUMAN FETAL TESTIS

Specific, high affinity binding of FSH is present in testes of human fetuses but not in fetal ovaries (Huhtaniemi *et al.*, 1987). The apparent dissociation constant (K_d) is 10^{-9} M. In a pool of seven pairs of fetal testis at weeks 9–11 of gestation, the concentration of FSH binding sites was found to be 10 fmol/g wet tissue; at 15 weeks of fetal age, this value is 29 fmol/g wet tissue and at 16 weeks, 37 fmol/g wet tissue. FSH binding appears to increase with fetal age. However, stimulation of cAMP production by FSH *in vitro* in minced fetal testis could not be demonstrated (Huhtaniemi *et al.*, 1987).

1.4. Primates

1.4.1. LH/HCG BINDING SITES IN FETAL TESTIS

In rhesus monkey (*Macaca mulatta*) fetuses of 140–160 days of gestation (length of pregnancy is 165 days), binding of ^{125}I-hCG was found to be between 31 and

102 pg/mg tissue (Huhtaniemi *et al.*, 1977b). The apparent dissociation constant was determined to be 0.5×10^{-10} M in one sample. No specific binding of radioactive hCG could be demonstrated in the fetal monkey ovary.

HCG stimulates testosterone production in fetal monkey testis in a dose-dependent manner *in vitro* (Huhtaniemi *et al.*, 1977b). Administration of hCG into the fetal circulation of chronically catheterized 129–145-day-old fetuses also causes as much as a six-fold increase in fetal serum testosterone levels.

The fetal monkey testis is sensitive to gonadotropic stimulation at least from day 129 of fetal age. In the rhesus monkey, chorionic gonadotropin levels are very low in the placenta or in the maternal circulation after the first third of gestation (Hodgen *et al.*, 1974; 1975). Fetal pituitary gonadotropins are, therefore, probably the source of the gonadotropic stimulation. In male monkey fetuses, the levels of circulating LH are relatively low (lower than the LH concentrations in female fetuses), but there is a slight increase by day 140 (Ellinwood and Resko, 1980). Fetal hypophysectomy after mid-gestation leads to hypoplasia of fetal gonads at birth (Gulyas *et al.*, 1977a,b). The fetal pituitary appears to be necessary for normal development of the gonads in rhesus monkeys.

1.4.2. FSH RECEPTORS IN FETAL TESTIS AND OVARIES

Huhtaniemi and co-workers (1987) described the characteristics of specific binding sites for FSH in the fetal monkey testis and ovary. The apparent dissociation constant of FSH binding in the fetal testis is 2.5×10^{-10} M. Table 2.49 indicates the concentrations of FSH binding sites found in fetal testis and ovary and their variations during development. In contrast to human fetal ovaries, the fetal ovaries of rhesus monkeys contain significant amounts of FSH receptors. In both the fetal testis and fetal ovary, FSH receptors seem to increase during development.

Incubations of fetal testis or ovaries with FSH failed to show increased cAMP production although immature (10-day-old) rat testis incubated under the same conditions responded to FSH with a 10-fold increase in cAMP. The role of FSH in gonadal function of primates still needs to be elucidated.

TABLE 2.49. *FSH Receptors in Fetal Testis and Ovary of the Rhesus Monkey*

	Testis fmol/g wet tissue	Ovary fmol/g wet tissue
Fetus		
112 days		19.6 ± 7.1
132 days		57.0 ± 9.9
135 days	12.7 ± 1.2	
154 days	139 ± 10.5	
Newborn	324 ± 4.7	

Means $\pm$ SE
Quoted from Huhtaniemi *et al.* (1987).

2. In the Maternal Compartment and During Lactation

The role of LH in preovulatory follicular development has been confirmed by studies using pregnant rats. During the first five days of pregnancy, changes in follicular cell function and gonadotropin receptors could be compared with those observed during the corresponding days of the estrous cycle. These events are presumably caused by the preceding gonadotropin surge and maintained in the presence of a developing corpus luteum and increasing concentrations of serum progesterone. Later, as gestation proceeds, the extent of differentiation of follicles at the small antral stage can be studied when serum progesterone concentrations are high and basal concentrations of gonadotropins are low. Since ovulation occurs spontaneously in the post-partum rat 18 h after parturition, the development of pre-ovulatory follicles on the last days of pregnancy appears to be induced by small but sustained increases in serum gonadotropins, especially LH (Cheng, 1976; Richards and Kersey, 1979; Bogovich *et al.*, 1981).

2.1. Rats

2.1.1. LH/hCG binding sites in the ovary during gestation

High affinity binding sites are present in rat ovaries during pregnancy (Cheng, 1976; Siebers *et al.*, 1977c). The dissociation constant for the binding of bovine ^{125}I-LH to rat ovaries is 3×10^{-9} M with a binding capacity of 1140 fmol/100 mg tissue on day 18 of gestation (Cheng, 1976). Binding affinity is not different from that of the LH receptor in the ovary at late diestrus or early pro-estrus, but the binding capacity on day 18 is 4–76 times greater (Cheng, 1976; Siebers *et al.*, 1977a). The binding of ^{125}I-hCG in the ovaries of the pregnant rat increases during the course of gestation (Fig. 2.49) (Siebers, 1977c) and tends to be inversely related to the serum LH concentrations (Cheng, 1976).

Autoradiographic studies have made it possible to localize the specific LH/hCG binding sites predominantly in the theca cell layer of small follicles while binding sites for FSH are localized exclusively in the membrana granulosa (Channing and Kammerman, 1973; Midgley, 1973; Zeleznik *et al.*, 1974; Amsterdam *et al.*, 1975; Richards *et al.*, 1976). The requirement for both LH and FSH in stimulating follicular growth is associated with the localization of their receptors and the compartmentalization of androgen and estrogen biosynthesis (Falck, 1959; Dorrington *et al.*, 1975; Erickson and Ryan, 1976). During days 3–6 of gestation LH receptor concentrations increase in both granulosa and theca cells (Richards and Kersey, 1979). Between days 3 and 5, LH stimulation of cAMP and accumulation of estradiol in whole follicles increases. Between days 8 and 19, LH receptors decrease and LH stimulation of cAMP is also reduced. The pre-ovulatory follicles developing between days 19 and 22 show increasing LH receptors in both granulosa and theca cells and an increase in estradiol accumulation and cAMP production in response to LH.

The administration of hCG to pregnant rats on days 14 and 15 of gestation leads to dose- and time-dependent increases in granulosa-cell and theca-cell LH receptors, follicular growth and estradiol accumulation similar to the changes observed during the pre-ovulatory follicular stage in the pregnant rat between days 20 and 23 (Bogovich *et al.*, 1981). At the same time, hCG treatment decreases the number of LH receptors in

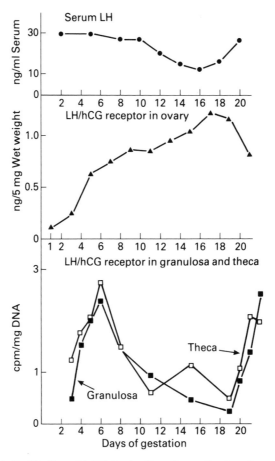

FIG 2.49. Binding of hCG in the Rat Ovary During Gestation.
[125]I-hCG binding in ovarian tissue homogenates adapted from Siebers *et al.* (1977c) and hCG binding in granulosa and theca cells of antral follicles and Richards and Kersey (1979). Serum LH concentrations quoted from Cheng (1976).

functional luteal cells present on days 14–16 of gestation suggesting that hCG triggers different cellular mechanisms in each ovarian cell type. The increase in LH receptors in preovulatory follicles may enable follicles to respond to the LH surge and luteinize.

2.1.2. FSH RECEPTORS IN THE RAT OVARY DURING GESTATION

Human FSH binds with higher affinity to its receptor than LH to its receptor in the pregnant rat ovary ($K_d = 1.6 \times 10^{-10}$ M), but the number of binding sites on day 18 of gestation is only 18 fmol/100 mg tissue (Cheng, 1976). However, in granulosa cells, the concentration of FSH binding sites is similar to that of LH (Fig. 2.50) and the variations in FSH and LH receptors in granulosa cells during gestation are similar.

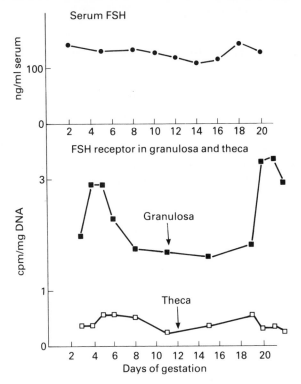

FIG 2.50. FSH Receptors in Granulosa and Theca Cells of Antral Follicles of the Rat
Ovary During Gestation.
Theca and granulosa cell FSH receptor data from Richards and Kersey (1979),
serum FSH concentrations from Cheng (1976).

However, the peaks in FSH receptors occur before the increase in LH receptors. In
contrast to the LH receptor, binding of FSH in theca cells is approximately five times
lower than the binding observed in granulosa cells.

Administration of human FSH to pregnant rats increases granulosa cell LH receptor content and aromatase activity but less effectively than hCG (Bogovich *et al.*,
1981). FSH does not increase theca cell LH receptors.

2.2. Humans

The binding of ^{125}I-hCG has been measured in a limited number of corpora
lutea obtained during the first trimester and at term pregnancy (Rajaniemi *et al.*,
1981). Specific binding of hCG up to 4 fmol/mg protein was observed; these concentrations are much lower than those found in corpora lutea during the menstrual
cycle. The low levels of receptors are probably caused by occupation and down-
regulation of the receptors by high serum levels of hCG (Conti *et al.*, 1977; Halme *et
al.*, 1978).

H. PROLACTIN RECEPTORS

1. In the Fetal Compartment

1.1. Rats

The physiologic role of prolactin in the developing fetus remains unknown. Prolactin is a polypeptide hormone whose best studied physiological function has been stimulation of milk production in adult mammary glands. Specific prolactin binding sites, therefore, have been most extensively studied in lactating mammary glands. Prolactin binding has, however, been demonstrated in fetal rhesus monkey liver, lungs and heart, in fetal rabbit liver and in fetal rat liver.

The binding of prolactin by fetal rat liver cell membrane fractions from days 17 to 21 of gestation has been studied (Dhanireddy and Ulane, 1984). Membranes obtained from fetal livers on days 17 to 20 of fetal age show no detectable specific prolactin binding. Kelly and co-workers (1974) reported low binding in livers from 20-day-old fetuses and up to 20 days after birth. On day 21 of fetal age, specific prolactin binding sites could clearly be detected. Freeze-thawing of membranes caused binding to be detected on day 20 of fetal age that had not been detectable in fresh, unfrozen membranes, but had no effect on membranes on days 17–19. Freeze-thawing also increased hormone binding by 45% in liver membranes from 21-day-old fetuses. The relative affinity constant (K_a) of the high affinity binding sites was found to be $2.1 \times 10^8 \, \text{M}^{-1}$. In the rat, prolactin receptors appear in liver only just before birth.

1.2. Rabbits

Prolactin receptors which are structurally and immunologically indistinguishable from the adult rabbit mammary gland prolactin receptor (Ymer and Herington, 1986) predominate in fetal and early neonatal rabbit liver (day 28 of fetal age) (Ymer *et al.*, 1989). Prolactin receptors were not found in fetal lung, kidney and heart and in the placenta. Prolactin receptors in fetal liver were detected by the binding of ^{125}I-human growth hormone (hGH) to macromolecules in the cytosol fraction. Growth hormone and prolactin receptors were separated by gel filtration on Ultrogel AcA44 and the specificity of each of the two peaks obtained was determined using specific monoclonal antibodies against the prolactin receptor and the growth hormone receptor. The molecular weight of the binding protein in the peak recognized by the prolactin receptor monoclonal antibody corresponded to the known molecular weight of the adult rabbit mammary gland cytosolic prolactin receptor (35 000 Da) (Ymer and Herington, 1986).

On day 28 of fetal age and the first few days of post-natal life, mostly high affinity prolactin receptors rather than growth hormone receptors were found to be present. Binding affinity is of high affinity $(K_a = 13.78 \pm 0.98 \times 10^{-9} \, \text{M}^{-1}(\text{SEM}))$ and low capacity $(127 \pm 24 \, \text{fmol/g}$ tissue or $5 \pm 0.4 \, \text{fmol/mg}$ protein). The quantity of specific prolactin binding sites increases four-fold between fetal day 28 and post-natal day 3 (Ymer *et al.*, 1989). Kelly and co-workers (1974) found similar low levels of ovine prolactin binding in livers of 20- and 30-day old rabbit fetuses.

1.3. Sheep

Chan and co-workers (1978) could only demonstrate small amounts of specific binding of ovine prolactin to fetal sheep adipose tissue, adrenal, kidney, spleen, pancreas, lung, heart, skeletal muscle, brain (cortex) and in the placenta between days 130 and 145 of gestation.

1.4. Rhesus Monkeys

The possible binding of prolactin in fetal tissues of the rhesus monkey was first observed when ^{125}I-prolactin was injected in the amniotic fluid and protein-bound radioactivity was found in fetal tissues and in the placenta (Josimovich *et al.*, 1974). Further studies showed that binding of ^{125}I-human prolactin is present in membrane preparations of fetal rhesus monkey lung, liver and heart and in the placenta from days 69 to 165 of gestation but not in fetal brain (Josimovich *et al.*, 1977). The apparent affinity constants were found to be of the same order of magnitude in all organs and over the range of fetal ages studied (K_a about 10^9 M^{-1}). Fetal heart had a somewhat higher binding capacity (111 fmol/mg cell membrane protein) than liver (10–67 fmol/mg protein), placenta (10–72 fmol/mg protein) and lungs (18 and 78 fmol/mg protein). No apparent relationship was found between binding capacity and gestational age (Josimovich *et al.*, 1977).

A deficiency or immaturity of plasma membrane receptors for prolactin may be a factor in the lack of apparent major effects of prolactin in fetal life despite the rise in fetal serum prolactin concentrations during fetal development (Aubert *et al.*, 1975; Winters *et al.*, 1975; Mueller *et al.*, 1979; Séron-Ferré *et al.*, 1979; Oliver *et al.*, 1980).

2. In the Maternal Compartment and During Lactation

Prolactin is important in the development of the mammary gland that leads to the initiation and maintenance of lactation (Lyons, 1958). Suppression of prolactin release by ergot alkaloids (Taylor and Peaker, 1975) or the sequestration of prolactin by antisera against prolactin (Shani *et al.*, 1975) decreases milk yield. Shiu and Friesen (1976) demonstrated that immunization of lactating rats with antibodies against prolactin receptor from rabbit mammary gland blocked several effects of prolactin, suggesting a functional role for the prolactin receptor in mediating the action of prolactin. The number of prolactin receptors in the rat mammary gland is related to the physiological state of the animal and is regulated in part by the endocrine system.

2.1. Rabbits

2.1.1. Mammary Gland

[125]I-Ovine prolactin binds to rabbit mammary tissue and autoradiographic studies have shown that the radioactive prolactin is bound on the surface of epithelial cells (Birkinshaw and Falconer, 1972). In 1988, Seddiki and co-workers were able to show with the use of a monoclonal antibody against the prolactin receptor the localization of prolactin receptors in the cytoplasm of mammary epithelial cells and on short portions of plasma membrane. The binding of prolactin to membranes prepared from mammary

TABLE 2.50. *Characteristics of ^{125}I-ovine Prolactin Binding in Mammary Gland of Pregnant Rabbits*

Number of sites	60 fmol/mg protein
	3 pmol/mg DNA
	40 pmol/mammary gland
K_d ($\times 10^{-10}$ M), 22° C	2–4
Trypsin proteolysis	Destroys 60% of binding
Phospholipase C	Destroys 40% of binding
Ribonuclease, DNAase, neuraminidase	No effect
Isoelectric point (pI)	5.0 and 5.9

Quoted from Shiu and Friesen (1974a) and Djiane *et al.* (1977).

glands and in isolated mammary epithelial cells has been extensively studied in the rabbit during gestation and lactation.

2.1.1.1. Characteristics of Prolactin Receptor in Mammary Glands

Shiu and Friesen (1974a) reported that ^{125}I-labeled human and ovine prolactin bind specifically and with high affinity to plasma membrane-containing subcellular particles isolated from mammary glands of the rabbit at the end of gestation and during the first days of lactation (Table 2.50). Binding is sensitive to proteolysis and phospholipase C, suggesting that proteins and phospholipids are functionally important for binding; the absence of effect of neuraminidase suggests that sialic acid is not essential (Shiu and Friesen, 1974a). A range of compounds such as estrogens, testosterone, progesterone, cortisol, mono-, di- and tri-phosphates of nucleotides, and thyroropin-releasing hormone do not affect prolactin binding to receptors *in vitro* (Shiu and Friesen, 1974a). Prolactin receptor has been solubilized by Triton X-100 from a crude particulate membrane fraction isolated from pregnant rabbit mammary glands and purified (Shiu and Friesen, 1974b).

2.1.1.2. Development of Prolactin Receptors During Pregnancy and Lactation

Prolactin binding is low in virgin, nonpregnant rabbit mammary glands and increases three to four times in the pregnant animal (McNeilly and Friesen, 1977; Richards *et al.*, 1984). During gestation, prolactin binding increases between day 14 and 22 and further increases after parturition, during lactation (Fig. 2.51) (Djiane *et al.*, 1977). Prolactin receptors seem to remain at a relatively low and constant level while mammary development takes place and serum prolactin levels are stable. A striking increase in receptors occur at the onset of milk secretion and the rise in serum prolactin after parturition.

High affinity binding of prolactin has also been characterized in dispersed mammary epithelial cells, free of interstitial cells (Suard *et al.*, 1979). The apparent affinity constant ($K_a = 10^{10}$ M^{-1}) does not change significantly throughout pregnancy and early lactation while binding capacity varies. In this study using preparations of epithelial cells rather than whole mammary glands, more binding was found in cells of

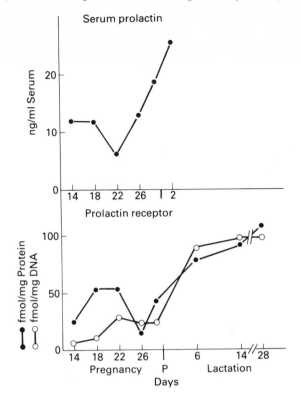

FIG 2.51. Variations in Prolactin Receptors in Rabbit Mammary Glands during Pregnancy and Lactation.
Prolactin receptor values quoted from Djiane *et al.* (1977) and serum prolactin concentrations from Suard *et al.* (1979).

virgin rabbits (1900 binding sites per cell) than at mid-pregnancy (850 sites/cell), but binding increased during lactation (1800 sites/cell). An inverse relation to serum progesterone concentrations was observed (Suard *et al.*, 1979). It has been demonstrated that progesterone antagonizes the induction by prolactin of milk specific proteins such as casein (Houdebine and Gaye, 1976; Josefsberg *et al.*, 1979; Rosen *et al.*, 1980).

Internalization of prolactin in mammary epithelial cells was visualized morphologically by electron microscopy (Suard *et al.*, 1979). At 37°C, a rapid and specific internalization of prolactin to intracellular organelles was observed. Autoradiographic labeling was found associated with vesicles, Golgi elements, lysosome-like structures and the nucleus.

2.2.2. OTHER TISSUES

Because of the diverse actions of prolactin (Nicoll and Bern, 1972), it is not surprising to find evidence of specific binding of prolactin in various organs of pregnant rabbits (Shiu and Friesen, 1974a). Besides the mammary gland and liver, kidney, adrenals, ovaries and uterus show significant amounts of binding of prolactin but brain and adipose tissue only have very low levels of binding (Grissom and Littleton, 1988).

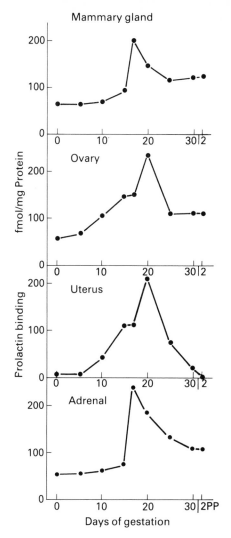

FIG 2.52. Prolactin Receptors in Mammary Gland, Ovary, Uterus and Adrenal
Gland of Rabbits during Gestation.
Quoted from Grissom and Littleton (1988).

Mammary gland and adrenals exhibit sharp increases in prolactin binding between
days 15 and 17 of gestation while ovarian and uterine receptors increase slowly after
day 5 and reach peak levels at day 20 (Fig. 2.52). Binding is essentially located in
adrenal cortex, nonluteal ovary (minus the corpus luteum) and in the endometrium
(Grissom and Littleton, 1988). Liver and kidney of pregnant rabbits showed no
variations in prolactin receptor concentrations during the course of gestation. Tissue-
specific differences in isoelectric points and immunoreactivity of prolactin receptors
have been observed in adrenal gland, kidney cortex, liver, mammary gland and ovary
of late pregnant and mid-lactating rabbits (Waters *et al.*, 1984).

2.2. Rats and Mice

2.2.1. MAMMARY GLAND

Saturable binding of high affinity and specificity for ^{125}I-prolactin has been character-ized in the mammary glands of lactating rats (Table 2.51) (Bohnet *et al.*, 1977; Hayden *et al.*, 1979). Mammary glands of lactating rats contain as much as six times more prolactin receptor than in nonlactating rats or in pregnant rats (Fig. 2.53). Prolactin receptor concentrations in lactating rat mammary glands rise sharply within two days after parturition and decline slowly with a further drop after weaning (Bohnet *et al.*, 1977; Hayden *et al.*, 1979). Receptor concentrations seem to be positively correlated with the serum prolactin levels (Fig. 2.53), but this is not always the case since estradiol treatment of lactating rats diminishes receptor concentrations in mammary glands without altering serum prolactin concentrations (Bohnet *et al.*, 1977). Prolactin autostim-ulates its own receptor in virgin rat mammary glands; this is accompanied by an increase in the number of epithelial cells (Hayden *et al.*, 1979). Bromocriptine treatment of lactating rats prevents the rise in serum prolactin and decreases prolactin receptor concentrations by 65% (Bohnet *et al.*, 1977). Hypophysectomy, thyroidectomy, ovariec-tomy and adrenalectomy of lactating rats also lead to significant reductions in prolactin receptor concentrations in the mammary gland (Hayden *et al.*, 1979).

As in the rat, prolactin receptors increase significantly immediately before and after parturition in mammary glands of mice (Sakai *et al.*, 1978). Glucocorticoids further stimulate the number of prolactin receptors in the mammary glands of mice at mid-gestation and during lactation (Sakai and Banerjee, 1979). Glucocorticoids may be acting in synergy with prolactin to stimulate lactogenesis in mice (Mills and Topper, 1969; Sakai *et al.*, 1979).

2.2.2. LIVER

Specific binding of prolactin occurs in livers of pregnant rats and mice (Posner, 1976; Hayden *et al.*, 1979). In pregnant and lactating rats, there is as much as 20 times more binding than in the mammary gland (Fig. 2.53) (Hayden *et al.*, 1979). In contrast to the mammary gland, liver prolactin receptors decrease after parturition in lactating rats and after lactation, binding increases to the levels found during pregnancy. The mechanism of control of prolactin receptor concentrations in the liver appear to differ from that of the mammary gland.

TABLE 2.51. *Characteristics of Prolactin Receptor in Mammary Gland of Lactating Rats*

Number of sites	11–50 fmol/mg protein
	190–300 fmol/g tissue
K_d ($\times 10^{-10}$ M), 6° C	2–6
Binding specificity	Binds ovine and rat prolactin
	No binding of rat FSH, TSH,
	LH or bovine insulin

Quoted from Bohnet *et al.* (1977) and Hayden *et al.* (1979).

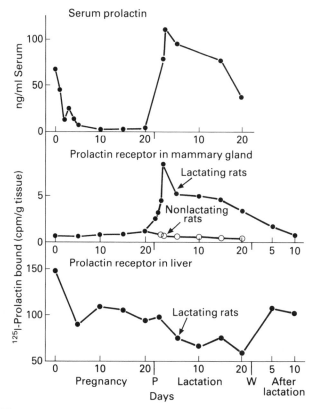

FIG 2.53. Variations in Prolactin Receptor Concentrations in Rat Mammary Gland
and Liver during Pregnancy, Lactation and after Lactation.
P = parturition; W = weaning. Prolactin receptor concentrations taken from Bohnet
et al. (1977) and Hayden *et al.* (1979). Serum prolactin levels adapted from
Morishige *et al.* (1973) and Bohnet *et al.* (1977).

2.2.3. OVARY

The binding capacity of pregnant rat ovarian tissues for ^{125}I-prolactin is highest
towards the end of gestation (15 fmol/100 mg tissue on day 18 of gestation) and is
comparable to that of the highest level attained in the ovary during the estrus cycle
(17 fmol/100 mg tissue at pro-estrus) (Cheng, 1976). The affinity constants (K_a) are
similar in the pregnant and pro-estrus ovaries $(1.1 \times 10^{10} \text{ M}^{-1})$. Receptor concentrations are highest when serum prolactin levels are also higher at late gestation and at
pro-estrus. Siebers and co-workers (1977c) showed that in the pregnant rat ovary LH
receptors already begin to increase from day 5 of gestation, which is before any change
in prolactin receptors (14–16 days) (Cheng, 1976).

2.3. Sheep

Specific binding of prolactin could be detected in membrane preparations of mammary gland, liver and adipose tissue of ewes during pregnancy and lactation (Emane *et
al.*, 1986). In the nonpregnant ewe, prolactin binding is lower in the mammary gland

than in liver, but between days 60 and 90 of gestation prolactin receptors increase abruptly in the mammary gland and decrease slightly in the liver. A second increase occurs in the mammary gland during early lactation. At parturition, prolactin binding returns to prepregnancy levels in the liver. Prolactin receptors in adipose tissue are low and do not vary (Emane *et al.*, 1986). It appears that prolactin receptor induction in the mammary gland occurs outside of the period of active cell multiplication. The highest level of prolactin receptors is found during lactation, when mammary cells are fully differentiated.

I. GROWTH HORMONE RECEPTORS

1. In the Fetal Compartment

Although fetal plasma concentrations of growth hormone are high, there is little evidence in a number of species including man that fetal growth hormone regulates fetal growth (Gluckman *et al.*, 1981). Growth hormone binding to specific receptors in the fetus was found to be very low or nondetectable in fetal livers of rats, rabbits, sheep and mice (Kelly *et al.*, 1974; Posner, 1976; Gluckman *et al.*, 1983; Freemark *et al.*, 1987).

On the other hand, specific binding of [^{125}I] human growth hormone has been observed in human fetal liver (Hill *et al.*, 1988). Two binding components are present, one with an affinity (K_d) of 1.6×10^{-9} M and a binding capacity of 79 fmol/mg protein and a second with a lower affinity (8.6×10^{-9} M) and greater capacity (160 fmol/mg protein).

2. In the Maternal Compartment

2.1. Rats and Mice

Radioiodinated growth hormone binds specifically to membrane preparations of livers of pregnant rats and mice (Kelly *et al.*, 1974; Posner, 1976). The apparent association constant (K_a) of human growth hormone binding in pregnant mouse livers is 6.2×10^8 M^{-1}. Binding is specific for growth hormone and not for lactogenic hormones. Pregnancy doubles the binding of growth hormone in both rat and mouse livers. Termination of pregnancy, either naturally or by hysterectomy, results in a rapid return of growth hormone receptor binding to levels seen in liver membranes of adult male and female mice (Posner, 1976).

2.2. Rabbits

Specific binding of growth hormone is high in the livers of pregnant rabbits (Kelly *et al.*, 1974; Cadman and Wallis, 1981). Binding capacities of liver membrane preparations increase from 225 fmol/mg protein in 10-day-old immature females to 707 fmol/mg protein in virgin, adult females to 1640 fmol/mg protein in pregnant females on day 30 of gestation. The apparent association constant (K_a) ranges from 0.8 to 1.5×10^9 M^{-1}.

J. PLACENTAL LACTOGEN RECEPTORS

Human placental lactogen or chorionic somatomammotropin is a polypeptide hormone with structural and functional similarities to human growth hormone and human prolactin (see *Hormones and the Fetus*, Volume I, Chapter 3 Chard, 1983). Placental lactogen binds to both somatotropic (growth hormone) and lactogenic (prolactin) receptors (Lesniak *et al.*, 1977) and also binds to unique placental lactogen binding sites (Freemark *et al.*, 1987).

1. In the Fetal Compartment

The biological actions of ovine placental lactogen in post-natal rat tissues are similar to those of ovine growth hormone (Chan *et al.*, 1976; Hurley *et al.*, 1977; Freemark and Handwerger, 1982; Butler *et al.*, 1978), but their actions are different in fetal rat tissues. Ovine placental lactogen has potent somatotropic and metabolic effects in fetal tissues while ovine growth hormone has little or no biological activity in the fetus (Freemark and Handwerger, 1983). Specific receptors in the fetus for placental lactogen could mediate metabolic effects in the fetus that are later controlled by growth hormone and growth hormone receptors in the post-natal period.

In hepatic membrane preparations from fetal lambs, specific binding of [^{125}I]ovine placental lactogen distinct from growth hormone and prolactin binding has been demonstrated (Chan *et al.*, 1978; Freemark and Handwerger, 1986; Freemark *et al.*, 1987). Maximal specific binding of placental lactogen is 26.3% (10.5 fmol/mg protein) while the maximal specific binding of growth hormone is only about 1%. Placental lactogen binds to a single class of receptors with a dissociation constant (K_d) of 1.1×10^{-10} M in livers of fetal lambs on days 90–95 of fetal age (Freemark and Handwerger, 1986). Growth hormone and prolactin compete only very weakly for placental lactogen binding sites in fetal liver (Freemark and Handwerger, 1986; Freemark *et al.*, 1987). Less than 3% specific binding of placental lactogen was also found in fetal adipose tissue, adrenal, kidney, spleen, pancreas, lung, heart, skeletal muscle and brain (cortex) (Chan *et al.*, 1978).

The relative binding of placental lactogen, prolactin and growth hormone for placental lactogen receptors is similar to the relative order of potencies of the three hormones in stimulating glycogen synthesis in fetal liver. Placental lactogen is 8 to 25 times more potent than growth hormone and prolactin in stimulating glycogen synthesis. Ovine placental lactogen stimulates fetal hepatic glycogen synthesis and binds to receptors in fetal liver at concentrations compatible with the fetal plasma concentration of ovine placental lactogen (Taylor *et al.*, 1980). The presence of specific, high affinity placental lactogen receptors in ovine fetal tissues suggests that placental lactogen may function as a growth hormone in the ovine fetus.

Hill and co-workers (1988) have reported the presence of specific binding sites for human placental lactogen in particulate cell membranes from human fetal liver and skeletal muscle at weeks 12–19 of gestation. Two classes of binding sites of differing affinities were observed in fetal liver: a K_d (dissociation constant) of 2.2×10^{-9} M and binding capacity of 81 fmol/mg protein for the high affinity binding sites and a K_d of 24×10^{-9} M and a capacity of 254 fmol/mg protein (Hill *et al.*, 1988). Binding of placental lactogen in muscle shows a single class of binding sites with a K_d of 5.6×10^{-9} M and a binding capacity of 146 fmol/mg protein. Some binding was also found in fetal adrenal gland, skin and lung (2.4–3.0%) and low levels of binding were detectable in heart, intestine, kidney and brain (0.8–1.9%). Placental lactogen has been shown to have direct anabolic effects in human fetal hepatocytes and skeletal muscle myoblasts (Hill *et al.*, 1986; Strain *et al.*, 1987).

2. In the Maternal Compartment

Ovine placental lactogen appears to bind with high affinity to two functionally and structurally distinct receptors in pregnant and nonpregnant sheep liver (Chan *et al.*, 1978; Freemark *et al.*, 1986; 1987). The ovine placental lactogen receptor has high affinity for ovine placental lactogen and low affinity for ovine growth hormone and ovine prolactin and the ovine growth hormone receptor has high affinity for both ovine growth hormone and placental lactogen and low affinity for prolactin. Growth hormone has low affinity for the hepatic placental lactogen receptor in the post-natal period.

In the pregnant sheep, besides the liver, adipose tissue, ovary, corpus luteum and uterus also contain significant quantities of specific binding of placental lactogen at early (22–27 days of gestation) and late stages of gestation (130–135 days) (Chan *et al.*, 1978). The binding affinity (K_a) in corpus luteum is $2.82 \times 10^9 \, M^{-1}$ with a binding capacity of 12.8 fmol/mg protein. In the uterus, the association constant is $1.65 \times 10^9 \, M^{-1}$ and the binding capacity is 40 fmol/mg protien. With the exception of the adipose tissue and uterus that showed decreased binding during pregnancy, no significant difference was observed in placental lactogen binding to tissues obtained from nonpregnant, early pregnant or late pregnant ewes (Chan *et al.*, 1978).

In the mouse, two placental lactogens have been identified; one is present at mid-pregnancy (mPL-I), and the other is present during the latter half of pregnancy (mPL-II) (Colosi *et al.*, 1982; 1987). Both are prolactin-like lactogenic glycoprotein hormones. Both mPL-I and mPL-II bind to day-17-pregnant mouse liver membranes (Colosi *et al.*, 1987; Harigaya *et al.*, 1988). Prolactin, but not growth hormone, competes for binding to these receptors. Hepatic binding of mPL-II increases from 0.75 fmol/mg protein in virgin mice to 169 fmol/mg protein on day 10 of gestation and 480 fmol/mg protein on day 17 (Harigaya *et al.*, 1988). Mouse placental lactogens are primarily lactogenic and seem to exert their effects through binding to receptors that also bind prolactin.

K. GONADOTROPIN-RELEASING HORMONE (GnRH) RECEPTORS

Gonadotropin-releasing hormone is associated with the ontogenesis of gonadotropin (LH and FSH) and gonadal sex steroid secretion (Warren *et al.*, 1975; Salisbury *et al.*, 1982). The presence of GnRH in the rat fetal hypothalamus on day 15 of gestation (Chiappa and Fink, 1977) suggests that GnRH may be involved in the appearance of LH secretion at 17 days (Salisbury *et al.*, 1982). Both *in vivo* and *in vitro* studies have shown that GnRH stimulates the fetal pituitary gland to secrete LH (Watanabe, 1981; Salisbury *et al.*, 1982; Mulchahey *et al.*, 1987).

GnRH has been demonstrated in the human fetal brain as early as 4.5 weeks (Winters *et al.*, 1974). *In vitro* studies with dispersed cells from mid-trimester human fetal pituitaries have shown that GnRH can elicit an LH-secretory response that is dose-dependent and that is potentiated by the addition of estradiol to the culture medium (Mulchahey *et al.*, 1987). GnRH appears early in the fetal brain and could play a role in the early stages of development of the pituitary anlage because, in the fetal rat, GnRH is present in the fetal hypothalamus long before the onset of LH secretion by the fetal pituitary (Aubert *et al.*, 1985).

1. In the Fetal Compartment

1.1. Fetal Rat Pituitary

Pituitary GnRH receptor binding sites were studied using a radioiodinated stable GnRH agonist as specific ligand ([DTrp^6,(N-Et)Pro^9,DesGly^{10}]GnRH). Significant amounts of binding of GnRH could be demonstrated in fetal pituitary even at day 12 of fetal age (Fig. 2.54) (Aubert *et al.*, 1985). The apparent dissociation constant (K_d) for binding in fetal and neonatal pituitaries is 10^{-10} M. After day 17 of fetal age, GnRH receptor concentrations increase in fetal pituitaries and continue to increase after birth (Aubert *et al.*, 1985). In fetuses and newborns, no statistically significant difference was observed between binding in females and males.

Immunoreactive GnRH could already be measured in fetal hypothalami on day 12 of fetal age (Fig. 2.54) (Aubert *et al.*, 1985). On day 19, hypothalamic GnRH increases

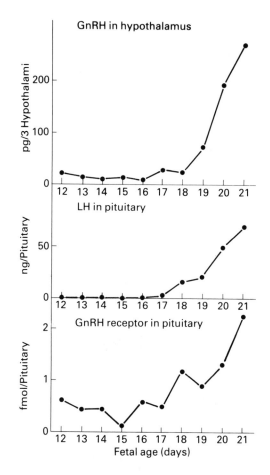

FIG 2.54. Ontogeny of Pituitary GnRH Receptors, Hypothalamic GnRH and Pituitary LH Content in Fetal Rats.
Adapted from Aubert *et al.* (1985).

significantly. GnRH could also be detected in fetal pituitary cells as early as day 14 by immunocytochemical localization of antigen–antibody complexes with electron microscopy (Aubert *et al.*, 1985). On the other hand, the presence of significant quantities of LH in fetal pituitary could only be demonstrated from day 17, after the appearance of hypothalamic GnRH and pituitary GnRH receptors (Fig. 2.54). It appears that GnRH is present in the fetal hypothalamus and pituitary and could be acting on the fetal pituitary through its receptors at least two days before LH production by the pituitary can be demonstrated.

1.2. Fetal Rat Testis

GnRH has inhibitory effects on androgen production by the testis that are mediated by the specific binding of GnRH to receptors in the Leydig cell (Clayton *et al.*, 1980). GnRH receptors are not detectable in homogenates of 20.5-day fetal testis or in freshly prepared fetal Leydig cells, but they are present from post-natal day 5 (Dufau and Knox, 1985). Fetal rat Leydig cells can be maintained in culture for up to 78 days and these cells show the presence of GnRH receptors on day 3 of culture ($K_a = 6.8 \times 10^9 \, \text{M}^{-1}$). GnRH and its agonist analogs increase GnRH receptor concentrations while LH reduces the basal, as well as the GnRH-stimulated levels of GnRH receptors (Dufau and Knox, 1985).

GnRH inhibits steroid production in LH-treated fetal Leydig cell cultures in a dose-dependent manner and abolishes the testosterone response to hCG (Dufau and Knox, 1985). GnRH receptors are either unmasked or synthesized during culture and LH exerts an inhibitory effect on GnRH receptors in fetal testis indicating that GnRH and its analogs can influence the actions of gonadotropins in fetal Leydig cells.

2. GnRH Binding in Pituitaries and Ovaries of Pregnant Rats

In the pituitary, binding sites for GnRH are higher during days 7 to 15 of gestation (66–98 fmol/mg protein), than afterwards (52–54 fmol/mg protein) (Blank *et al.*, 1983). The concentration of GnRH receptors in the ovary remains relatively constant between days 9 and 20 of gestation (about 60 fmol/mg protein) (Blank *et al.*, 1983). The progressive decline in pituitary GnRH receptors during gestation in the rat suggests that decreased hypothalamic secretion of GnRH leads to reduced circulating LH during gestation.

3. GnRH Receptors in Human Placenta

Human term placenta contains significant amounts of GnRH that is similar to hypothalamic GnRH (Siler-Khodr and Khodr, 1978; Lee *et al.*, 1981) and exogenous GnRH stimulates hCG production and release from placental tissue (Siler-Khodr and Khodr 1981). GnRH receptors are also present in term placenta (Currie *et al.*, 1981; Guévin *et al.*, 1985; Iwashita *et al.*, 1986).

Iwashita and co-workers (1986) have described some properties of binding of GnRH membrane receptors in human term placenta. Binding is of relatively low affinity ($K_a = 1.1 \times 10^6 \, \text{M}^{-1}$), lower than the affinity of GnRH receptors in the pituitary (Clayton and Catt, 1981). The low binding affinity is appropriate considering that

GnRH is produced in abundance at close proximity to its receptor sites in the placenta (Iwashita *et al.*, 1986). The human placental receptor for GnRH could be a low affinity regulatory site for locally formed GnRH within the placenta and has possible importance in the regulation of hCG production during pregnancy analogous to the action of the pituitary GnRH receptor on LH secretion. Placental GnRH could play a role in the maintenance of pregnancy.

L. ADRENOCORTICOTROPIC HORMONE (ACTH) RECEPTORS

The plasma concentrations of corticoids often increase during late pregnancy in many mammalian species and are involved in the maturation of some fetal organ systems (see Section D above). In the fetal sheep, increased cortisol levels during the last two weeks of gestation occur at the same time as the enlargement of the adrenal glands (Bassett and Thorburn, 1969; Liggins *et al.*, 1973). Moreover, in the sheep as well as in other domestic ruminants, this rise in fetal plasma cortisol triggers the onset of parturition (Liggins *et al.*, 1973). Fetal adrenocortical function is influenced by hypophyseal factors since removal of the fetal pituitary abolishes the increase in cortisol (Challis *et al.*, 1977) while perfusion with adrenocorticotropic hormone (ACTH) stimulates the fetal adrenals, resulting in premature parturition (Liggins, 1969).

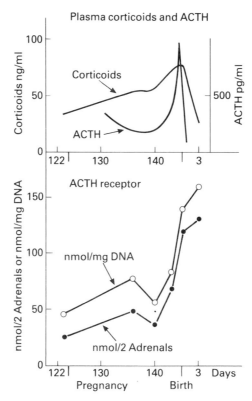

FIG 2.55. Ontogeny of ACTH Receptors in Fetal Lamb Adrenals and Fetal Plasma Concentrations of Corticoids and ACTH.
Adapted from Durand (1979) and Durand *et al.* (1980).

Specific, saturable binding of ^{125}I-ACTH$_{1-24}$ was demonstrated in membrane preparations from fetal lamb adrenals in late gestation (Durand, 1979). Binding affinity ($K_d = 1.9-2.6 \, 10^{-7} \, M$) is similar to that found in human, rat and sheep (adult) adrenals (Saez *et al.*, 1974). Figure 2.55 shows that the concentration of ACTH receptors (expressed per two adrenal glands or per mg DNA) increases five-fold between day 123 of gestation and birth (Durand, 1979). ACTH receptors seem to increase at the same time as the pre-partum rise in fetal plasma corticoids (Fig. 2.55). ACTH stimulates corticoid secretion and adenylate cyclase activity in ovine fetal adrenals, and this response develops during the period when ACTH receptors are also increasing (Madill and Bassett, 1973; Wintour *et al.*, 1975; Durand *et al.*, 1980, 1981). However, as seen in Fig. 2.55, fetal plasma ACTH increases after cortisol levels are already high. ACTH receptors are present in ovine fetal adrenals at an appropriate time during fetal development and can be correlated with some responsiveness to ACTH, but the regulation of steroidogenic function of the fetal adrenal probably involves other modulatory factors besides ACTH.

M. INSULIN AND GLUCAGON RECEPTORS

During intra-uterine life, the fetus is in a state of continual anabolism. In the presence of a supply of maternally derived glucose and amino acids, a high insulin to glucagon ratio and limited fetal responsiveness to catabolic hormones such as glucagon, the fetus is primarily concerned with fuel storage and organ growth (Girard *et al.*, 1973; Blazquez *et al.*, 1976; Vinicor *et al.*, 1976; Hay, 1979).

Insulin appears to be an important anabolic hormone for the developing fetus, exerting specific effects on growth and enzyme activity (Hill, 1976). The human embryo synthesizes and secretes insulin as early as week 8 of fetal age (Adesanya *et al.*, 1966; Adam *et al.*, 1969). Increased somatic growth occurs in infants of diabetic mothers because of an excess of fetal insulin (Hill, 1978). Fetal hyperinsulinemia also seems to play an important role in the increased perinatal mortality and morbidity of these infants (Robert *et al.*, 1976).

Insulin resistance at the cellular level and increase in the rate and amount of insulin release to maintain glucose control are characteristic features of glucose metabolism in the maternal compartment during late pregnancy (Spellacy and Goetz, 1963; Burt and Davidson, 1974). The etiology of this insulin resistance is not clear.

1. In the Fetal Compartment

1.1. Rats

1.1.1. LIVER

Specific binding of [^{125}I] insulin can be demonstrated in fetal liver from at least day 15 of fetal age (Kelly *et al.*, 1974; Blazquez *et al.*, 1976; Vinicor and Kiedrowski, 1982). Kelly *et al.* (1974) and Blazquez *et al.* (1976) have reported an increase in receptor concentrations between the fetal and the adult periods, but Vinicor and Kiedrowski

(1982) observed a seven-fold decrease; there is no evident explanation for this difference. Lowe and co-workers (1986) also observed a small increase in the amount of specific binding of insulin between fetuses (day 19 of fetal age) and newborns (1-day-old) in crude membrane preparations of livers. Mulay and co-workers (1983) reported a concentration of about 10 pmol/mg protein and an apparent affinity constant (K_a) of 2.6×10^8 M^{-1} for insulin binding to hepatic membranes of fetal rats (days 20–21 of fetal age). Alvarez and Blazquez (1987) found a concentration of insulin bound to isolated hepatocytes of fetal rats (day 21 of fetal age) of 3.2 ± 0.3 (SEM) fmol/10^6 cells or 181.8 ± 35.9 fmol/mg protein.

In contrast, specific binding of glucagon, is less than 1% of adult levels of binding on day 15 of fetal age and remains low during fetal development (Blazquez *et al.*, 1976). The stimulatory effect of glucagon on adenylate cyclase activity in the livers of 15-day-old fetal rats is only 7% of the response in the adult liver, suggesting glucagon resistance in the fetal period that is possibly due to the reduced number of glucagon receptor binding sites (Blazquez *et al.*, 1976). The higher concentrations of insulin binding sites in fetal liver would seem to favor the anabolic actions of insulin and the lower concentrations of glucagon binding would discriminate against the catabolic actions of glucagon.

1.1.2. LUNG

As seen in the Section D (see above), fetal lung maturation is regulated principally by glucocorticoids, but other hormones such as thyroid hormones and insulin also affect this fetal organ. The incidence of respiratory distress syndrome in infants of diabetic mothers is high (Robert *et al.*, 1976). Insulin can antagonize the glucocorticoid-induced incorporation of radioactive choline into phosphatidylcholine (Kikkawa *et al.*, 1971; Gross *et al.*, 1980). The biosynthesis of phosphatidylcholine is decreased in fetal lung of diabetic rats (Tyden *et al.*, 1980).

Mulay and co-workers (1983) reported values of insulin receptor binding in fetal rat lungs (days 20–21 of fetal age) of 20.4 pmol/mg protein in untreated, control rats and 10.6 pmol/mg protein in genetically diabetic BB Wistar rats. Down-regulation of insulin receptor by high endogenous concentrations of circulating insulin is the reason for this observed decrease (Soll *et al.*, 1975).

1.1.3. BRAIN

Specific insulin binding is present on membrane preparations from whole brains of fetal rats on day 19 of fetal age (Lowe *et al.*, 1986). Binding is lower in the fetus than in 1-day-old newborns.

1.2. Rabbits

1.2.1. LUNG

Membrane preparations as well as Type II pneumocytes from fetal rabbit lungs (day 27 of fetal age) show high affinity, specific binding of insulin (Neufeld *et al.*, 1981;

Kaplan *et al.*, 1984). Binding capacity is $11\,800 \pm 1400$ (SEM) sites per cell and the apparent dissociation constant (K_d) of the high affinity binding site is 4.5×10^{-10} M (Kaplan *et al.*, 1984).

1.2.2. BRAIN

Fetal rabbit brain (days 27 and 30 of gestation) contains specific insulin binding sites (Devaskar *et al.*, 1985). The binding capacity of the high affinity binding sites is 15.2 ± 2.4 (SEM) $\times 10^4$ sites per mg protein with an association constant of $8.6 \pm 0.9 \times 10^8$ M^{-1}. Maternal administration of thyroxine or betamethasone (a synthetic glucocorticoid) has no effect on insulin binding in fetal brain.

1.2.3. HEART

Insulin binding sites are also present in fetal rabbit heart (Devaskar *et al.*, 1985). The number of binding sites was found to be 11 ± 4 (SEM) $\times 10^4$ sites per mg protein and the association constant $8.5 \pm 1.6 \times 10^8$ M^{-1}. Thyroxine treatment increases the low affinity, high capacity receptor sites from 126 to 233×10^4 sites per mg protein. Betamethasone treatment elicits no effect on insulin binding.

1.3. Guinea-pigs

Both insulin and glucagon receptors are present in fetal guinea-pig livers at late gestation (Kelly *et al.*, 1974; Ganguli *et al.*, 1984). Receptor binding capacity for insulin and receptor affinity $(K_a = 7.53 \times 10^9$ M^{-1} on day 65 and 2.94×10^9 M^{-1} on day 56–58) is higher in the day-65 fetus than in the day-56–58 fetus (Ganguli *et al.*, 1984). Glucagon receptors show similar ontogenic variations in receptor number and receptor affinity in fetal guinea-pig liver (Ganguli *et al.*, 1984).

1.4. Sheep

Specific binding of insulin to partially purified ovine fetal liver membranes is present as early as day 110 of fetal age and increases in male fetuses with fetal age due to an increase in affinity of the receptor for insulin (Morriss *et al.*, 1986). Insulin binding in female liver membranes does not vary significantly during fetal development.

As in the liver, insulin binding could also be demonstrated in ovine fetal kidney membranes from at least day 110 of fetal age (Morriss *et al.*, 1986).

1.5. Humans

Insulin receptors are present from as early as week 14 of gestation in cerebrum, cerbellum and hypothalamus of human fetuses. Before week 20 of gestation, the mean receptor concentration is 6 pmol/mg protein and decreases at week 30 of gestation and after birth (0.6 pmol/mg protein) (Potau *et al.*, 1984).

2. In the Maternal Compartment and During Lactation

2.1. Rats and Mice

2.1.1. ADIPOSE TISSUE

Adipocytes prepared from parametrial fat pads bind insulin in the 16- and 20-day pregnant rat (Sutter-Dub *et al.*, 1984). The group found that the amount of high affinity, specific binding is not significantly different between the adipocytes from pregnant rats on day 20 of gestation and the nonpregnant rats. Flint and co-workers (1979) reported a decrease in binding at parturition. Binding is increased in the 16-day pregnant rats (Sutter-Dub *et al.*, 1984). Dissociation constants (K_d) for the high affinity binding sites do not vary significantly in the nonpregnant and pregnant rats ($1.04-1.5 \times 10^{-9}$ M). The ability of pregnant rat adipocytes to oxidize ^{14}C-glucose in the presence of insulin is reduced compared to the nonpregnant rat (Sutter-Dub *et al.*, 1984) indicating insulin resistance of this tissue despite normal insulin binding. A post-receptor defect in insulin action has been suggested.

2.1.2. MAMMARY GLAND

In the mouse, specific binding of insulin to dissociated mammary cells decreases progressively during gestation (from 2500 to 300 sites per cell) and increases sharply before parturition to culminate on day 3 of lactation (1000 sites per cell) (Inagaki and Kohmoto, 1982). An increase in insulin receptors in the mammary epithelial cell at parturition has also been observed in the rat (O'Keefe and Cuatrecasas, 1974). Apparent dissociation constants are lower during early pregnancy (about 10^{-8} M) than during late pregnancy and during lactation (about 10^{-7} M) (Inagaki and Kohmoto, 1982). Bromocriptine treatment of lactating rats, or removal of the litter, produces a decrease in serum prolactin, a decrease in the number of insulin receptors in the mammary gland and an increase in the concentration of insulin in the serum (Flint, 1982).

2.1.3. UTERUS

During pregnancy, the glycogen content of the myometrium increases until term then decreases post-partum (Chew and Renard, 1979). Insulin stimulates glucose uptake or amino acid uptake in the myometrium (Smith and Gorski, 1968; Mohri *et al.*, 1974). Specific binding of insulin has been demonstrated in the myometrium of pregnant rats (Sakamoto *et al.*, 1987). Binding increases from 160 fmol/mg protein on day 15 of gestation to 255 fmol/mg protein on day 21 of gestation. By 12 h post-partum, binding decreases to about one-third of the pre-partum levels. The apparent dissociation constant (K_d) for the higher affinity insulin binding component is 1×10^{-11} M (Sakamoto *et al.*, 1987). Myometrial glycogen content parallels the increase in insulin receptors.

2.2. Sheep

Insulin receptor concentrations increase in isolated hepatocytes of pregnant ewes when compared with unmated animals (Gill and Hart, 1982). At the end of gestation

(140 days), receptor concentrations are doubled (about 12 000 sites per cell) while binding affinity is relatively unchanged ($K_d = 1.3-1.7 \times 10^{-10}$ M). In contrast, glucagon receptor binding decreases by day 140 of gestation to half the concentration present in hepatocytes from unmated ewes. Binding affinity remains similar ($K_d = 3-4 \times 10^{-10}$ M).

2.3. Humans

Insulin receptors have been studied during human pregnancy mainly in circulating blood cells (monocytes and erythrocytes) (Jarrett *et al.*, 1984). The presence of specific binding of insulin to blood cells is confirmed, but no consistent changes can be correlated with pregnancy (either normal or diabetic).

Pagano and co-workers (1980) also reported binding of insulin in human adipocytes whose number and affinity decreased during pregnancy. Jarrett and co-workers (1984) correlated changes in the binding affinity of insulin in isolated human adipocytes at term with the opposing effects of prolactin and relaxin. Prolactin decreases and relaxin increases the binding affinity of insulin.

3. In the Placenta

3.1. Rats

Wang and co-workers (1987) characterized insulin receptors in the rat placenta on day 11 and day 19 of gestation. Binding capacity decreases with gestation while the affinity of insulin for the high affinity binding sites increases (Table 2.52). Total binding capacity per placenta is comparable in day 11 and day 19 placentas.

TABLE 2.52. *Variations in Properties of Insulin Receptors in Placentas of Rats During Gestation*

	Day 11	Day 19
Number of sites		
fmol/mg protein	270	40
K_d ($\times 10^{-9}$ M)	23.8	5.6

Quoted from Wang *et al.* (1987).

3.2. Humans

Binding of insulin to membranes is particularly high in the human placenta (Table 2.53) and increases during gestation (Demers *et al.*, 1972; Marshall *et al.*, 1974; Posner, 1974; Takano *et al.*, 1975). The insulin receptor from human placental membranes has been solubilized (Harrison *et al.*, 1978; Kohanski and Lane, 1983), and the human placenta has been used as a rich source of insulin receptor for purification and studies of the purified receptor protein (Williams and Turtle, 1979; Siegel *et al.*, 1981).

TABLE 2.53. *Properties of Insulin Receptors in Particulate Membrane Preparations of Human Term Placenta*

Number of sites	5400 pmol/mg protein
K_d ($\times 10^{-8}$ M)	0.26
Specificity	Porcine insulin = bovine insulin >
	glucagon > somatomedins A or C
Effect of pH	Optimal binding between pH 7 and 8
Phospholipase C	Slightly increases binding
Neuraminidase	No effect
Pronase and trypsin	Binding destroyed

Quoted from Marshall *et al.* (1974), Takano *et al.* (1975), and Harrison *et al.* (1978).

Placental insulin receptors have been found to be localized on the microvillus brush border membrane which is exposed to maternal blood in the intervillous space (Whitsett *et al.*, 1979). Short term monolayer cultures have been established from trypsinized chorionic villi predominantly of syncytial origin (Deal and Guyda, 1983). The insulin receptors in these cells conserve their insulin binding properties and show maximal binding of insulin between days 2 and 4 of culture.

N. OXYTOCIN RECEPTORS

The neurohypophysial hormone, oxytocin, causes myometrial contraction and has been used to induce labor. Since oxytocin concentrations in blood increase significantly only during the expulsive phase of labor (see Volume I, Chapter 5), oxytocin secretion may not be essential for the initiation of labor. However, this does not exclude an increase in the sensitivity of the myometrium at the time of parturition that may be attributed to an increase in the concentration of oxytocin receptors.

Oxytocin also stimulates the expulsion of milk in lactating animals by provoking the contractions of the myoepithelial cells surrounding the alveoli in mammary glands (Cross and Harris, 1952). Oxytocin receptors play a role in the sensitivity of the mammary gland to oxytocin.

1. Rats

Specific binding of ^{3}H-oxytocin is present in rat myometrium and mammary gland during gestation, parturition and lactation (Soloff *et al.*, 1979). It is interesting to compare these two tissues because the profiles of oxytocin binding are different. Oxytocin receptors from both tissues bind oxytocin with comparable affinity ($K_d = 1-3 \times 10^{-9}$ M) (Soloff *et al.*, 1979; Pearlmutter and Soloff, 1979). In the myometrium, oxytocin binding increases abruptly and reaches peak values during labor and decreases rapidly from day 1 post-partum (Fig. 2.56). In contrast, oxytocin binding in mammary glands increases steadily throughout gestation and reaches maximal values during lactation (Fig. 2.56). These observations can be correlated with the response to oxytocin in pregnant rats. Oxytocin does not induce parturition in rats earlier than

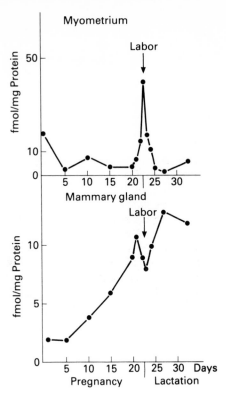

FIG 2.56. Oxytocin Receptors in Myometrium and Mammary Gland of Rats during
Gestation, Labor and Lactation.
Adapted from Soloff *et al.* (1979).

6–8 h before spontaneous delivery (Fuchs and Poblete, 1970) and the mammary gland becomes more sensitive to smaller doses of oxytocin between day 9 and day 18 of gestation and between days 1 and 10 post-partum during lactation (Sala and Freire, 1974). The threshold dose of oxytocin that significantly increases contractile activity of the uterus above the prevailing spontaneous activity is inversely proportional to the concentration of oxytocin receptors in the myometrium (Fuchs *et al.*, 1983a). A linear correlation exists between the concentration of oxytocin binding sites in the myometrium and the uterine activity induced by oxytocin infusion of pregnant rats on days 21–23 of gestation (Fuchs *et al.*, 1983a).

Estrogens have a stimulatory effect on the concentrations of myometrial oxytocin receptors and the responsiveness of the uterus to oxytocin (Robson, 1937; Soloff, 1975; Nissenson *et al.*, 1978; Fuchs *et al.*, 1983b). In the perinatal period, the change in oxytocin receptor concentration is proportional to the ratio of plasma estradiol to progesterone levels, and a proportional increase in myometrial estrogen receptor concentration precedes the appearance of oxytocin receptors (Fig. 2.57) (Alexandrova and Soloff, 1980). Estrogen and progesterone receptor concentrations are also higher when plasma progesterone levels decline since progesterone is an estrogen antagonist and progesterone down-regulates its own receptor. The myometrial oxytocin receptor

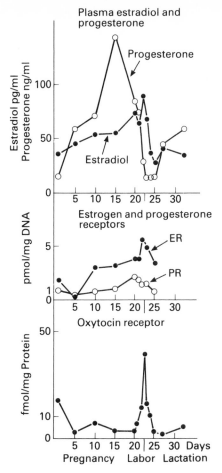

FIG 2.57. Comparison of Concentrations of Myometrial Estrogen, Progesterone and Oxytocin Receptors and Plasma Ovarian Steroid Concentrations in Rats during Pregnancy, Labor and Lactation.
Oxytocin receptor values taken from Soloff *et al.* (1979) and estrogen (ER) and progesterone (PR) receptors from Alexandrova and Soloff (1980). Plasma estradiol and progesterone concentrations quoted from Soloff *et al.* (1979).

appears to be an estrogen-induced, progesterone-inhibited receptor. On the other hand, oxytocin receptors in the mammary glands do not seem to be regulated by these abrupt changes in plasma estradiol and progesterone (Soloff *et al.*, 1979; Soloff and Wieder, 1983).

In the rat, at least part of the process of parturition seems to involve a drop in plasma progesterone levels that releases the antagonistic effect of progesterone on estrogen receptors and, consequently, causes an increase in estrogen receptors that mediate the stimulation of oxytocin receptor concentrations that lead to increased sensitivity of the myometrium to oxytocin (Alexandrova and Soloff, 1980; Fuchs *et al.*, 1983a,b; Soloff *et al.*, 1983).

2. Rabbits

Binding of ^{3}H-oxytocin is present in myometrium of pregnant rabbits (Riemer *et al.*, 1986). The equilibrium dissociation constant for the high affinity, saturable class of binding sites is approximately 1.6×10^{-9} M. The concentrations of oxytocin receptors increase from about 20 fmol/mg protein on days 22–27 of gestation to 700 fmol/mg protein on day 31. Contractile sensitivity of isolated uterine strips also increases at least four-fold between days 30 and 31 of gestation. These observations confirm that oxytocin plays an important role in the initiation of parturition through changes in oxytocin receptor concentrations.

3. Guinea-pigs

The concentration of oxytocin receptors in the myometrium of the pregnant guinea-pig rises during gestation and reaches 400 fmol/mg DNA between day 60 of gestation and 12 h after parturition (Alexandrova and Soloff, 1980). After this time, there is a sharp drop in receptor concentrations. The concentration of estrogen receptors (cytosol plus nuclear) vary in a similar manner. Plasma progesterone levels remain relatively high prior to labor, but plasma estradiol concentrations rise between days 50 and 60 of gestation, causing an increased estradiol to progesterone ratio (Challis *et al.*, 1971). Despite the absence of a fall in plasma progesterone levels prior to parturition, the guinea-pig resembles the rat in that the concentrations of oxytocin and estrogen receptors increase in the myometrium. The change in oxytocin receptor concentration corresponds to the increased myometrial sensitivity to oxytocin in the guinea-pig (Bell, 1941).

4. Humans

Oxytocin receptors are present in both the myometrium and parietal decidua of pregnant women (Fuchs *et al.*, 1982; 1984). The apparent dissociation constant in both myometrium and decidua is in the range of $1-2 \times 10^{-9}$ M and does not vary significantly during pregnancy and labor. The concentrations of receptors are relatively low in mid-gestation and are maximal during labor (Table 2.54).

TABLE 2.54. *Oxytocin Receptor Concentrations in Myometrium and Decidua of Human Uteri During Pregnancy and Labor*

	Myometrium fmol/mg DNA	Decidua fmol/mg DNA
Pregnant (13–17 weeks)	172 ± 67	629
Before Labor (37–43 weeks)	1391 ± 180	1510 ± 382
Preterm Labor (28–36 weeks)	2352 ± 358	3673 ± 947
Early Labor (37–43 weeks)[a]	3468 ± 886	3177 ± 1426
Advanced Labor (37–43 weeks)[b]	257 ± 104	786

Means $\pm$ SEM; [a]Patients scheduled for cesarean section when labor began; [b]Emergency cesarean sections
Quoted from Fuchs *et al.* (1982).

Decidua has high levels of prostaglandin synthetase activity (Willman and Collins, 1978). Oxytocin increases prostaglandin production *in vitro* in decidua but not in myometrium (Fuchs *et al.*, 1982). Oxytocin binding in decidua could mediate the stimulation of prostaglandin synthesis that would enhance the oxytocin-induced contractions of the myometrium.

Similar to the observations in rats, rabbits and guinea-pigs, the finding that women in spontaneous labor have higher oxytocin receptor concentrations than women before the onset of labor suggests that when myometrial oxytocin receptor concentrations reach a certain threshold level, effective uterine contractions are triggered. Decidual oxytocin receptors may be involved in the concomitant production of prostaglandins that could act in synergy with oxytocin in the myometrium.

O. RELAXIN RECEPTORS

Relaxin is produced by the pregnant ovary (Anderson *et al.*, 1973; Sherwood *et al.*, 1980). It inhibits myometrial activity and induces softening of the uterine cervix (Schwabe *et al.*, 1978; Downing and Sherwood, 1985a,b,c). Relaxin acts directly on the uterine myometrium and this activity is mediated by the presence of relaxin receptors in the myometrium (Sherwood, 1988).

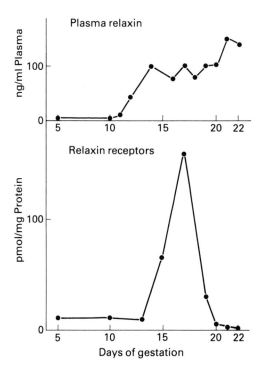

FIG 2.58. Relaxin Receptor Concentrations in the Myometrium of Rats during Gestation (Comparison with Plasma Relaxin Concentrations).
Relaxin receptor values taken from Mercado-Simmen *et al.* (1982) and plasma relaxin concentrations from Sherwood *et al.* (1980).

In the myometrium of the pregnant rat, relaxin receptor concentrations rise by day 15 of gestation and are maximal on day 17 (Fig. 2.58) (Mercado-Simmen et al., 1980; 1982). The binding affinity of relaxin does not vary during gestation ($K_d = 0.3-0.8 \times 10^{-10}$ M). The decrease after day 17 of gestation occurs when plasma relaxin is high and is probably due to the binding of endogenous unlabeled relaxin to receptor binding sites and a down-regulation of relaxin receptors by relaxin (Mercado-Simmen et al., 1982).

P. ANGIOTENSIN RECEPTORS

1. In the Fetal Compartment

The octapeptide angiotensin II acts on vasoconstriction, stimulation of mineralocorticoid secretion, stimulation of thirst and control of renal sodium and water transport. Renin and angiotensin are present in placenta and amniotic fluid, and the renin-angiotensin system is known to be active during fetal life (Skinner et al., 1968).

Autoradiographic analysis of the retention of radioiodinated angiotensin II in 17-day-old fetal mice revealed high density of radioactive labeling widely distributed throughout the body (Zemel et al., 1989). More radioactivity was found to be localized in primitive mesenchymal tissue under the epidermis and surrounding muscle and cartilage, in skeletal and smooth muscle, and in all layers of the adrenal cortex. Less labeling was seen in the kidney, liver and lungs. The localization of angiotensin in the mesenchymal tissue and skeletal muscle of the fetus is not observed in the adult. This distribution of labeled angiotensin was confirmed by Millan and co-workers (1989) in the fetal rat; particularly intense autoradiographic labeling was seen in the tongue. Little or no binding was observed in brain, spinal cord, cartilage, bone, fat and heart.

Angiotensin II receptor binding was characterized in membranes from skin and lingual skeletal muscle of the rat fetus (Millan et al., 1989). Angiotensin II receptor concentrations in skin decrease from 44 pmol/mg protein in the 19-day-old fetus to 9 pmol/mg protein one day after birth and is undetectable in the adult. The dissociation constant (K_d) of binding in fetal skin is 6.2×10^{-9} M. Angiotensin II binding is also high in the fetal tongue (24 pmol/mg protein) and declines to 11 pmol/mg protein by day 5 after birth. Some binding is still detectable in the adult rat tongue.

Cultured skin fibroblasts from fetal rats are able to respond to angiotensin II (Millan et al., 1989). Angiotensin II increases inositol phosphate formation and cytosolic calcium in the cultured cells.

The exact function of angiotensin II in the fetus remains to be elucidated, but the presence of functional receptors at unique sites in the fetus and the response elicited in fetal skin fibroblasts suggest a role in fetal growth and development.

2. In the Maternal Compartment

2.1. Rats

It has been postulated that angiotensin II could be a factor in provoking uterine contractions during parturition and receptor sites for angiotensin II have been found in the uterus of pregnant rats (Schirar *et al.*, 1980). Uterine angiotensin II receptor binding capacity rises from day 2 of gestation and peaks on day 9 (200 fmol/mg protein). From day 14 of gestation, receptor values are lower than control, nonpregnant values until one day after delivery. The dissociation constant (K_d) is 2.5×10^{-9} M on days 8 and 9 of gestation, not significantly different from the binding affinity in nonpregnant rat uterus. Most of the variation in uterine angiotensin II receptors occurs in the implantation area and could be related to the decidualization process. The low receptor concentration observed at the time of delivery indicates that angiotensin II does not play an important role in the process of parturition in the rat.

2.2. Rabbits

During human pregnancy, circulating levels of angiotensin II are high (Wilson *et al.*, 1980); nevertheless, renal and peripheral vascular blood flows increase (Atherton and Green, 1983) and the systemic blood pressure and the pressor response to exogenous angiotensin II fall (Gant *et al.*, 1973).

Both vascular (glomeruli and mesenteric arteries) and nonvascular (adrenal glomerulosa) tissues from rabbits from days 24 to 28 of gestation contain binding sites for angiotensin II (Brown and Venuto, 1986). Receptor concentrations in vascular tissue are lower in pregnant than in nonpregnant rabbits but binding affinity is not affected ($K_d = 1-2 \times 10^{-9}$ M). Binding in adrenal glomerulosa is 10 to 40 times higher (4 pmol/mg protein) than in vascular tissue, but no change occurs during gestation. It is suggested that the control of angiotensin receptor concentrations differ between vascular tissue and adrenal glomerulosa and that the receptor levels in vascular tissue are decreased by the elevated circulating levels of angiotensin II. Reduced concentrations of receptors may lead to refractoriness of the tissues during pregnancy.

References

ABE, K. (1973) Concentration of [^{14}C]aldosterone by various tissues in pregnant rats. *J. Endocr.* **56:** 611–612.

ADAM, P. A. J., TERAMO, K., RAIHA, N., GITLAIN, D. and SCHWARTZ, R. (1969) Human fetal insulin metabolism early in the gestation. Response to acute elevation of the fetal glucose concentrations and placental transfer of human insulin-^{131}I. *Diabetes* **18:** 409–415.

ADESANYA, T., GRILLO, I. and SHIMA, K. (1966) Insulin content and enzyme histochemistry of the human foetal pancreatic islet. *J. Endocr.* **36:** 151–158.

ALEXANDROVA, M. and SOLOFF, M. S. (1980) Oxytocin receptors and parturition. I. Control of oxytocin receptor concentration in the rat myometrium at term. *Endocrinology* **106:** 730–735.

ALLFREY, V. G. (1980) Molecular aspects of the regulation of eukaryotic transcription: nucleosomal proteins and their postsynthetic modifications in the control of DNA conformation and template function. In: *Cell Biology*, Vol. 3, Goldstein, L. and Prescott D. M. (Eds), Academic Press, New York, London, pp. 347–437.

ALVAREZ, E. and BLAZQUEZ, E. (1987) Lack of insulin effect on its own receptors in fetal rat hepatocytes. *Horm. Metab. Res.* **19:** 458–463.

AMSTERDAM, A., KOCH, Y., LIEBERMAN, M. E. and LINDNER, H. E. (1975) Distribution of binding sites for human chorionic gonadotropin in the preovulatory follicle of the rat. *J. Cell Biol.* **67:** 894–900.

ANDERSON, A. B. M., FLINT, A. P. F. and TURNBULL, A. C. (1975) Mechanism of action of glucocorticoids in induction of ovine parturition: effect on placental steroid metabolism. *J. Endocr.* **66:** 61–70.

ANDERSON, J. N., PECK, E. J. Jr. and CLARK, J. H. (1975) Estrogen-induced uterine responses and growth: relationship to receptor estrogen binding by uterine nuclei. *Endocrinology* **96:** 160–167.

ANDERSON, L. L., BAST, J. D. and MELAMPY, R. M. (1973) Relaxin in ovarian tissue during different reproductive stages in the rat. *J. Endocr.* **59:** 371–372.

ANDERSON, W., KANG, Y.-H., PEROTTI, M. E., BRAMLEY, T. A. and RYAN, R. J. (1979) Interactions of gonadotropins with corpus luteum membranes. III. Electron microscopic localization of [^{125}I]-hCG binding to sensitive and desensitizied ovaries seven days after PMSG-hCG. *Biol. Reprod.* **20:** 362–376.

ANDERSSON, S. M., RAIHA, N. C. R. and OHISALO J. J. (1980) Regulation of tyrosine aminotransferase in foetal rat liver. *Biochem. J.* **186:** 609–612.

ANDREW, F. D., BOWEN, D. and ZIMMERMAN, E. F. (1972) Glucocorticoid inhibition of RNA synthesis and the critical period for cleft palate induction in inbred mice. *Teratology* **7:** 167–176.

ANDREWS, W. V. and CONN, P. M. (1986) Gonadotropin-releasing hormone stimulates mass changes in phosphoinositides and diacylglycerol accumulation in purified gonadotrope cell cultures. *Endocrinology* **118:** 1148–1158.

ANTAKLY, T. and EISEN, H. J. (1984) Immunocytochemical localization of glucocorticoid receptor in target cells. *Endocrinology* **115:** 1984–1989.

ARMSTRONG, E. G. Jr., TOBERT, J. A., TALLEY, D. J. and VILLEE, C. A. (1977) Changes in progesterone receptor levels during deciduomata development in the pseudopregnancy rat. *Endocrinology* **101:** 1545–1551.

ARRIZA, J. L., WEINBERGER, C., CERELLI, G., GLASER, T. M., HANDELIN, B. L., HOUSMAN, D. E. and EVANS, R. M. (1987) Cloning of human mineralocorticoid receptor cDNA: structural and functional kinship with the glucocorticoid receptor. *Science* **237:** 268–275.

ARTHUR, A. T. and DANIEL, J. C., Jr. (1972) Progesterone regulation of blastokinin production and maintenance of rabbit blastocysts transferred into uteri of castrated recipients. *Fertil. Steril.* **23:** 115–122.

ASANTILA, T., VAHALA, J. and TOIVANEN, P. (1974) Response of human fetal lymphocytes in xenogeneic mixed leukocyte culture: phylogenetic and ontogenetic aspects. *Immunogenetics* **3:** 272–290.

ASTWOOD, E. B. (1939) An assay method for progesterone based upon the decidual reaction in the rat. *J. Endocr.* **1:** 49–55.

ATHERTON, J. C. and GREEN, R. (1983) Renal function in pregnancy. *Clin. Sci.* **65:** 449–455.

AUBERT, M. L., GRUMBACH, M. M. and KAPLAN, S. L. (1975) The ontogenesis of human fetal hormones. III. Prolactin. *J. Clin. Invest.* **56:** 155–164.

AUBERT, M. L., BEGEOT, M., WINIGER, B. P., MOREL, G., SIZONENKO, P. C. and DUBOIS, P. M. (1985) Ontogeny of hypothalamic luteinizing hormone-releasing hormone (GnRH) and pituitary GnRH receptors in fetal and neonatal rats. *Endocrinology* **116:** 1565–1576.

AURICCHIO, F., ROTONDI, A. and BRESCIANI, F. (1976) Oestrogen receptor in mammary gland cytosol of virgin, pregnant and lactating mice. *Mol. Cell. Endocr.* **4:** 55–60.

AVERY, M. E. and MEAD, J. (1959) Surface properties in relation to atelectasis and hyaline membrane disease. *Am. J. Dis. Child.* **97:** 517–523.

BALINSKY, B. I. (1949) On the developmental process in mammary glands and other epidermal structures. *Trans. Roy. Soc. Edinburgh* **62:** 1–31.

BALLARD, P. L. (1989) Hormonal regulation of pulmonary surfactant. *Endocrine Rev.* **10:** 165–181.

BALLARD, P. L. and BALLARD, R. A. (1972) Glucocorticoid receptors and the role of glucocorticoids in fetal lung development. *Proc. Natl. Acad. Sci. USA* **69:** 2668–2672.

BALLARD, P. L. and BALLARD, R. A. (1974) Cytoplasmic receptor for glucocorticoids in lung of the human fetus and neonate. *J. Clin. Invest.* **53:** 477–486.

BALLARD, P. L., BAXTER, J. D., HIGGINS, S. J., ROUSSEAU, G. G. and TOMKINS, G. M. (1974) General presence of glucocorticoid receptors in mammalian tissues. *Endocrinology* **94**: 998–1002.

BALLARD, P. L., CARTER, J. P., GRAHAM, B. S. and BAXTER, J. D. (1975) A radioreceptor assay for evaluation of the plasma glucocorticoid activity of natural and synthetic steroids in man. *J. Clin. Endocr. Metab.* **41**: 290–304.

BALLARD, P. L., MASON, R. J. and DOUGLAS, W. H. J. (1978) Glucocorticoid binding by isolated lung cells. *Endocrinology* **102**: 1570–1575.

BALLARD, P. L., BALLARD, R. A., GRANBERG, J. P., SNIDERMAN, S., GLUCKMAN, P. D., KAPLAN, S. L. and GRUMBACH, M. M. (1980a) Fetal sex and prenatal betamethasone therapy. *J. Pediatr.* **97**: 451–454.

BALLARD, P. L., BENSON, B. J., BREHIER, A., CARTER, J. P., KRIZ, B. M. and JORGENSEN, E. C. (1980b) Transplacental stimulation of lung development in the fetal rabbit by 3,5-dimethyl-3′-iso-propyl-L-thyronine. *J. Clin. Invest.* **65**: 1407–1417.

BALLARD, P. L., BALLARD, R. A., GONZALES, L. K., HÜMMELINK, R., WILSON, C. M. and GROSS, I. (1984a) Early events in the action of glucocorticoids in developing tissues. *J. Steroid Biochem.* **21**: 117–126.

BALLARD, P. L., HOVEY, M. L. and GONZALES, L. K. (1984b) Thyroid hormone stimulation of phosphatidylcholine synthesis in cultured fetal rabbit lung. *J. Clin. Invest.* **74**: 898–905.

BALLARD, P. L., HAWGOOD, S., LILEY, H., WELLENSTEIN, G., GONZALES, L. W., BENSON, B., CORDELL, B. and WHITE, R. T. (1986) Regulation of pulmonary surfactant apoprotein SP 28–36 gene in fetal human lung. *Proc. Natl. Acad. Sci. USA* **83**: 9527–9531.

BANERJEE, M. R. (1976) Responses of mammary cells to hormones. *Int. Rev. Cytol.* **47**: 1–97.

BANERJEE, M. R. and BANERJEE, D. N. (1971) Hormonal regulation of RNA synthesis and membrane ultrastructure in mouse mammary gland. *Exp. Cell Res.* **64**: 307–316.

BARDIN, C. W., BROWN, T. R., MILLS, N. C., GUPTA, C. and BULLOCK, L. P. (1978) The regulation of the beta-glucuronidase gene by androgens and progestins. *Biol. Reprod.* **18**: 74–83.

BARILE, G., GIANI, S., MONTEMURRO, A., MANGO, D. and SCIRPA, P. (1979) Evidence for a testosterone binding macromolecule in human placental cytosol. *J. Steroid Biochem.* **11**: 1247–1252.

BARKLEY, M. S., MICHAEL, S. D., GESCHWIND, I. I. and BRADFORD, G. E. (1977) Plasma testosterone during pregnancy in the mouse. *Endocrinology* **100**: 1472–1475.

BARLOW, R. M. (1969) The foetal sheep: morphogenesis of the nervous system and histochemical aspects of myelination. *J. Comp. Neurol.* **135**: 249–262.

BARLOW, S. M., MORRISON, P. J. and SULLIVAN, F. M. (1974) Plasma corticosterone levels during pregnancy in the mouse—the relative contributions of the adrenal glands and foeto-placental units. *J. Endocr.* **60**: 473–483.

BARR, H. A., LUGG, M. A. and NICHOLAS, T. E. (1980) Cortisone and cortisol in maternal and fetal blood and in amniotic fluid during the final ten days of gestation in the rabbit. *Biol. Neonate* **38**: 214–220.

BASSETT, J. M. and THORBURN, G. D. (1969) Foetal plasma corticosteroids and the initiation of parturition in the sheep. *J. Endocr.* **44**: 285–286.

BAST, J. D. and MELAMPY, R. M. (1972) Luteinizing hormone, prolactin and ovarian 20α-hydroxy-steroid dehydrogenase levels during pregnancy and pseudopregnancy in the rat. *Endocrinology* **91**: 1499–1505.

BAYARD, F., DAMILANO, S., ROBEL, P. and BAULIEU, E-E. (1978) Cytoplasmic and nuclear estradiol and progesterone receptors in human endometrium. *J. Clin. Endocr. Metab.* **46**: 635–648.

BAZER, F. W. and THATCHER, W. W. (1977) Theory of maternal recognition of pregnancy in swine based on estrogen controlled endocrine versus exocrine secretion of prostaglandin F2α by the uterine endometrium. *Prostaglandins* **14**: 397–401.

BEARN, J. G. (1973) In: *Hormones in Development*, Hamburgh, M. and Barrington, E. J. W. (Eds), Appleton-Century-Croft, New York, p. 121.

BEIER, H. M. (1968) Uteroglobin: a hormone sensitive endometrial protein involved in blastocyst development. *Biochim. Biophys. Acta* **160**: 289–291.

BEIER, H. M. (1976) Uteroglobin and related biochemical changes in the reproductive tract during early pregnancy in the rabbit. *J. Reprod. Fertil. (Suppl.)* **25**: 53–69.

BELL, G. H. (1941) The behaviour of the pregnant uterus of the guinea-pig. *J. Physiol.* **100**: 263–274.

BERNAL, J. and PEKONEN, F. (1984) Ontogenesis of the nuclear 3,5,3′-triiodothyronine receptor in the human fetal brain. *Endocrinology* **114**: 677–679.

BHATT, B. M. and BULLOCK, D. W. (1974) Binding of oestradiol to rabbit blastocysts and its possible role in implantation. *J. Reprod. Fertil.* **39**: 65–70.

BHATT, B. M. and BULLOCK, D. W. (1978) Non-specific effects of passive immunization on implantation in the rabbit. *J. Reprod. Fertil.* **54**: 177–181.

BILLAT, C., NAGEL, M.-D., NAGEL, J. and JACQUOT, R. (1980) Early reactivity of liver erythropoietic tissue of the rat foetus towards glucocorticoids. *Biol. Cell.* **38**: 187–194.

BILLAT, C., FELIX, J. M., MAYEUX, P. and JACQUOT, R. (1981) Binding of glucocorticosteroids to hepatic erythropoietic cells of the rat fetus. *J. Endocr.* **89**: 307–315.

BIRGE, C. A., PEAKE, G. T., MARIZ, I. K., and DAUGHADAY, W. H. (1967) Radioimmunoassayable growth hormone in the rat pituitary gland: effects of age, sex and hormonal state. *Endocrinology* **81**: 195–204.

BIRKINSHAW, M. and FALCONER, I. R. (1972) The localization of prolactin labelled with radioactive iodine in rabbit mammary tissue. *J. Endocr.* **55**: 323–334.

BLACKBURN, W. R., TRAVERS, H. and POTTER, D. M. (1972) The role of the pituitary-adrenal-thyroid axis in lung differentiation. I. Studies on the cytology and physical properties of anancephalic fetal rat lung. *Lab. Invest.* **26**: 306–318.

BLANK, M. S., LOUMAYE, E., CATT, K. J. and DUFAU, M. L. (1983) Role of gonadotropins in the hormonal regulation of pregnancy in the rat. In: *Factors Regulating Ovarian Function*, Greenwald, G. S. and Terranova, P. F. (Eds), Raven Press, New York, pp. 11–16.

BLAZQUEZ, E., SIMON, F. A., BLAZQUEZ, M. and FOA, P. P. (1974) Changes in serum growth hormone levels from fetal to adult age in the rat. *Proc. Soc. Exp. Biol. Med.* **147**: 780–783.

BLAZQUEZ, E., RUBALCAVA, B., MONTESANO, R., ORCI, L. and UNGER, R. H. (1976) Development of insulin and glucagon binding and the adenylate cyclase response in liver membranes of the prenatal, postnatal, and adult rat: evidence of glucagon "resistance". *Endocrinology* **98**: 1014–1023.

BLOCH, E., BENIRSCHKE, K. and ROSEMBERG, E. (1956) C19 steroids, 17alpha-hydroxycorticosterone and a sodium retaining factor in human fetal adrenal glands. *Endocrinology* **58**: 626–633.

BOCHSKANL, R. and KIRCHNER, C. (1981) Uteroglobin and the accumulation of progesterone in the uterine lumen of the rabbit. *Wilhelm Roux Arch. Dev. Biol.* **190**: 127–131.

BOCHSKANL, R., THIE, M. and KIRCHNER, C. (1984) Progesterone dependent uptake of uteroglobin by rabbit endometrium. *Histochemistry* **80**: 581–589.

BOGGARAM, V. and MENDELSON, C. R. (1988) Transcriptional regulation of the gene encoding the major surfactant protein (SP-A) in rabbit fetal lung. *J. Biol. Chem.* **263**: 19060–19065.

BOGGARAM, V., QING, K. and MENDELSON, C. R. (1988) The major apoprotein of rabbit pulmonary surfactant. Elucidation of primary sequence and cyclic AMP and developmental regulation. *J. Biol. Chem.* **263**: 2939–2947.

BOGOVICH, K., RICHARDS, J. S. and REICHERT, L. E. Jr. (1981) Obligatory role of luteinizing hormone (LH) in the initiation of preovulatory follicular growth in the pregnant rat: specific effects of human chorionic gonadotropin and follicle-stimulating hormone on LH receptors and steroidogenesis in theca, granulosa, and luteal cells. *Endocrinology* **109**: 860–867.

BOHNET, H. G., GOMEZ, F. and FRIESEN, H. G. (1977) Prolactin and estrogen binding sites in the mammary gland of the lactating and non-lactating rat. *Endocrinology* **101**: 1111–1121.

BOLANDER, F. F. and TOPPER, Y. T. (1981) Loss of differentiative potential of the mammary gland in ovariectomized mice; identification of a biochemical lesion. *Endocrinology* **108**: 1649–1653.

BORLAND, R. M., ERICKSON, G. F. and DUCIBELLA T. (1977) Accumulation of steroids in rabbit preimplantation blatocysts. *J. Reprod. Fertil.* **49:** 219–224.

BOURBON, J., GILBERT, M. and JOST, A. (1979) Glucocorticosteroid receptors in the liver of normal and decapitated rabbit foetuses. *J. Endocr.* **81:** 291–297.

BOURBON, J. R., FARRELL, P. M., DOUCET, E., BROWN, D. J. and VALENZA, C. (1987) Biochemical maturation of fetal rat lung: a comprehensive study including surfactant determination. *Biol. Neonate* **52:** 48–60.

BRANHAM, W. S., SHEEHAN, D. M., ZEHR, D. R., RIDLON, E. and NELSON, C. J. (1985) The postnatal ontogeny of rat uterine glands and age-related effects of 17β-estradiol. *Endocrinology* **117:** 2229–2237.

BRESCIANI, F. (1965) Effect of ovarian hormones on duration of DNA synthesis of the C3H mouse mammary gland. *Exp. Cell Res.* **38:** 13–32.

BRINKMANN, A. O. and VAN STRAALEN, R. J. C. (1979) Development of the LH-response in fetal guinea pig testes. *Biol. Reprod.* **21:** 991–997.

BRODIE, J. Y. and GREEN, B. (1978) Progesterone binding in rat uterine cytosol during early pregnancy. *Biochem. Soc. Trans.* **6:** 773–775.

BRÖNNEGARD, M. and OKRET, S. (1988) Characterization of the glucocorticoid receptor in fetal rat lung during development: Influence of proteolytic activity. *J. Steroid Biochem.* **31:** 809–817.

BROWN, G. P. and VENUTO, R. C. (1986) Angiotensin II receptor alterations during pregnancy in rabbits. *Am. J. Physiol.* **251:** E58–E64.

BROWN-GRANT, K. and SHERWOOD, M. R. (1971) The "early androgen syndrome" in the guinea pig. *J. Endocr.* **49:** 277–291.

BROWNE, C. A. and THORBURN, G. D. (1989) Endocrine control of fetal growth. *Biol. Neonate* **55:** 331–346.

BUDY, A. M. (1955) Metabolism, excretion and retention of ^{14}C-labeled estrone in immature mice. *Arch. Int. Pharmacodyn.* **103:** 435–452.

BULLOCK, D. W. (1980) Uterine proteins as markers of progesterone action. In: *Steroid Induced Uterine Proteins. Developments in Endocrinology*, Vol. 8, Beato, M. (Ed.), Elsevier North Holland Biomedical Press, Amsterdam, pp. 315–350.

BURT, R. L. and DAVIDSON, I. W. F. (1974) Insulin half-life and utilization in normal pregnancy. *Obstet. Gynecol.* **43:** 161–170.

BURWEN, S. J. and JONES, A. L. (1987) The association of polypeptide hormones and growth factors with the nuclei of target cells. *Trends in Biochem. Sci.* **12:** 159–162.

BUTCHER, R. L., COLLINS, W. E. and FUGO, N. W. (1974) Plasma concentration of LH, FSH, prolactin, progesterone and estradiol-17β throughout the 4-day estrous cycle of the rat. *Endocrinology* **94:** 1704–1708.

BUTLER, S. R., HURLEY, T. W., SCHANBERG, S. M. and HANDWERGER, S. (1978) Ovine placental lactogen stimulation of ornithine decarboxylase activity in brain and liver of neonatal rats. *Life Sci.* **22:** 2073–2078.

CADMAN, H. F. and WALLIS, M. (1981) An investigation of sites that bind human somatotropin (growth hormone) in the liver of the pregnant rabbit. *Biochem. J.* **198:** 605–614.

CAKE, M. H., YEOH, G., OLIVER, I. T. and LITWACK, G. (1980) Developmental changes in the glucocorticoid induction of hepatic tyrosine aminotransferase. In: *The Development of Responsiveness to Steroid Hormones, Advances in the Biosciences*, Vol. 25, Kaye, A. M. and Kaye, M. (Eds), Pergamon Press, Oxford, pp. 263–272.

CAKE, M. H., YEOH, G. C. T. and OLIVER, I. T. (1981) Ontogeny of the glucocorticoid receptor and its relationship to tyrosine aminotransferase induction in cultured foetal hepatocytes. *Biochem. J.* **198:** 301–307.

CAMPICHE, M. A., GAUTIER, A., HERNANDEZ, E. I. and REYMOND, A. (1963) An electron microscope study of the fetal development of human lung. *Pediatrics* **32:** 976–994.

CAPUCO, A. V., FELDHOFF, P. A., AKERS, R. M., WITTLIFF, J. L. and TUCKER, H. A. (1982)

Progestin binding in mammary tissue of prepartum, nonlactating and postpartum, lactating cows. *Steroids* **40:** 503–517.

CARR, D. and FRIESEN, H. G. (1976) Growth hormone and insulin binding to human liver. *J. Clin. Endo. Metab.* **42:** 482–493.

CARTER, J. (1976) The effect of progesterone, oestradiol and HCG on cell mediated immunity in pregnant mice. *J. Reprod. Fertil.* **46:** 211–216.

CATT, K. J., DUFAU, M. L. and TSURUHARA, T. (1971) Studies on a radioligand-receptor assay system for luteinizing hormone and chorionic gonadotropin. *J. Clin. Endocr. Metab.* **32:** 860–863.

CATT, K. J., DUFAU, M. L. and TSURUHARA, T. (1972) Radioligand-receptor assay of luteinizing hormone and chorionic gonadotropin. *J. Clin. Endocr. Metab.* **34:** 123–132.

CATT, K. J., DUFAU, M. L., NEAVES, W. B., WALSH, P. C. and WILSON, J. D. (1975) LH-hCG receptors and testosterone content during differentiation of the testis in the rabbit embryo. *Endocrinology* **97:** 1157–1165.

CHAFOULEAS, J. G., GUERRIERO, V. and MEANS, A. R. (1982) Possible regulatory roles of calmodulin and myosin light chain kinase in secretion. In: *Cellular Regulation of Secretion and Release*, Conn, P. M. (Ed.), Academic Press, New York, pp. 445–458.

CHALLIS, J. R. G., HEAP, R. B. and ILLINGWORTH, D. V. (1971) Concentrations of oestrogen and progesterone in the plasma of non-pregnant, pregnant and lactating guinea-pigs. *J. Endocr.* **51:** 333–345.

CHALLIS, J. R. G., DAVIES, I. J. and RYAN, K. J. (1973) The concentrations of progesterone, estrone and estradiol-17β in the plasma of pregnant rabbits. *Endocrinology* **93:** 971–976.

CHALLIS, J. R. G., KENDALL, J. Z., ROBINSON, J. S. and THORBURN, G. D. (1977) The regulation of corticosteroids during late pregnancy and their role in parturition. *Biol. Reprod.* **16:** 57–69.

CHALLIS, J. R. G., HUHTANEN, D., SPRAGUE, C., MITCHELL, B. F. and LYE, S. J. (1985) Modulation by cortisol of adrenocorticotropin-induced activation of adrenal function in fetal sheep. *Endocrinology* **116:** 2267–2272.

CHAMBON, Y. (1949) Besoins endocriniens qualitatifs et quantitatifs de l'ovoimplantation chez la lapine. *C. R. Soc. Biol. d'Alger* **143:** 1172–1175.

CHAN, J. S. D., ROBERTSON, H. A. and FRIESEN, H. G. (1978) Distribution of binding sites for ovine placental lactogen in the sheep. *Endocrinology* **102:** 632–640.

CHANG, C., KOKONTIS, J. and LIAO, S. (1988) Molecular cloning of human and rat complementary DNA encoding androgen receptors. *Science* **240:** 324–326.

CHANNING, C. P. and KAMMERMAN, S. (1973) Characteristics of gonadotropin receptors of porcine granulosa cells during follicle maturation. *Endocrinology* **92:** 531–540.

CHAPMAN, R. G., HOPKINS, P. S. and THORBURN, G. D. (1974) The effects of foetal thyroidectomy and thyroxine administration on the development of the skin and wool follicles of sheep foetuses. *J. Anat.* **117:** 419–432.

CHARD, T. (1983) Human placental lactogen. In: *The Endocrinology of Pregnancy and Parturition*, Martini, L. and James, V. H. T. (Eds), Academic Press, London, pp. 167–191.

CHATELAIN, A., DUPOUY, J. P. and DUBOIS, M. P. (1979) Ontogenesis of cells producing polypeptide hormones (ACTH, MSH, LPH, GH, prolactin) in the fetal hypophysis of the rat: influence of the hypothalamus. *Cell Tissue Res.* **196:** 409–427.

CHATTERTON, R. T. Jr., HARRIS, J. A., KING, W. J. and WYNN, R. M. (1979) Ultrastructural alterations in mammary glands of pregnant rats after ovariectomy and hysterectomy: effects of adrenal steroids and prolactin. *Am. J. Obstet. Gynecol.* **133:** 694–702.

CHENG, K. W. (1976) Changes in rat ovaries of specific binding for LH, FSH and prolactin during the oestrous cycle and pregnancy. *J. Reprod. Fert.* **48:** 129–135.

CHEW, C. S. and RENARD, G. A. (1979) Glycogen levels in the rat myometrium at the end of pregnancy and immediately postpartum. *Biol. Reprod.* **20:** 1111–1114.

CHIAPPA, S. A. and FINK, G. (1977) Releasing factor and hormonal changes in the hypothalamic-pituitary gonadotrophin and adrenocorticotrophin systems before and after birth and puberty in male, female, and androgenized rats. *J. Endocr.* **72:** 211–224.

CHILTON B. S., WILLIAMS N. D., COBB A. D. and LEAVITT W. W. (1987) Ligand-receptor dissociation: a potential mechanism for the attenuation of estrogen action in the juvenile rabbit uterus. *Endocrinology* **120:** 750–757.

CHOPRA, I. J., SACK, J. and FISHER, D. A. (1975) 3,3',5'-Triiodothyronine (reverse T3) and 3,3',5-triiodothyronine (T3) in fetal and adult sheep: studies of metabolic clearance rates, production rates, serum binding, and thyroidal content relative to thyroxine. *Endocrinology* **97:** 1080–1088.

CHOWDHURY, M. and STEINBERGER, E. (1976) Pituitary and plasma levels of gonadotrophins in foetal and newborn male and female rats. *J. Endocr.* **69:** 381–384.

CHRISTENSEN, L. W. and GORSKI, R. A. (1978) Independent masculinization of neuroendocrine systems by intracerebral implants of testosterone or estradiol in the neonatal female rat. *Brain Res.* **146:** 325–340.

CLAPPER, D. L. and CONN, P. M. (1985) Gonadotropin-releasing hormone stimulation of pituitary gonadotrope cells produces an increase in intracellular calcium. *Biol. Reprod.* **32:** 269–278.

CLARK, J. H. and GORSKI, J. (1970) Ontogeny of the estrogen receptor during early uterine development. *Science* **169:** 76–78.

CLARK, J. H. and MARKAVERICH, B. M. (1988) Actions of ovarian steroid hormones. In: *The Physiology of Reproduction*, Vol. 1, Knobil, E. and Neill, J. D. (Eds), Raven Press, New York, pp. 675–724.

CLARK, J. H. and PECK, E. J. Jr. (1979) *Female Sex Steroids. Receptors and Function. Monographs on Endocrinology*, Vol. 14, Gross, F., Grumbach, M. M., Labhard, A., Lipsett, M. B., Mann, T., Samuels, L. T. and Zander, J. (Eds), Springer-Verlag, Berlin, pp. 70–134.

CLARK, J. H., ANDERSON, J. and PECK, E. J. Jr. (1972) Receptor-estrogen complex in the nuclear fraction of rat uterine cells during the estrous cycle. *Science* **176:** 528–530.

CLARK, J. H., HSUEH, A. J. W. and PECK, E. J. Jr. (1977a) Regulation of estrogen receptor replenishment by progesterone. *Ann. N. Y. Acad. Sci.* **286:** 161–179.

CLARK, J. H., PASZKO, Z. and PECK, E. J. Jr. (1977b) Nuclear binding and retention of the receptor estrogen complex: relation to the agonistic and antagonistic properties of estriol. *Endocrinology* **100:** 91–96.

CLAYTON, R. N. and CATT, K. J. (1981) Gonadotropin-releasing hormone receptors: characterization, physiological regulation, and relationship to reproductive function. *Endocr. Rev.* **2:** 186–209.

CLAYTON, R. N., KATIKINEMI, M., CHAN, V., DUFAU, M. L. and CATT, K. J. (1980) Direct inhibition of testicular function by gonadotropin-releasing hormone mediation by specific gonadotropin releasing hormone receptors in interstitial cells. *Proc. Natl Acad. Sci. USA* **77:** 4459–4463.

CLEMENTS, J. A., REYES, F. I., WINTER, J. S. D. and FAIMAN, C. (1976) Studies on human sexual development. III. Fetal pituitary and serum, and amniotic fluid concentrations of LH, CG, and FSH. *J. Clin. Endocr. Metab.* **42:** 9–19.

COIRO, V., BRAVERMAN, L. E., CHRISTIANSON, D., FANG, S. L. and GOODMAN H. M. (1979) Effect of hypothyroidism and thyroxine replacement on growth hormone in the rat. *Endocrinology* **105:** 641–646.

COLOSI, P., MARR, G., LOPEZ, J., HARO, L., OGREN, L. and TALAMANTES, F. (1982) Isolation, purification, and characterization of mouse placental lactogen. *Proc. Natl Acad. Sci. USA* **79:** 771–775.

COLOSI, P., OGREN, L., THORDARSON, G. and TALAMANTES, F. (1987) Purification and partial characterization of two prolactin-like glycoprotein hormone complexes from the midpregnant mouse conceptus. *Endocrinology* **120:** 2500–2511.

COMB, M., BIRNBERG, N. C., SEASHOLTZ, A., HERBERT, E. and GOODMAN, H. M. (1986) A cyclic AMP- and phorbol ester-inducible DNA element. *Nature* **323:** 353–356.

CONN, P. M. (1986) The molecular basis of gonadotropin-releasing hormone action. *Endocrine Rev.* **7:** 3–10.

CONTI, M., HARWOOD, J. P., DUFAU, M. L. and CATT, K. J. (1977) Regulation of luteinizing hormone receptors and adenylate cyclase activity by gonadotropin in the rat ovary. *Mol. Pharmacol.* **13:** 1024–1032.

CORVOL, P., FALK, R., FREIFELD, M. and BARDIN, C. W. (1972) In vitro studies of progesterone binding protein in guinea pig uterus. *Endocrinology* **90:** 1464–1469.

CRABBÉ, J. (1977) The mechanism of action of aldosterone. In: *Receptors and Mechanism of Action of Steroid Hormones, Part II, Modern Pharmacology-Toxicology*, Vol. 8, Pasqualini, J. R. (Ed.), Marcel Dekker, Inc., New York, pp. 513–568.

CROSS, B. A. and HARRIS, G. W. (1952) The role of the neurohypophysis in the milk-ejection reflex. *J. Endocr.* **8:** 148–161.

CSAPO, A. I. and TAKEDA, H. (1965) Effect of progesterone on the electrical activity and intrauterine pressure of pregnant and parturient rabbits. *Am. J. Obstet. Gynecol.* **91:** 221–231.

CUATRECASAS, P. (1972) Isolation of the insulin receptor of liver and fat-cell membranes. *Proc. Natl Acad. Sci. USA* **69:** 318–322.

CUNHA, G. R. and FUJII, H. (1981) Stromal-parenchymal interactions in normal and abnormal development of the genital tract. In: *Developmental Effects of Diethylstilbestrol (DES) in Pregnancy*, Herbst, A. and Bern, H. A. (Eds), Thieme-Stratton, Inc., New York, pp. 179–193.

CUNHA, G. R. and LUNG, B. (1978) The possible influence of temporal factors in androgenic responsiveness of urogenital tissue recombinants from wild-type and androgen-insensitive (TFM) mice. *J. Exp. Zool.* **205:** 181–194.

CUNHA, G. R., CHUNG, L. W. K., SHANNON, J. M. and REESE, B. A. (1980a) Stromal-epithelial interactions in sex differentiation. *Biol. Reprod.* **22:** 19–42.

CUNHA, G. R., LUNG, B. and REESE, B. (1980b) Glandular epithelial induction by embryonic mesenchyme in adult bladder epithelium of Balb/c mice. *Invest. Utrol.* **17:** 302–304.

CUNHA, G. R., REESE, B. A. and SEKKINGSTAD, M. (1980c) Induction of nuclear androgen-binding sites in epithelium of the embryonic urinary bladder by mesenchyme of the urogenital sinus of embryonic mice. *Endocrinology* **107:** 1767–1770.

CUNHA, G. R., SHANNON, J. M., NEUBAUER, B. L., SAWYER, L. M., FUJII, H., TAGUCHI, O. and CHUNG, L. W. K. (1981) Mesenchymal-epithelial interactions in sex differentiation. *Human Genet.* **56:** 68–77.

CUNHA, G. R., SHANNON, J. M., VANDERSLICE K. D., SEKKINGSTAD, M. and ROBBOY, S. J. (1982) Autoradiographic analysis of nuclear estrogen binding sites during postnatal development of the genital tract of female mice. *J. Steroid Biochem.* **17:** 281–286.

CUNHA, G. R., BIGSBY R. M., COOKE, P. S. and SUGIMURA Y. (1985) Stromal-epithelial interactions in the determination of hormonal responsiveness. In: *Estrogens in the Environment. II. Influences on Development*, J. A. McLachlan (Ed.), Elsevier, New York, pp. 273–287.

CURLEWIS, J. D. and STONE, G. M. (1986) Effects of oestradiol, the oestrous cycle and pregnancy on weight, metabolism and cytosol receptors in the uterus of the brush-tail possum (*Trichosurus vulpecula*). *J. Endocr.* **198:** 201–210.

CURRIE, A. J., FRASER, H. M. and SHARPE, R. M. (1981) Human placental receptors for luteinizing hormone releasing hormone. *Biochem. Biophys. Res. Commun.* **99:** 332–338.

DALLE, M. and DELOST, P. (1976) Plasma and adrenal cortisol concentrations in foetal, newborn and mother guinea pigs during the perinatal period. *J. Endocr.* **70:** 207–214.

DARBEIDA, J. and DURAND, P. (1987) Glucocorticoid enhancement of adrenocorticotropin-induced 3′,5′-cyclic adenosine monophosphate production by cultured ovine adrenocortical cells. *Endocrinology* **121:** 1051–1055.

DAVIES, I. J. and RYAN, K. J. (1972) Comparative endocrinology of gestation. *Vit. Horm.* **30:** 223–279.

DAVIES, I. J., CHALLIS, J. R. G. and RYAN, K. J. (1974) Progesterone receptors in the myometrium of pregnant rabbits. *Endocrinology* **95:** 165–173.

DAVIES, I. J., NAFTOLIN, F., RYAN, K. J. and SIU, J. (1975) A specific, high-affinity, limited-capacity estrogen binding component in the cytosol of human fetal pituitary and brain tissues. *J. Clin. Endocr. Metab.* **40:** 909–912.

DAVIS, J. W., WIKMAN-COFFELT, J. and EDDINGTON, C. L. (1972) The effect of progesterone on biosynthetic pathways in mammary tissue. *Endocrinology* **91:** 1011–1019.

DEAL, C. L. and GUYDA, H. J. (1983) Insulin receptors of human term placental cells and choriocarcinoma (JEG-3) cells: characteristics and regulation. *Endocrinology* **112:** 1512–1523.

DEAVER, D. R. and GUTHRIE, H. D. (1980) Cytoplasmic estrogen receptor, estradiol and progesterone concentrations in endometrium of nonpregnant and pregnant pigs. *Biol. Reprod.* **23:** 72–77.

DeCICCO NARDONE, F., D'AURIZIO, G. M., MORI, P., LUPI, G., VITALE, A. M. and DELL' ACQUA, S. (1984) Androgen binding in human fetal amnion. *J. Steroid Biochem.* **20:** 495–499.

DeFESI, C. E. R., ASTIER, H. S. and SURKS, M. I. (1979) Kinetics of thyrotrophs somatotrophs during development of hypothyroidism and L-triiodothyronine treatment of hypothyroid rats. *Endocrinology* **104:** 1172–1180.

DeHERTOGH R., EKKA E., VANDERHEYDEN I. and GLORIEUX B. (1986) Estrogen and progestogen receptors in the implantation sites and interembryonic segments of rat uterus endometrium and myometrium. *Endocrinology* **119:** 680–684.

DeKRESTER, D. M., CATT, K. J., BURGER, H. G. and SMITH, G. C. (1969) Radioautographic studies on the localization of ^{125}I-labelled human luteinizing and growth hormone in immature male rats. *J. Endocr.* **43:** 105–111.

DeKRESTER, D. M., CATT, K. J. and PAULSEN, C. A. (1971) Studies on the in vitro testicular binding of iodinated luteinizing hormone in rats. *Endocrinology* **88:** 332–337.

De LAUZON, S., UHRICH, F., VANDEL, S., CITTANOVA, N. and JAYLE, M. F. (1974) Determination of progesterone and of free and conjugated estrogens in pregnant and pseudo-pregnant rats. *Steroids* **24:** 31–40.

DEMERS, L. M., GABBE, S. G., VILLEE, C. A. and GREEP, R. O. (1972) The effects of insulin on human placental glycogenesis. *Endocrinology* **91:** 270–275.

DENAMUR, R. (1971) Hormonal control of lactogenesis. *J. Dairy Res.* **38:** 237–264.

DENAMUR, R. and DeLOUIS, C. (1972) Effects of progesterone and prolactin on the secretory activity and the nucleic acid content of the mammary gland of pregnant rabbits. *Acta Endocr. (Copenh.)* **70:** 603–618.

DENIS, M., POELLINGER, L., WIKSTRÖM, A. C. and GUSTAFSSON, J. A. (1988) Requirement of hormone for thermal conversion of the glucocorticoid receptor to a DNA-binding state. *Nature* **333:** 686–688.

DEVASKAR, S. U., GRIM, P. F. III and DEVASKAR, U. P. (1985) A differential effect of thyroxine and glucocorticoids on fetal brain and heart insulin receptor. *Pediatric Res.* **19:** 192–198.

DEY, S. K., DICKMANN, Z. and GUPTA, J. S. (1976) Evidence that the maintenance of early pregnancy in the rabbit requires "blastocyst estrogen". *Steroids* **28:** 481–485.

DHANIREDDY, R. and ULANE, R. E. (1984) Prolactin binding in the developing rat fetal liver. *Life Sci.* **35:** 733–740.

DHINDSA, D. S. and DZIUK, P. J. (1968) Effect on pregnancy in the pig after killing embryos or fetuses in one uterine horn in early gestation. *J. Anim. Sci.* **27:** 122–126.

DIAMOND, M., RUST, N. and WESTPHAL, U. (1969) High affinity binding of progesterone, testosterone and cortisol in normal and androgen-treated guinea-pigs during various reproductive stages (relationship to masculinization). *Endocrinology* **84:** 1143–1151.

DICKEY, R. P. and ROBERTSON, A. F. (1969) Newborn estrogen excretion. Its relationship to sex, birth weight, maternal complications, and idiopathic respiratory distress syndrome. *Am. J. Obstet. Gynecol.* **104:** 551–555.

DICKMANN, Z., DEY, S. K. and SEN GUPTA, J. (1975) Steroidogenesis in rabbit pre-implantation embryos. *Proc. Natl Acad. Sci. U.S.A.* **72:** 298–300.

DICKMANN, Z., DEY, S. K. and SEN GUPTA, J. (1976) A new concept: control of early pregnancy by steroid hormones originating in the pre-implantation embryo. *Vit. Horm.* **34:** 215–242.

DJIANE, J., DURAND, P. and KELLY, P. A. (1977) Evolution of prolactin receptors in rabbit mammary gland during pregnancy and lactation. *Endocrinology* **100:** 1348–1356.

DOBBING, J. and SANDS, J. (1970) Timing of neuroblast multiplication in developing human brain. *Nature* **226:** 639–640.

DÖHLER, K. D. and WUTTKE, W. (1975) Changes with age in levels of serum gonadotropins, prolactin, and gonadal steroids in prepubertal male and female rats. *Endocrinology* **97:** 898–907.

DORRINGTON, J. H., MOON, Y. S. and ARMSTRONG, D. T. (1975) Estradiol-17 beta biosynthesis in cultured granulosa cells from hypophysectomized immature rats: stimulation by follicle stimulating hormone. *Endocrinology* **97:** 1328–1331.

DOWNING, S. J. and SHERWOOD, O. D. (1985a) The physiological role of relaxin in the pregnant rat. I. The influence of relaxin on parturition. *Endocrinology* **116:** 1200–1205.

DOWNING, S. J. and SHERWOOD, O. D. (1985b) The physiological role of relaxin in the pregnant rat. II. The influence of relaxin on uterine contractile activity. *Endocrinology* **116:** 1206–1214.

DOWNING, S. J. and SHERWOOD, O. D. (1985c) The physiological role of relaxin in the pregnant rat. III. The influence of relaxin on cervical extensibility. *Endocrinology* **116:** 1215–1220.

DREWS, U. and DREWS, U. (1977) Regression of mouse mammary gland anlagen in recombinants of TFM and wild-type tissues: testosterone acts via the mesenchyme. *Cell* **10:** 401–404.

DUFAU, M. L. and CATT, K. J. (1978) Gonadotropin receptors and regulation of steroidogenesis in testis and ovary. *Vit. Horm.* **36:** 461–592.

DUFAU, M. L. and KNOX, G. F. (1985) Fetal Leydig cell culture—an in vitro system for the study of trophic hormone and GnRH receptors and actions. *J. Steroid Biochem.* **23:** 743–755.

DUFAU, M. L. and KUSUDA, S. (1987) Purification and characterization of ovarian LH/hCG and prolactin receptors. *J. Receptor Res.* **7:** 167–193.

DUFAU, M. L. and VILLÉE, D. B. (1969) Aldosterone biosynthesis by human fetal adrenals "in vitro". *Biochim. Biophys. Acta* **176:** 637–640.

DUFAU, M. L., WINTERS, C. A., HATTORI, M., AQUILANO, D., BARANAO, L., NOZU, K., BAUKAL, A. and CATT, K. J. (1984) Hormonal regulation of androgen production by the Leydig cell. *J. Steroid Biochem.* **20:** 161–173.

DUPOUY, J. P., COFFIGNY, H. and MAGRE, S. (1975) Maternal and foetal corticosterone levels during late pregnancy in rats. *J. Endocr.* **65:** 347–352.

DURAND, P. (1979) ACTH receptor levels in lamb adrenals at late gestation and early neonatal stages. *Biol. Reprod.* **20:** 837–845.

DURAND, P., BOSC, M. J. and LOCATELLI, A. (1980) Adrenal maturation of the sheep fetus during late pregnancy. *Reprod. Nutr. Dévelop.* **20:** 339–347.

DURAND, P., CATHIARD, A.-M., MORERA, A.-M., DAZORD, A. and SAEZ, J. M. (1981) Maturation of adrenocorticotropin-sensitive adenylate cyclase of ovine fetal adrenal during late pregnancy. *Endocrinology* **108:** 2114–2119.

DÜRNBERGER, H. and KRATOCHWIL, K. (1980) Specificity of tissue interaction and origin of mesenchymal cells in the androgen response of the embryonic mammary gland. *Cell* **19:** 465–471.

DUVAL, D., DARDENNE, M., DAUSSE, J. P. and HOMO, F. (1977) Glucocorticoid receptors in corticosensitive and corticoresistant thymocyte subpopulations. II. Studies with hydrocortisone treated mice. *Biochim. Biophys. Acta* **496:** 312–320.

DUVAL, D., DARDENNE, M. and HOMO, F. (1979) Glucocorticoid receptors in thymocytes of fetus, newborn, and adult CBA mice. *Endocrinology* **104:** 1152–1157.

EHRLICH, P. (1913) Chemotherapeutics: scientific principles, methods, and results. *Lancet* **ii:** 445–451.

EIDE, A., HOISAETER, P. Å. and KVINNSLAND, S. (1975) Estradiol receptor in uterine tissue from neonatal mice. Influence by cyclic AMP. *J. Steroid Biochem.* **6:** 1121–1125.

EKELUND, L., ARVIDSON, G. and ASTEDT, B. (1975a) Cortisol-induced accumulation of phospholipids in organ culture of human fetal lung. *Scand. J. Clin. Lab. Invest.* **35:** 419–423.

EKELUND, L., ARVIDSON, G., EMANUELSSON, H., MYHRBERG, H. and ASTEDT, B. (1975b)

Effect of cortisol on human fetal lung in organ culture. A biochemical, electron-microscopic and autoradiographic study. *Cell Tissue Res.* **163**: 263–272.

ELIAS, J. J. (1957) Cultivation of adult mouse mammary gland in hormone-enriched synthetic medium. *Science* **126**: 842–843.

ELLINWOOD, W. E. and RESKO, J. A. (1980) Sex differences in biologically active and immunoreactive gonadotropins in the fetal circulation of rhesus monkeys. *Endocrinology* **107**: 902–907.

ELLIS, D., TUROCY, J. F., SWEENEY, W. E. Jr. and AVNER, E. D. (1986) Partial characterization and ontogeny of renal cytosolic glucocorticoid receptors in mouse kidney. *J. Steroid Biochem.* **24**: 997–1003.

EMANE, P. N'G., DeLOUIS, C., KELLY, P. A. and DJIANE, J. (1986) Evolution of prolactin and placental lactogen receptors in ewes during pregnancy and lactation. *Endocrinology* **118**: 695–700.

ERDOS, T. and FRIÈS, J. (1979) The endometrial nuclear estradiol receptor of the pregnant cow has a molecular weight of 53 000 in 6 M guanidine-HCl. *Mol. Cell. Endocr.* **13**: 203–209.

ERENBERG, A., OMORI, K., MENKES, J. H., OH, W. and FISHER, D. A. (1974) Growth and development of the thyroidectomized ovine fetus. *Pediat. Res.* **8**: 783–789.

ERICKSON, G. F. and RYAN, K. J. (1976) Stimulation of testosterone production in isolated rabbit thecal tissue by LH/FSH, dibutyryl cyclic AMP, PGF 2α and PGE2. *Endocrinology* **99**: 452–458.

EVANS, R. M. (1988) The steroid and thyroid hormone receptor superfamily. *Science* **240**: 889–895.

EVANS, R. W., CHEN, T. J., HENDRY, W. J. III and LEAVITT, W. W. (1980) Progesterone regulation of estrogen receptor in the hamster uterus during the estrous cycle. *Endocrinology* **107**: 383–390.

FAJER, A. B. and BARRACLOUGH, C. A. (1967) Ovarian secretion of progesterone and 20α-hydroxy-pregn-4-en-3-one during pseudopregnancy and pregnancy in rats. *Endocrinology* **81**: 617–622.

FALCK, B. (1959) Site of production of oestrogen in rat ovary as studied by microtransplants. *Acta Physiol. Scand.* **47** (Suppl. 163): 1–101.

FANG, S., ANDERSON, K. M. and LIAO S. (1969) Receptor proteins for androgens. On the role of specific proteins in selective retention of 17β-hydroxy- 5a-androstan-3-one by rat ventral prostate in vivo and in vitro. *J. Biol. Chem.* **244**: 6584–6595.

FARRELL, P. M. (1977) Fetal lung development and the influence of glucocorticoids on pulmonary surfactant. *J. Steroid Biochem.* **8**: 463–470.

FARRELL, P. M. and AVERY, M. E. (1975) Hyaline membrane disease. *Am. Rev. Resp. Dis.* **3**: 657–688.

FARRELL, P. M. and HAMOSH, M. (1978) The biochemistry of lung development. *Clin. Perinatol.* **5**: 197–229.

FARRELL, P. M. and WOOD, R. E. (1976) Epidemiology of hyaline membrane disease in the United States: Analysis of national mortality statistics. *Pediatrics* **58**: 167–176.

FARRELL, P. M. and ZACHMAN, R. D. (1973) Induction of choline phosphotransferase and lecithin synthesis in the fetal lung by corticosteroids. *Science* **179**: 297–298.

FARRELL, P. M., LUNDGREN, D. W. and ADAMS, A. J. (1974) Choline kinase and choline phosphotransferase in developing rat lung. *Biochem. Biophys. Res. Commun.* **57**: 696–701.

FEHERTY, P., ROBERTSON, D. M., WAYNWORTH, H. B. and KELLIE, A. E. (1970) Changes in the concentration of high affinity oestradiol receptors in rat uterine supernatant preparations during the oestrous cycle, pseudopregnancy, pregnancy, maturation and after ovariectomy. *Biochem. J.* **120**: 837–844.

FEIL, P. D., GLASSER, S. R., TOFT, D. O. and O'MALLEY, B. W. (1972) Progesterone binding in the mouse and rat uterus. *Endocrinology* **91**: 738–746.

FELDMAN, D. (1974) Ontogeny of rat hepatic glucocorticoid receptors. *Endocrinology* **95**: 1219–1227.

FELDMAN, S. C. and BLOCH, E. (1978) Developmental pattern of testosterone synthesis by fetal rat testes in response to luteinizing hormone. *Endocrinology* **102**: 999–1007.

FERREIRO, B., BERNAL, J. and POTTER, B. J. (1987) Ontogenesis of thyroid hormone receptor in foetal lambs. *Acta Endocr. (Copenh.)* **116**: 205–210.

FINN, C. A. and MARTIN, L. (1970) The role of the oestrogens secreted before oestrus in the preparation of the uterus for implantation in the mouse. *J. Endocr.* **47:** 431–438.

FINN, C. A. and MARTIN, L. (1973) Endocrine control of gland proliferation in the mouse uterus. *Biol. Reprod.* **8:** 585–588.

FINN, R., St. HILL, C. A., GOVAN, A. J., RALFS, I. G., GURNEY, F. J. and DENYE, V. (1972) Immunological responses in pregnancy and survival of foetal homograft. *Br. Med. J.* **3:** 150–152.

FISHER, D. A. and KLEIN, A. H. (1981) Thyroid development and disorders of thyroid function in the newborn. *New Eng. J. Med.* **304:** 702–712.

FLINT, A. P. F. and BURTON, R. D. (1984) Properties and ontogeny of the glucocorticoid receptor in the placenta and fetal lung of the sheep. *J. Endocr.* **103:** 31–42.

FLINT, D. J. (1982) Regulation of insulin receptors by prolactin in lactating rat mammary gland. *J. Endocr.* **93:** 279–285.

FLINT, D. J., SINNETT-SMITH, P. A., CLEGG, R. A. and VERNON, R. G. (1979) Role of insulin receptors in the changing metabolism of adipose tissue during pregnancy and lactation in the rat. *Biochem. J.* **182:** 421–427.

FLOCKHARD, D. A. and CORBIN, J. D. (1982) Regulatory mechanisms in the control of protein kinases. *CRC Crit. Rev. Biochem.* **12:** 133–186.

FLUG, F., COPP, R. P., CASANOVA, J., HOROWITZ, Z. D., JANOCKO, L., PLOTNICK, M., SAMUELS, H. H. (1987) Cis-acting elements of the rat growth hormone gene which mediate basal and regulated expression by thyroid hormone. *J. Biol. Chem.* **262:** 6373–6382.

FRAWLEY, L. S., HOEFFLER, J. P. and BOOCKFOR, F. R. (1985) Functional maturation of somatotropes in fetal rat pituitaries: analysis by reverse hemolytic plaque assay. *Endocrinology* **116:** 2355–2360.

FREEMAN, C. S. and TOPPER, Y. J. (1978) Progesterone is not essential to the differentiative potential of mammary epithelium in the male mouse. *Endocrinology* **103:** 186–192.

FREEMARK, M. and HANDWERGER, S. (1982) Ovine placental lactogen stimulates amino acid transport in rat diaphragm. *Endocrinology* **110:** 2201–2203.

FREEMARK, M. and HANDWERGER, S. (1983) Ovine placental lactogen, but not growth hormone, stimulates amino acid transport in fetal rat diaphragm. *Endocrinology* **112:** 402–404.

FREEMARK, M. and HANDWERGER, S. (1986) The glycogenic effects of placental lactogen and growth hormone in ovine fetal liver are mediated through binding to specific fetal ovine placental lactogen receptors. *Endocrinology* **118:** 613–618.

FREEMARK, M., COMER, M. and HANDWERGER, S. (1986) Placental lactogen and growth hormone receptors in sheep liver: striking differences in ontogeny and function. *Am. J. Physiol.* **251:** E328–E333.

FREEMARK, M., COMER, M., KORNER, G. and HANDWERGER, S. (1987) A unique placental lactogen receptor: implications for fetal growth. *Endocrinology* **120:** 1865–1872.

FRIEDMAN, W. J., McEWEN, B. S., TORAN-ALLERAND, C. D. and GERLACH, J. L. (1983) Perinatal development of hypothalamic and cortical estrogen receptors in mouse brain: methodological aspects. *Devel. Brain Res.* **11:** 19–28.

FUCHS, A-R. (1978) Hormonal control of myometrial function during pregnancy and parturition. *Acta endocr. (Copenh.)* **89:** (Suppl. 221) 3–70.

FUCHS, A.-R. and POBLETE, V. F. Jr. (1970) Oxytocin and uterine function in pregnant and parturient rats. *Biol. Reprod.* **2:** 387–400.

FUCHS, A.-R., FUCHS, F., HUSSLEIN, P., SOLOFF, M. S. and FERNSTRÖM, M. J. (1982) Oxytocin receptors and human parturition: a dual role for oxytocin in the initiation of labor. *Science* **215:** 1396–1398.

FUCHS, A.-R., PERIYASAMY, S. and SOLOFF, M. S. (1983a) Systemic and local regulation of oxytocin receptors in the rat uterus, and their functional significance. *Can. J. Biochem. Cell Biol.* **61:** 615–624.

FUCHS, A.-R., PERIYASAMY, S., ALEXANDROVA, M. and SOLOFF, M. S. (1983b) Correlation between oxytocin receptor concentration and responsiveness to oxytocin in pregnant rat myometrium: effects of ovarian steroids. *Endocrinology* **113**: 742–749.

FUCHS, A.-R., FUCHS, F., HUSSLEIN, P. and SOLOFF, M. S. (1984) Oxytocin receptors in the human uterus during pregnancy and parturition. *Am. J. Obst. Gynec.* **150**: 734–741.

FUENTEALBA, B., VERA, R., NIETO, M. and CROXATTO, H. B. (1982) Changes in nuclear estrogen receptor level in the rat oviduct during ovum transport. *Biol. Reprod.* **27**: 12–16.˙

FUJIMORI, K. and YAMADA, M. (1977) In vitro evidence for 17β-estradiol receptor in the human placenta. *Cell. Mol. Biol.* **22**: 357–365.

FUNDER, J. W., FELDMAN, D. and EDELMAN, I. S. (1973) The roles of plasma binding and receptor specificity in the mineralocorticoid action of aldosterone. *Endocrinology* **92**: 994–1004.

FUNKENSTEIN, B., NIMROD, A. and LINDNER, H. R. (1980) The development of steroidogenic capability and responsiveness to gonadotropins in cultured neonatal rat ovaries. *Endocrinology* **106**: 98–106.

GANGNERAU, M-N., FUNKENSTEIN, B. and PICON, R. (1982) LH/hCG receptors and stimulation of testosterone biosynthesis in the rat testis: changes during foetal development in vivo and in vitro. *Mol. Cell. Endocr.* **28**: 499–512.

GANGULI, S., SINHA, M. and SPERLING, M. A. (1984) Ontogeny of insulin and glucagon receptors and the adenylate cyclase system in guinea pig liver. *Pediatric Res.* **18**: 558–565.

GANT, N. F., DALEY, G. L., CHAND, S., WHALLEY, P. J. and MacDONALD, P. C. (1973) A study of angiotensin II pressor response throughout primigravid pregnancy. *J. Clin. Invest.* **52**: 2682–2689.

GARDNER, D. G. and WITTLIFF, J. L. (1973a) Specific estrogen receptors in the lactating mammary gland of the rat. *Biochemistry* **12**: 3090–3096.

GARDNER, D. G. and WITTLIFF, J. L. (1973b) Characterization of distinct glucocorticoid-binding protein in the lactating mammary gland of the rat. *Biochim. Biophys. Acta* **320**: 617–627.

GAUBERT, C-M., BIANCUCCI, S. and SHYAMALA, G. (1982) A comparison of the cytoplasmic estrogen receptors of mammary gland from virgin and lactating mice. *Endocrinology* **110**: 683–685.

GAUBERT, C-M., CARRIERO, R. and SHYAMALA, G. (1986) Relationships between mammary estrogen receptor and estrogenic sensitivity. Molecular properties of cytoplasmic receptor and its binding to deoxyribonucleic acid. *Endocrinology* **118**: 1504–1512.

GELATO, M., MARSHALL, S., BOUDREAU, M., BRUNI, J., CAMPBELL, G. A. and MEITES, J. (1975) Effects of thyroid and ovaries on prolactin binding in rat liver. *Endocrinology* **96**: 1292–1296.

GELLY, C., SUMIDA, C., GULINO, A. and PASQUALINI, J. R. (1981) Concentrations of oestradiol and oestrone in plasma, uterus and other tissues of fetal guinea-pigs: their relationship to uptake and specific binding of ³H-oestradiol. *J. Endocr.* **89**: 71–77.

GEORGE, F. W. and NOBLE, J. F. (1984) Androgen receptors are similar in fetal and adult rabbits. *Endocrinology* **115**: 1451–1458.

GEORGE, F. W. and PETERSON, K. G. (1988) 5α-Dihydrotestosterone formation is necessary for embryogenesis of the rat prostate. *Endocrinology* **122**: 1159–1164.

GEORGE, F. W. and WILSON, J. D. (1978) Estrogen formation in the early rabbit embryo. *Science* **199**: 200–201.

GEORGE, F. W. and WILSON, J. D. (1979) The regulation of androgen and estrogen formation in fetal gonads. *Ann. Biol. Anim. Biochim. Biophys.* **19** (4B): 1297–1306.

GEORGE, F. W., CATT, K. J., NEAVES, W. B. and WILSON, J. D. (1978) Studies on the regulation of testosterone synthesis in the fetal rabbit testis. *Endocrinology* **102**: 665–673.

GERLACH, J. L., McEWEN, B. S., TORAN-ALLERAND, C. D. and FRIEDMAN, W. J. (1983) Perinatal development of estrogen receptors in mouse brain assessed by radioautography, nuclear isolation and receptor assay. *Devel. Brain Res.* **11**: 7–18.

GEYER, H., de GREGORIO, G. and LERNBECHER, G. (1982) Oestrogen and progesterone receptors in the involuting rat uterus. *Acta Endocr. (Copenh.)* **100**: 450–454.

GHOSH, D. and SENGUPTA, J. (1988) Patterns of estrogen and progesterone receptors in rhesus monkey endometrium during secretory phase of normal menstrual cycle and preimplantation stages of gestation. *J. Steroid Biochem.* **31**: 223–229.

GIAMBIAGI, N. and PASQUALINI, J. R. (1982) Immunorecognition of cytosol and nuclear estradiol receptor of fetal guinea pig uterus using monoclonal antibody. *Endocrinology* **110**: 1067–1069.

GIAMBIAGI, N. and PASQUALINI, J. R. (1985) Immunorecognition of the active form of the oestrogen receptor by using a monoclonal antibody. *Biochem. J.* **230**: 203–210.

GIAMBIAGI, N. and PASQUALINI, J. R. (1987) Immunological difference between ribonuclease and temperature, time and salt-induced forms of the estrogen receptor detected by a monoclonal antibody. *Biochem. Biophys. Acta* **931**: 87–93.

GIAMBIAGI, N. and PASQUALINI, J. R. (1988) Interaction of the 8–9 S form of the estrogen receptor with monoclonal antibodies. *8th Intl Cong. of Endocrinology*, July 17–23, 1988, Kyoto, Japan, Abst. No. 16–18–030.

GIAMBIAGI, N. and PASQUALINI, J. R. (1989) RNA-induced transformation of the estrogen receptor detected by a monoclonal antibody which recognizes the activated receptor. *Life Sci.* **44**: 2067–2074.

GIAMBIAGI, N. and PASQUALINI, J. R. (1990) Interaction of three monoclonal antibodies with the nonactivated forms of the estrogen receptor. *Endocrinology* **126**: 1263–1270.

GIAMBIAGI, N. and PASQUALINI, J. R., GREENE, G. and JENSEN, E. V. (1984) Recognition of two forms of the estrogen receptor in the guinea-pig uterus at different stages of development by a monoclonal antibody to the human estrogen receptor. Dynamics of the translocation of these two forms to the nucleus. *J. Steroid Biochem.* **20**: 397–400.

GIANNOPOULOS, G. (1973) Glucocorticoid receptors in lung. I. Specific binding of glucocorticoids to cytoplasmic components of rabbit fetal lung. *J. Biol. Chem.* **248**: 3876–3883.

GIANNOPOULOS, G. (1974a) Variations in the levels of cytoplasmic glucocorticoid receptors in lungs of various species and different developmental stages. *Endocrinology* **94**: 450–458.

GIANNOPOULOS, G. (1974b) Uptake and metabolism of cortisone and cortisol by the fetal rabbit lung. *Steroids* **23**: 845–853.

GIANNOPOULOS, G. (1975a) Early events in the action of glucocorticoids in developing tissues. *J. Steroid Biochem.* **6**: 623–631.

GIANNOPOULOS, G. (1975b) Ontogeny of glucocorticoid receptors in rat liver. *J. Biol. Chem.* **250**: 5847–5851.

GIANNOPOULOS, G. (1976) A comparative study of receptors for natural and synthetic glucocorticoids in fetal rabbit lung. *J. Steroid Biochem.* **7**: 553–559.

GIANNOPOULOS, G. (1980) Glucocorticoids and fetal lung development. In: *The Development of Responsiveness to Steroid Hormones, Advances in the Biosciences*, Vol. 25, Kaye, A. M. and Kaye, M. (Eds), Pergamon Press, Oxford, pp. 241–261.

GIANNOPOULOS, G. and KEICHLINE, D. (1981) Species-related differences in steroid-binding specificity of glucocorticoid receptors in lung. *Endocrinology* **108**: 1414–1419.

GIANNOPOULOS, G. and SMITH, S. K. S. (1982) Androgen receptors in fetal rabbit lung and the effect of fetal sex on the levels of circulating hormones and pulmonary hormone receptors. *J. Steroid Biochem.* **17**: 461–465.

GIANNOPOULOS, G. and TULCHINSKY, D. (1979) Cytoplasmic and nuclear progestin receptors in human myometrium during the menstrual cycle and in pregnancy at term. *J. Clin. Endocr. Metab.* **49**: 100–106.

GIANNOPOULOS, G., HASSAN, Z. and SOLOMON, S. (1974) Glucocorticoid receptors in fetal and adult rabbit tissues. *J. Biol. Chem.* **249**: 2424–2427.

GIANNOPOULOS, G., GOLDBERG, P., SHEA, T. B. and TULCHINSKY, D. (1980) Unoccupied and occupied estrogen receptors in myometrial cytosol and nuclei from nonpregnant and pregnant women. *J. Clin. Endocr. Metab.* **51**: 702–710.

GIANNOPOULOS, G., PHELPS, D. S. and MUNOWITZ, P. (1982) Heterogeneity and ontogenesis of progestin receptors in rabbit lung. *J. Steroid Biochem.* **17**: 503–510.

GIANNOPOULOS, G., JACKSON, K. and TULCHINSKY, D. (1983) Specific glucocorticoid binding in human uterine tissues, placenta and fetal membranes. *J. Steroid Biochem.* **19:** 1375–1378.

GILL, R. D. and HART, I. C. (1982) Hepatic receptors for insulin and glucagon in relation to plasma hormones and metabolites in pregnant and unmated ewes. *J. Endocr.* **93:** 231–238.

GILL, T. J. and REPETTI, C. F. (1979) Immunologic and genetic factors influencing reproduction. *Am. J. Pathol.* **95:** 465–570.

GIRARD, J. R., CUENDET, G. S., MARLISS, E. B., KERVRAN, A., RIEUTORT, M. and ASSAN, R. (1973) Fuels, hormones and liver metabolism at term and during the early postnatal period in the rat. *J. Clin. Invest.* **52:** 3190–3200.

GIRY, J. and DELOST, P. (1977) Changes in the concentrations of aldosterone in the plasma and adrenal glands of the foetus, the newborn and the pregnant guinea-pig during the perinatal period. *Acta Endocr. (Copenh.)* **84:** 133–141.

GLASCOCK, R. F. and HOEKSTRA, W. G. (1959) Selective accumulation of tritium-labelled hexoestrol by the reproductive organs of immature female goats and sheep. *Biochem. J.* **72:** 673–682.

GLASSER, S. R. and CLARK J. H. (1975) A determinant role for progesterone in the development of uterine sensitivity to decidualization and ovo-implantation. In: *The Developmental Biology of Reproduction*, Markert, C. L. and Papaconstantinou, J. (Eds), Academic Press, New York, pp. 311–345.

GLUCK, L., MOTOYAMA, E. K., SMITS, H. L. and KULOVICH, M. V. (1967a) The biochemical development of surface activity in mammalian lung. I. The surface-active phospholipids; the separation and distribution of surface-active lecithin in the lung of the developing rabbit fetus. *Pediatric Res.* **1:** 237–246.

GLUCK, L., SRIBNEY, M. and KULOVICH, M. V. (1967b) The biochemical development of surface activity in mammalian lung. II. The biosynthesis of phospholipids in the lung of the developing rabbit fetus and newborn. *Pediatric Res.* **1:** 247–265.

GLUCK, L., LANDOWNE, R. A. and KULOVICH, M. V. (1970) Biochemical development of surface activity in mammalian lung. III. Structural changes in lung lecithin during development of the rabbit fetus and newborn. *Pediatric Res.* **4:** 352–364.

GLUCKMAN, P. D., GRUMBACH, M. M. and KAPLAN, S. L. (1981) The neuroendocrine regulation and function of growth hormone and prolactin in the mammalian fetus. *Endocr. Rev.* **2:** 363–395.

GLUCKMAN, P. D., BUTLER, J. H. and ELLIOTT, T. B. (1983) The ontogeny of somatotropic binding sites in ovine hepatic membranes. *Endocrinology* **112:** 1607–1612.

GODOWSKI, P. J., RUSCONI, S., MIESFELD, R. and YAMAMOTO, K. R. (1987) Glucocorticoid receptor mutants that are constitutive activators of transcriptional enhancement. *Nature* **325:** 365–368.

GOERKE, J. (1974) Lung surfactant. *Biochim. Biophys. Acta* **344:** 241–261.

GOLDMAN, A. S., SHAPIRO, B. H. and NEUMANN, F. (1976) Role of testosterone and its metabolites in the differentiation of the mammary gland in rats. *Endocrinology* **99:** 1490–1495.

GONZALES, L. W. and BALLARD, P. L. (1981) Identification and characterization of nuclear 3,5,3′-triiodothyronine-binding sites in fetal human lung. *J. Clin. Endocr. Meta.* **53:** 21–28.

GONZALES, L. W. and BALLARD, P. L. (1982) Nuclear 3,5,3′-triiodothyronine receptors in rabbit lung: characterization and developmental changes. *Endocrinology* **111:** 542–552.

GONZALES, L. W., BALLARD, P. L., ERTSEY, R. and WILLIAMS, M. C. (1986) Glucocorticoids and thyroid hormones stimulate biochemical and morphological differentiation of human fetal lung in organ culture. *J. Clin. Endocr. Metab.* **62:** 678–691.

GOODMAN, R. L. (1978) The site of positive feedback action of estradiol in the rat. *Endocrinology* **102:** 151–159.

GOY, R. W., PHOENIX, G. H. and MEIDINGER, R. (1967) Postnatal development of sensitivity to estrogen and androgen in male, female and pseudohermaphrodite guinea pigs. *Anat. Rec.* **157:** 87–96.

GRAY, B. and GALTON, V. A. (1974) The transplacental passage of thyroxine and foetal thyroid function in the rat. *Acta Endocr. (Copenh).* **75:** 725–733.

GREEN, S. and CHAMBON, P. (1988) Nuclear receptors enhance our understanding of transcription regulation. *Trends Genet* **4:** 309–314.

GREEN, S., WALTER, P., KUMAR, V., KRUST, A., BORNERT, J. M., ARGOS, P. and CHAMBON, P. (1986) Human estrogen receptor cDNA: sequence, expression and homology to v-erbA. *Nature* **320:** 134–139.

GREENE, G. L., NOLAN, C., ENGLER, J. P. and JENSEN, E. V. (1980) Monoclonal antibodies to human estrogen receptor. *Proc. Natl Acad. Sci. U.S.A.* **77:** 5115–5119.

GREENGARD, O. (1970) The developmental formation of enzymes in rat liver. In: *Biochemical Actions of Hormones*, Vol. I. Litwack, G. (Ed.), Academic Press, New York, pp. 53–87.

GREENGARD, O. (1971) Enzymatic differentiation in mammalian tissues. *Essays Biochem.* **7:** 159–205.

GREENGARD, O., FEDERMAN, M. and KNOX, W. E. (1972) Cytomorphometry of developing rat liver and its application to enzymic differentiation. *J. Cell Biol.* **52:** 261–272.

GREENWAY, B., IQBAL, M. J., JOHNSON, P. J. and WILLIAMS, R. (1981) Oestrogen receptor proteins in malignant and fetal pancreas. *Br. Med. J.* **283:** 751–753.

GRINSTED, J. (1982) Influence of mesonephros on foetal and neonatal rabbit gonads. II. Sex-steroid release by the ovary in vitro. *Acta Endocr. (Copenh.)* **99:** 281–287.

GRISSOM, F. E. and LITTLETON, G. K. (1988) Evolution of lactogen receptors in selected rabbit tissues during pregnancy. *Endocr. Res.* **14:** 1–19.

GRODY, W. W., SCHRADER, W. T. and O'MALLEY, B. W. (1982) Activation, transformation and subunit structure of steroid hormone receptors. *Endocrine Reviews* **3:** 141–163.

GROSS, I., WILSON, C. M., INGELSON, L. D., BREHIER, A. and ROONEY, S. A. (1979) The influence of hormones on the biochemical development of fetal rat lung in organ culture. I. Estrogen. *Biochim. Biophys. Acta* **575:** 375–383.

GROSS, I., SMITH, G. J. W., WILSON, C. M., MANISCALCO, W. M., INGLESON, L. D., BREHIER, A. and ROONEY, S. A. (1980) The influence of hormones on the biochemical development of fetal rat lung in organ culture. II. Insulin. *Pediatric Res.* **14:** 834–838.

GROSS, I., BALLARD, P. L., BALLARD, R. A., JONES, C. T. and WILSON, C. M. (1983) Corticosteroid stimulation of phosphatidylcholine synthesis in cultured fetal rabbit lung. Evidence for de novo protein synthesis mediated by glucocorticoid receptors. *Endocrinology* **112:** 829–837.

GROSS, I., WILSON, C. M., FLOROS, J., and DYNIA, D. W. (1989) Initiation of fetal rat lung phospholipid and surfactant-associated protein A mRNA synthesis. *Pediat. Res.* **25:** 239–244.

GUERNE, J-M. and STUTINSKY, F. (1978) Estradiol and progesterone binding in rabbit placenta during gestation. *Horm. Metab. Res.* **10:** 548–553.

GUÉVIN, J.-F., BELISLE, S., LEHOUX, J.-G., BELLABARBA, D. and GALLO-PAYET, N. (1985) Characterization and ontogenesis of LHRH binding sites in human placental cells. *67th Meeting American Endocrine Society*, Abst. 348.

GULINO, A. and PASQUALINI, J. R. (1980) Dynamic studies on the selective uptake of 3H-estradiol by the fetal uterus and other fetal organs of guinea pig. *Biol. Reprod.* **23:** 336–344.

GULINO, A. and PASQUALINI, J. R. (1982) Heterogeneity of binding sites for tamoxifen and tamoxifen derivatives in estrogen target and non target fetal organs of guinea pig. *Cancer Res.* **42:** 1913–1921.

GULINO, A. and PASQUALINI, J. R. (1983) Modulation of tamoxifen-specific binding sites and estrogen receptors by estradiol and progesterone in the neonatal uterus of guinea pig. *Endocrinology* **112:** 1871–1873.

GULINO, A., SUMIDA, C., GELLY, C., GIAMBIAGI, N. and PASQUALINI, J. R. (1981) Comparative dynamic studies on the biological responses to estriol and 17β-estradiol in the fetal uterus of guinea pig: relationship to circulating estrogen concentrations. *Endocrinology* **109:** 748–756.

GULINO A., SCREPANTI, I. and PASQUALINI, J. R. (1983) Estrogen and antiestrogen effects on different lymphoid cell populations in the developing fetal thymus of guinea pig. *Endocrinology* **113:** 1754–1762.

GULINO A., SCREPANTI, I. and PASQUALINI, J. R. (1984) Differential estrogen and antiestrogen responsiveness of uterine epithelium during development from the fetal to the immature age in the guinea pig. *Biol. Reprod.* **31:** 371–381.

GULINO, A., SCREPANTI, I., TORRISI, M. R. and FRATI, L. (1985) Estrogen receptors and estrogen sensitivity of fetal thymocytes are restricted to blast lymphoid cells. *Endocrinology* **117:** 47–54.

GULYAS, B. J., TULLNER, W. W. and HODGEN, G. D. (1977a) Fetal or maternal hypophysectomy in rhesus monkeys (*Macaca mulatta*): effects on the development of testes and other endocrine organs. *Biol. Reprod.* **17:** 650–660.

GULYAS, B. J., HODGEN, G. D., TULLNER, W. W. and ROSS, G. T. (1977b) Effects of fetal or maternal hypophysectomy on endocrine organs and body weight in infant rhesus monkeys (*Macaca mulatta*): with particular emphasis on oogenesis. *Biol. Reprod.* **16:** 216–227.

GUPTA, C. and BLOCH, E. (1976) Testosterone-binding protein in reproductive tracts of fetal rats. *Endocrinology* **99:** 389–399.

HABERT, R. and PICON, R. (1982) Control of testicular steroidogenesis in foetal rat: effect of decapitation on testosterone and plasma luteinizing hormone-like activity. *Acta Endocr. (Copenh.)* **99:** 466–473.

HABERT, R. and PICON, R. (1984) Testosterone, dihydrotestosterone and estradiol-17β levels in maternal and fetal plasma and in fetal testes in the rat. *J. Steroid Biochem.* **21:** 193–198.

HAGE, E. (1973) The morphological development of the pulmonary epithelium of human foetuses studied by light and electron microscopy. *Z. Anat. Entwickl. Gesch.* **140:** 271–279.

HALME, J. IKONEN, M., RUTANEN, E. M. and SEPPÄLÄ, M. (1978) Gonadotropin receptors of human corpus luteum during menstrual cycle and pregnancy. *Am. J. Obstet. Gynecol.* **131:** 728–734.

HAMOSH, M. and HAMOSH, P. (1977) The effect of prolactin on the lecithin content of fetal rabbit lung. *J. Clin. Invest.* **59:** 1002–1005.

HANAHAN, D. J., DASKALAKIS, E. G., EDWARDS, T. and DAUBEN, H. J. Jr. (1953) The metabolic pattern of ^{14}C-diethylstilbestrol. *Endocrinology* **53:** 163–170.

HANDA, R. J., CONNOLLY, P. B. and RESKO, J. A. (1988) Ontogeny of cytosolic androgen receptors in the brain of the fetal rhesus monkey. *Endocrinology* **122:** 1890–1896.

HARIGAYA, T., SMITH, W. C. and TALAMANTES, F. (1988) Hepatic placental lactogen receptors during pregnancy in the mouse. *Endocrinology* **122:** 1366–1372.

HARRISON, L. C., BILLINGTON, T., EAST, I. J., NICHOLS, R. J. and CLARK, S. (1978) The effect of solubilization on the properties of the insulin receptor of human placental membranes. *Endocrinology* **102:** 1485–1495.

HASLAM, S. Z. (1986) Mammary fibroblast influence on normal mouse mammary epithelial cell responses to estrogen in vitro. *Cancer Res.* **46:** 310–316.

HASLAM, S. Z. and SHYAMALA, G. (1979a) Effect of oestradiol on progesterone receptors in normal mammary glands and its relationship with lactation. *Biochem. J.* **182:** 127–131.

HASLAM, S. Z. and SHYAMALA, G. (1979b) Progesterone receptors in normal mammary glands of mice: characterization and relationship to development. *Endocrinology* **105:** 786–795.

HASLAM, S. Z. and SHYAMALA, G. (1981) Relative distribution of estrogen and progesterone receptors among the epithelial, adipose, and connective tissue components of the normal mammary gland. *Endocrinology* **108:** 825–830.

HASLAM, S. Z., GALE, K. J. and DACHTLER, S. L. (1984) Estrogen receptor activation in normal mammary gland. *Endocrinology* **114:** 1163–1172.

HATIER, R., MALAPRADE, D., ROUX, M., NGUYEN, B-L., GRIGNON, G. and PASQUALINI, J. R. (1990) Autoradiographic location of ^{3}H estradiol in epididymis, seminal vesicles and prostate of fetal guinea pig. *Intern. J. Andr.* **13:** 147–154.

HAUKKAMAA, M. (1974) Binding of progesterone by rat myometrium during pregnancy and by human myometrium in late pregnancy. *J. Steroid Biochem.* **5:** 73–79.

HAY, W. W. Jr. (1979) Fetal glucose metabolism. *Sem. Perinat.* **3:** 157–176.

HAYDEN, T. J. and SMITH, S. V. (1981) Effects of bromocriptine and occlusion of nipples on prolactin receptor and lactose synthetase activity in the mammary gland of the lactating rat. *J. Endocr.* **91:** 225–232.

HAYDEN, T. J., BONNEY, R. C. and FORSYTH, I. A. (1979) Ontogeny and control of prolactin receptors in the mammary gland and liver of virgin, pregnant and lactating rats. *J. Endocr.* **80:** 259–269.

HAZUM, E. and CONN, P. M. (1988) Molecular mechanism of gonadotropin releasing hormone (GnRH) action. I. The GnRH receptor. *Endocrine Rev.* **9:** 379–386.

HAZUM, E., SCHVARTZ, I. and POPLIKER, M. (1987) Production and characterization of antibodies to gonadotropin-releasing hormone receptor. *J. Biol. Chem.* **262:** 531–534.

HEAP, R. B., PERRY, J. S., GADSBY, J. E. and BURTON, R. D. (1975) Endocrine activities of the blastocyst and early embryonic tissue in the pig. *Biochem. Soc. Trans.* **3:** 1183–1188.

HEATH, M. F. and JACOBSON, W. (1984) Developmental changes in enzyme activities in fetal and neonatal rabbit lung. Cytidylytransferase, cholinephosphotransferase, phospholipase A1, phospholipase A2, beta-galactosidase. *Prog. Resp. Res.* **18:** 170–175.

HELLER, C., COIRINI, H. and De NICOLA, A. F. (1981) Binding of ^{3}H-dexamethasone by rat placenta. *Endocrinology* **108:** 1697–1702.

HEMMING, F. J., AUBERT, M. L. and DUBOIS, P. M. (1988) Differentiation of fetal rat somatotropes in vitro: effects of cortisol, 3,5,3′-triiodothyronine, and glucagon, a light microscopic and radioimmunological study. *Endocrinology* **123:** 1230–1236.

HENRICKS, D. M. and HARRIS, R. B. Jr. (1978) Cytoplasmic estrogen receptors and estrogen concentrations in bovine uterine endometrium. *Endocrinology* **103:** 176–185.

HERMAN, T. S., FIMOGNARI, G. M. and EDELMAN, I. S. (1968) Studies on renal aldosterone-binding proteins. *J. Biol. Chem.* **243:** 3849–3856.

HERRERA, R. and ROSEN, O. M. (1987) Regulation of the protein kinase activity of the human insulin receptor. *J. Receptor Res.* **7:** 405–415.

HEUBERGER, B., FITZKA, I., WASNER, G. and KRATOCHWIL, K. (1982) Induction of androgen receptor formation by epithelial-mesenchymal interaction in embryonic mouse mammary gland. *Proc. Natl Acad. Sci. U.S.A.* **79:** 2957–2961.

HILL, D. E. (1976) Insulin and fetal growth. In: *Diabetes and Other Endocrine Disorders during Pregnancy in the Newborn*, Alan R. Liss, New York, pp. 127–139.

HILL, D. E. (1978) Effect of insulin on fetal growth. *Sem Perinatol* **2:** 319–328.

HILL, D. J., CRACE, C. J., STRAIN, A. J. and MILNER, R. D. G. (1986) Regulation of amino acid uptake and deoxyribonucleic acid synthesis in isolated human fetal fibroblasts and myoblasts: effect of human placental lactogen, somatomedin-C, multiplication stimulating activity, and insulin. *J. Clin. Endocr. Metab.* **62:** 753–760.

HILL, D. J., FREEMARK, M., STRAIN, A. J., HANDWERGER, S. and MILNER, R. D. G. (1988) Placental lactogen and growth hormone receptors in human fetal tissues: relationship to fetal plasma human placental lactogen concentrations and fetal growth. *J. Clin. Endocr. Metab.* **66:** 1283–1290.

HILLIARD, J. and EATON, L. W. (1971) Estradiol-17β, progesterone and 20α-hydroxypregn-4-en-3-one in rabbit ovarian venous plasma. II. From mating through implantation. *Endocrinology* **89:** 522–527.

HITCHCOCK, K. R. (1979) Hormones and the lung. I. Thyroid hormones and glucocorticoids in lung development. *Anat. Rec.* **194:** 15–40.

HOCHNER-CELNIKIER, D., MARANDICI, A., IOHAN, F. and MONDER, C. (1986) Estrogen and progesterone receptors in the organs of prenatal cynomolgus monkey and laboratory mouse. *Biol. Reprod.* **35:** 633–640.

HODGEN, G. D., TULLNER, W. W., VAITUKAITIS, J. L., WARD, D. N. and ROSS, G. T. (1974) Specific radioimmunoassay of chorionic gonadotropin during implantation in rhesus monkeys. *J. Clin. Endocr. Metab.* **39:** 457–464.

HODGEN, G. D., NIEMANN, W. H. and TULLNER, W. W. (1975) Duration of chorionic gonadotropin production by the placenta of the rhesus monkey. *Endocrinology* **96:** 789–791.

HOEFFLER, J. P., DEUTSCH, P. J., LIN, J. and HABENER, J. F. (1989) Distinct adenosine 3′,5′-monophosphate and phorbol ester-responsive signal transduction pathways converge at the level of transcriptional activation by the interactions of DNA-binding proteins. *Mol. Endocr.* **3:** 868–880.

HOLCOMB, H. H., COSTLOW, M. E., BUSCHOW, R. A. and McGUIRE, W. L. (1976) Prolactin binding in rat mammary gland during pregnancy and lactation. *Biochim. Biophys. Acta* **428:** 104–112.

HOLLENBERG, S. M., WEINBERGER, C., ONG, E. S., CERELLI, G., ORO, A., LEBO, R., THOMPSON, E. B., ROSENFELD, M. G. and EVANS, R. M. (1985) Primary structure and expression of a functional human glucocorticoid receptor cDNA. *Nature* **318:** 635–641.

HOLT, A. B., KERR, G. R. and CHEEK, D. B. (1975) Prenatal hypothyroidism and brain composition. In: *Fetal and Postnatal Cellular Growth. Hormones and Nutrition*, Cheek, D. B. (Ed.), J. Wiley and Sons, New York, pp. 141–153.

HOLT, P. G. and OLIVER, I. T. (1968) Plasma corticosterone concentrations in the perinatal rat. *Biochem. J.* **108:** 339–341.

HOPKINS, P. S. and THORBURN, G. D. (1972) The effects of fetal thyroidectomy in the development of the ovine fetus. *J. Endocr.* **54:** 55–66.

HORWITZ, K. B. and McGUIRE, W. L. (1978) Estrogen control of progesterone receptor in human breast cancer. Correlation with nuclear processing of estrogen receptor. *J. Biol. Chem.* **253:** 2223–2228.

HOUDEBINE, L. M. and GAYE, P. (1976) Regulation of casein synthesis in the rabbit mammary gland. Titration of mRNA activity for casein under prolactin and progesterone treatments. *Mol. Cell. Endocr.* **3:** 37–55.

HSUEH, A. J. W., PECK, E. J. Jr. and CLARK, J. H. (1973) Oestrogen receptors in the mammary gland of the lactating rat. *J. Endocr.* **58:** 503–511.

HSUEH, A. J. W., DUFAU, M. L. and CATT, K. J. (1976a) Regulation of luteinizing hormone receptors in testicular interstitial cells by gonadotropin. *Biochem. Biophys. Res. Commun.* **72:** 1145–1152.

HSUEH, A. J. W., PECK, E. J. Jr. and CLARK, J. H. (1976b) Control of uterine estrogen receptor levels by progesterone. *Endocrinology* **98:** 438–444.

HUHTANIEMI, I. T., KORENBROT, C. C. and JAFFE, R. B. (1977a) hCG Binding and stimulation of testosterone biosynthesis in the human fetal testis. *J. Clin. Endocr. Metab.* **44:** 963–967.

HUHTANIEMI, I. T., KORENBROT, C. C., SÉRON-FERRÉ, M., FOSTER, D. B., PARER, J. T. and JAFFE, R. B. (1977b) Stimulation of testosterone production in vivo and in vitro in the male rhesus monkey fetus in late gestation. *Endocrinology* **100:** 839–844.

HÜMMELINK, R. and BALLARD, P. L. (1986) Endogenous corticoids and lung development in the fetal rabbit. *Endocrinology* **118:** 1622–1629.

HUNT, M.E. and MULDOON, T. G. (1977) Factors controlling estrogen receptor levels in normal mouse mammary tissue. *J. Steroid Biochem.* **8:** 181–186.

HURLEY, T. W., D'ERCOLE, A. J., HANDWERGER, S., UNDERWOOD, L. E., FURLANETTO, R. W. and FELLOWS, R. E. (1977) Ovine placental lactogen induces somatomedin: a possible role in fetal growth. *Endocrinology* **101:** 1635–1638.

IMPERATO-McGINLEY, J., BINIENDA, Z., GEDNEY, J. and VAUGHAN, E. D., Jr. (1986) Nipple differentiation in fetal male rats treated with an inhibitor of the enzyme 5α-reductase: definition of a selective role for dihydrotestosterone. *Endocrinology* **118:** 132–137.

INAGAKI, Y. and KOHMOTO, K. (1982) Changes in Scatchard plots for insulin binding to mammary epithelial cells from cycling, pregnant, and lactating mice. *Endocrinology* **110:** 176–182.

IWASHITA, M., EVANS, M. I. and CATT, K. J. (1986) Characterization of a gonadotropin-releasing hormone receptor site in term placenta and chorionic villi. *J. Clin. Endocr. Metab.* **62:** 127–133.

JACOBS, S. and CUATRECASAS, P. (1981) Insulin: structure and function. *Endocr. Rev.* **2:** 251–263.

JACQUOT, R. (1959) Recherches sur le contrôle endocrinien de l'accumulation de glycogène dans le foie chez le foetus de rat. *J. Physiol (Paris)* **51:** 655–692.

JACQUOT, R. and KRETCHMER, N. (1964) Effect of fetal decapitation on enzymes of glycogen metabolism. *J. Biol. Chem.* **239:** 1301–1304.

JACQUOT, R. L., PLAS, C. and NAGEL, J. (1973) Two examples of physiological maturations in rat fetal liver. *Enzyme* **15:** 296–303.

JARRETT, J. C. II, BALLEJO, G., SALEEM, T. H., TSIBRIS, J. C. M. and SPELLACY, W. N. (1984) The effect of prolactin and relaxin on insulin binding by adipocytes from pregnant women. *Am. J. Obstet. Gynec.* **149**: 250–255.

JELTSCH, J. M., KROZOWSKI, Z., QUIRIN-STRICKER, C., GRONEMEYER, H., SIMPSON, R. J., GARNIER, J. M., KRUST, A., JACOB, F. and CHAMBON, P. (1986) Cloning of the chicken progesterone receptor. *Proc. Natl Acad. Sci. USA* **83**: 5424–5428.

JENNES, L., BRONSON, D., STUMPF, W. E. and CONN, P. M. (1985) Evidence for an association between calmodulin and membrane patches containing gonadotropin-releasing hormone-receptor complexes in cultured gonadotropes. *Cell Tissue Res.* **239**: 311–315.

JENSEN, E. V. and JACOBSON, H. I. (1960) Biological activities of steroids in relation to cancer. In: *Fate of Steroid Estrogens in Target Tissues*, Pincus, G. and Vollmer, E. P. (Eds), Academic Press, New York, pp. 161–178.

JOHNSON, J. A., DAVIS, J. O., BAUMBER, J. S. and SCHNEIDER, E. G. (1970) Effects of estrogens and progesterone on electrolyte balances in normal dogs. *Am. J. Physiol* **219**: 1691–1697.

JONES, C. T., BODDY, K. and ROBINSON, J. S. (1977) Changes in the concentration of adrenocorticotrophin and corticosteroid in the plasma of foetal sheep in the latter half of pregnancy and during labour. *J. Endocr.* **72**: 293–300.

JOSEFSBERG, Z., POSNER, B. I., PATEL, B. and BERGERON, J. J. M. (1979) The uptake of prolactin into female rat liver. Concentration of intact hormone in the Golgi apparatus. *J. Biol. Chem.* **254**: 209–214.

JOSIMOVICH, J. B., WEISS, G. and HUTCHINSON, D. L. (1974) Sources and disposition of pituitary prolactin in maternal circulation, amniotic fluid, fetus and placenta in the pregnant rhesus monkey. *Endocrinology* **94**: 1364–1371.

JOSIMOVICH, J. B., MERISKO, K., BOCCELLA, L. and TOBON, H. (1977) Binding of prolactin by fetal rhesus cell membrane fractions. *Endocrinology* **100**: 557–563.

JOST, A. (1961) The role of fetal hormones in prenatal development. *Harvey Lect.* **55**: 201–226.

JOST, A. (1966a) Anterior pituitary function in foetal life. In: *The Pituitary Gland*, Vol. 2, Harris, G. W. and Donovan, B. T. (Eds), University of California Press, Berkeley, Los Angeles, pp. 299–323.

JOST, A. (1966b) Problems of fetal endocrinology: the adrenal glands. *Rec. Prog. Horm. Res.* **22**: 541–574.

JOST, A. (1985) Sexual organogenesis. In: *Handbook of Behavioral Neurobiology. Reproduction.* Vol. 7, Adler, N., Pfaff, D. and Goy, R. W. (Eds), Plenum Press, New York, pp. 3–19.

JOST, A. and HATEY, J. (1949) Influence de la décapitation sur la teneur en glycogène du foie du foetus de lapin. *C. R. Soc. Biol.* **143**: 146–147.

JOST, A. and JACQUOT, R. (1955) Recherches sur les facteurs endocriniens de la charge en glycogène du foie foetal chez le lapin (avec des indications sur le glycogène placentaire). *Ann. Endocrl. (Paris)* **16**: 849–872.

JOST, A. and JACQUOT, R. (1958) Sur le rôle de l'hypophyse, des surrénales et du placenta dans la synthèse de glycogène par le foie foetal du lapin et du rat. *C. R. Acad. Sci. (Paris)* **247**: 2459–2462.

JOST, A. and PICON, L. (1970) Hormonal control of fetal development and metabolism. *Adv. Metab. Disord.* **4**: 123–184.

JOST, J. P., GEISER M. and SELDRAN M. (1985) Specific modulation of the transcription of cloned avian vitellogenin II gene by estradiol-receptor complex in vitro. *Proc. Natl Acad. Sci. (USA)* **82**: 988–991.

JUNGMANN, R. A. and HUNZICKER-DUNN, M. (1978) Mechanism of action of gonadotropins and the regulation of gene expression. In: *Structure and Function of the Gonadotropins*, McKerns, K. W. (Ed.), Plenum, New York, pp. 1–29.

KALIMI, M. and GUPTA, S. (1982) Physicochemical characterization of rat liver glucocorticoid receptor during development. *J. Biol. Chem.* **257**: 13324–13328.

KALLAND, T. (1980) Decreased and disproportionate T-cell population in adult mice after neonatal exposure to diethylstilbestrol. *Cell. Immunol.* **51**: 55–63.

KALLAND, T., STRAND, Ø. and FORSBERG, J.-G. (1979) Long-term effects of neonatal estrogen treatment on mitogen responsiveness of mouse spleen lymphocytes. *J. Natl Cancer Inst.* **63:** 413–421.

KALTER, H. (1965) Interplay of intrinsic and extrinsic factors. In: *Teratology, Principles and Techniques*, Wilson, J. G. and Warkany, J. (Eds), Univ. of Chicago Press, Chicago, Illinois, pp. 57–80.

KAPLAN, S. A., BARRETT, C. T., SCOTT, M. L. and WHITSON, R. H. (1984) Insulin receptors in fetal rabbit lung Type II cells. *Endocrinology* **114:** 2199–2204.

KASUGA, M., FUJITA-YAMAGUCHI, Y., BLITHE, D. L. and KAHN, C. R. (1983) Tyrosine-specific protein kinase activity is associated with the purified insulin receptor. *Proc. Natl Acad. Sci. USA* **80:** 2137–2141.

KATZENELLENBOGEN, B. S. and GREGER, N. G. (1974) Ontogeny of uterine responsiveness to estrogen during early development in the rat. *Mol. Cell. Endocr.* **2:** 31–42.

KAWAOI, A. and TSUNEDA, M. (1985) Functional development and maturation of the rat thyroid gland in the foetal and newborn periods: an immunohistochemical study. *Acta Endocr. (Copenh.)* **108:** 518–524.

KELLY, P. A., POSNER, B. I., TSUSHIMA, T. and FRIESEN, H. G. (1974) Studies of insulin, growth hormone and prolactin binding: ontogenesis, effects of sex and pregnancy. *Endocrinology* **95:** 532–539.

KELLY, P. A., DJIANE, J. and MALANCON, R. (1983) Characterization of estrogen, progesterone and glucocorticoid receptors in rabbit mammary glands and their measurement during pregnancy and lactation. *J. Steroid Biochem.* **18:** 215–221.

KERO, P. O. and PULKKINEN, M. O. (1979) Plasma progesterone in the respiratory distress syndrome. *Eur. J. Pediat.* **132:** 7–10.

KHAN-DAWOOD, F. S. and DAWOOD, M. Y. (1984) Estrogen and progesterone receptor and hormone levels in human myometrium and placenta in term pregnancy. *Am. J. Obstet. Gynecol.* **150:** 501–505.

KHOSLA, S. S. and ROONEY, S. A. (1979) Stimulation of fetal lung surfactant production by administration of 17β-estradiol to the maternal rabbit. *Am. J. Obstet. Gynecol.* **133:** 213–216.

KHOSLA, S. S., GOBRAN, L. I. and ROONEY, S. A. (1980) Stimulation of phosphatidylcholine synthesis by 17β-estradiol in fetal rabbit lung. *Biochim. Biophys. Acta* **617:** 282–290.

KHOSLA, S. S., BREHIER, A., EISENFELD, A. J., INGLESON, L. D., PARKS, P. A. and ROONEY, S. A. (1983) Influence of sex hormones on lung maturation in the fetal rabbit. *Biochim. Biophys. Acta* **750:** 112–126.

KIKKAWA, T., KAIBARA, M., MOTOYAMA, E. K., ORZALESI, M. M. and COOK, C. D. (1971) Morphologic development of fetal rabbit lung and its acceleration with cortisol. *Am. J. Pathol.* **64:** 423–442.

KIMMEL, G. L. and HARMON, J. R. (1980) Characteristics of estrogen binding in uterine cytosol during the perinatal period in the rat. *J. Steroid Biochem.* **12:** 73–75.

KIMMEL, G. L., HARMON, J. R., OLSON, M. E. and SHEEHAN, D. M. (1981) Transplacental estrogen (E) stimulation of ornithine decarboxylase (ODC) in fetal rat uterus. *Teratology* **23:** 46A.

KIMMEL, G. L., HARMON, J. R. and SLIKKER, W. Jr. (1983) Characterization of estrogen binding in uterine cytosol from the fetal Rhesus monkey. *Teratogen. Carcinogen. Mutagen.* **3:** 355–365.

KING, R. J., RUCH, J., GIKAS, E. G., PLATZKEN, A. C. G. and CREASY, R. K. (1975) Appearance of apoproteins of pulmonary surfactant in human amniotic fluid. *J. Appl. Physiol.* **39:** 735–741.

KING, R. J. B. and MAINWARING, W. I. P. (1974) *Steroid-Cell Interactions*, Butterworth and Co., London.

KING, W. J. and GREENE, G. L. (1984) Monoclonal antibodies localize oestrogen receptor in the nuclei of target cells. *Nature* **307:** 745–747.

KITRAKI, E., ALEXIS, M. N. and STYLIANOPOULOU, F. (1984) Glucocorticoid receptors in developing rat brain and liver. *J. Steroid Biochem.* **20:** 263–269.

KNEUSSL, E. S., ANCES, I. G. and ALBRECHT, E. D. (1982) A specific cytosolic estrogen receptor in human term placenta. *Am. J. Obstet. Gynecol.* **144:** 803–809.

KNOBIL, E. (1974) On the control of gonadotropin secretion in the Rhesus monkey. *Rec. Prog. Horm. Res.* **30:** 1–46.

KOHANSKI, R. A. and LANE, M. D. (1983) Binding of insulin to solubilized insulin receptor from human placenta. Evidence for a single class of noninteracting binding sites. *J. Biol. Chem.* **258:** 7460–7468.

KÖHLER, G. and MILSTEIN, C. (1975) Continuous cultures of fused cells secreting antibody of predefined specificity. *Nature* **256:** 495–497.

KOLIGIAN, K. B. and STORMSHAK, F. (1977) Progesterone inhibition of estrogen receptor replenishment in ovine endometrium. *Biol. Reprod.* **17:** 412–416.

KOLODNY, J. M., LEONARD, J. L., LARSEN, P. R. and SILVA, J. E. (1985) Studies of nuclear 3,5,3′-triiodothyronine binding in primary cultures of rat brain. *Endocrinology* **117:** 1848–1857.

KOTAS, R. V. and AVERY, M. E. (1980) The influence of sex on fetal rabbit lung maturation and on the response to glucocorticoid. *Am. Rev. Resp. Dis.* **121:** 377–380.

KRATOCHWIL, K. (1969) Organ specificity in mesenchymal induction demonstrated in the embryonic development of the mammary gland of the mouse. *Devel. Biol.* **20:** 46–71.

KRATOCHWIL, K. (1972) I. Tissue interaction during embryonic development: general properties. In: *Tissue Interactions in Carcinogenesis*, Tanin, D. (Ed.), Academic Press, New York, pp. 1–47.

KRATOCHWIL, K. (1977) Development and loss of androgen responsiveness in the embryonic rudiment of the mouse mammary gland. *Dev. Biol.* **61:** 358–365.

KRATOCHWIL, K. and SCHWARTZ, P. (1976) Tissue interaction in androgen response of embryonic mammary rudiment of the mouse: identification of target tissue for testosterone. *Proc. Natl Acad. Sci. U.S.A.* **73:** 4041–4044.

KREITMANN, B. and BAYARD, F. (1979) Oestrogen and progesterone receptor concentrations in human endometrium during gestation. *Acta Endocr. (Copenh.)* **92:** 547–552.

KREITMANN-GIMBAL, B., BAYARD, F. and HODGEN, G. D. (1981) Changing ratios of nuclear estrone to estradiol binding in endometrium at implantation: regulation by chorionic gonadotropin and progesterone during rescue of the primate corpus luteum. *J. Clin. Endocr. Metab.* **52:** 133–137.

KRISHNAN, R. S. and DANIEL, J. C. Jr. (1967) Blastokinin: inducer and regulator of blastocyst development in the rabbit uterus. *Science* **158:** 490–492.

KROZOWSKI, Z. S., RUNDLE, S. E., WALLACE, C., CASTELL, M. J., SHEN, J-H., DOWLING, J., FUNDER, J. W. and SMITH, A. I. (1989) Immunolocalization of renal mineralocorticoid receptors with an antiserum against a peptide deduced from the complementary deoxyribonucleic acid sequence. *Endocrinology* **125:** 192–198.

KUHN, N. J. (1969) Specificity of progesterone inhibition of lactogenesis. *J. Endocr.* **45:** 615–616.

KUMAR, V., GREEN, S., STACK, G., BERRY, M., JIN, J-R. and CHAMBON, P. (1987) Functional domains of the human estrogen receptor. *Cell* **51:** 941–951.

KUO, J. F. and GREENGARD, P. (1969) Cyclic nucleotide-dependent protein kinase. IV. Widespread occurrence of adenosine 3′,5′-monophosphate-dependent protein kinase in various tissues and phyla of the animal kingdom. *Proc. Natl Acad. Sci. USA* **64:** 1349–1353.

KUROKI, Y., TAKAHASHI, H., FUKADA Y., MIKAWA M., INAGAWA A., FUJIMOTO S. and AKINO T. (1985) Two site "simultaneous" immunoassay with monoclonal antibodies for the determination of surfactant apoproteins in human amniotic fluid. *Pediatric Res.* **19:** 1017–1020.

LAGESON, J. M., SPELSBERG, T.C. and COULAM, C. B. (1983) Glucocorticoid receptor in human placenta: studies of concentration and functional differences of preterm and term tissue. *Am. J. Obstet. Gynecol.* **145:** 515–523.

LANGLEY, J. N. (1905) On the reaction of cells and of nerve-endings to certain poisons chiefly as regards the reaction of striated muscle to nicotine and to curare. *J. Physiol.* **33:** 374–413.

LANZONE, A., NGUYEN, B. L. and PASQUALINI, J. R. (1983) Uptake, receptor and biological response of estrone in the fetal uterus of guinea pig. *Horm. Res.* **17:** 168–180.

LARSEN, P. R., HARNEY, J. W. and MOORE, D. D. (1986) Sequences required for cell-type specific thyroid hormone regulation of rat growth hormone promoter activity. *J. Biol. Chem.* **261:** 14373–14376.

LAURÉ, F. and PASQUALINI, J. R. (1983) Effect of oestradiol on RNA polymerase of foetal guinea pig uterus. *Experientia* **39**: 209–210.

LAX, E. R., TAMULEVICIUS, P., MULLER, A. and SCHRIEFERS, H. (1983) Hepatic nuclear estrogen receptor concentrations in the rat—influence of age, sex, gestation, lactation and estrous cycle. *J. Steroid Biochem.* **19**: 1083–1088.

Le HOANG, P., PAPIERNIK, M., BERRIH, S. and DUVAL, D. (1981a) Thymic involution in pregnant mice. I. Characterization of the remaining thymocyte subpopulations. *Clin. Exp. Immunol.* **44**: 247–252.

Le HOANG, P., PAPIERNIK, M., DARDENNE, M. (1981b) Thymic involution in pregnant mice. II. Functional aspects of the remaining thymocytes. *Clin. Exp. Immunol.* **44**: 253–261.

LEAVITT, W. W. (1985) Hormonal regulation of myometrial estrogen, progesterone, and oxytocin receptors in the pregnant and pseudopregnant hamster. *Endocrinology* **116**: 1079–1084.

LEAVITT, W. W. and OKULICZ, W. C. (1985) Occupied and unoccupied estrogen receptor during estrous cycle and pregnancy. *Am. J. Physiol.* **249**: E589–E594.

LEAVITT, W. W. and REUSS, B. J. (1975) Progesterone receptors in different uterine compartments during pregnancy and pseudopregnancy in the hamster. *57th Ann. Meeting American Endocrine Soc.*, p. 273.

LEAVITT, W. W., TOFT, D. O., STROTT, C. A. and O'MALLEY, B. W. (1974) A specific progesterone receptor in the hamster uterus: physiologic properties and regulation during the estrous cycle. *Endocrinology* **94**: 1041–1053.

LEE, D. K. H. and SOLOMON, S. (1978) Characteristics and ontogeny of nuclear receptor for glucocorticoids in the rabbit fetal small intestine. *Endocrinology* **102**: 312–320.

LEE, D. K. H., STERN, M. and SOLOMON, S. (1976) Cytoplasmic glucocorticoid receptors in the developing small intestine of the rabbit fetus. *Endocrinology* **99**: 379–388.

LEE, J. N., SEPPÄLÄ, M. and CHARD, T. (1981) Characterization of placental luteinizing hormone-releasing factor-like material. *Acta Endocr. (Copenh.)* **96**: 394–397.

LEINONEN, P. J. and JAFFE, R. B. (1985) Leydig cell desensitization by human chorionic gonadotropin does not occur in the human fetal testis. *J. Clin. Endocr. Metab.* **61**: 234–238.

LERNER, L. J. (1964) Hormone antagonists: inhibitors of specific activities of estrogen and androgen. *Rec. Prog. Horm. Res.* **20**: 435–490.

LEOSCAT, D., JAVRÉ, J. L. and CHAMBON, Y. (1985) Changes in cytosolic estradiol receptor concentrations in embryonic and interembryonic segments of the rabbit uterus before and after ovoimplantation. *IRCS Med. Sci.* **13**: 372–373.

LESNIAK, M. A., ROTH, J., GORDEN, P. and GAVINE J. R. III (1973) Human growth hormone radioreceptor assay using cultured human lymphocytes. *Nature (London), New Biol.* **241**: 20–22.

LESNIAK, M. A., GORDEN, P. and ROTH, J. (1977) Reactivity of non-primate growth hormones and prolactins with human growth hormone receptors on cultured human lymphocytes. *J. Clin. Endocr. Metab.* **44**: 838–849.

LEUNG, B. S. and SASAKI, G. H. (1973) Prolactin and progesterone effect on specific estradiol binding in uterine and mammary tissues in vitro. *Biochem. Biophys. Res. Comm.* **55**: 1180–1187.

LEUNG, B. S., JACK, W. M. and REINEY, C. G. (1976) Estrogen receptor in mammary glands and uterus of rats during pregnancy, lactation and involution. *J. Steroid Biochem.* **7**: 89–95.

LIEBERBURG, I., MacLUSKY, N. and McEWEN, B. S. (1980) Androgen receptors in the perinatal rat brain. *Brain Res.* **196**: 125–138.

LIGGINS, G. C. (1969) Premature delivery of foetal lambs infused with glucocorticoids. *J. Endocr.* **45**: 515–523.

LIGGINS, G. C. (1976) Adrenocortical-related maturational events in the fetus. *Am. J. Obstet. Gynecol.* **126**: 931–941.

LIGGINS, G. C., FAIRCLOUGH, R. J., GRIEVES, S. A., KENDALL, J. Z. and KNOX, B. S. (1973) The mehanism of initiation of parturition in the ewe. *Rec. Prog. Horm. Res.* **29**: 111–150.

LILEY, H. G., HAWGOOD, S., WELLENSTEIN, G. A., BENSON, B., WHITE, R. T. and BALLARD,

P. L. (1987) Surfactant protein of molecular weight 28,000–36,000 in cultured human fetal lung: cellular localization and effect of dexamethasone. *Mol. Endocr.* **1**: 205–215.

LIMPAPHAYOM, K., LEE, C., JACOBSON, H. I. and KING, T. M. (1971) Estrogen receptor in human endometrium during the menstrual cycle and early pregnancy. *Am. J. Obstet. Gynecol.* **111**: 1064–1068.

LINDENBAUM, M. and CHATTERTON, R. T. Jr. (1981) Interaction of steroids with dexamethasone-binding receptor and corticosteroid-binding globulin in the mammary gland of the mouse in relation to lactation. *Endocrinology* **109**: 363–375.

LINDENBERG, J. A., BREHIER, A. and BALLARD, P. L. (1978) Triiodothyronine nuclear binding in fetal and adult rabbit lung and cultured lung cells. *Endocrinology* **103**: 1725–1731.

LITWACK, G. and SINGER, S. (1972) In: *Biochemical Actions of Hormones*, Vol. 2, Litwack, G. (Ed.), Academic Press, New York, pp. 114.

LOGEAT, F., SARTOR, P., VU HAI, M. T. and MILGROM, E. (1980) Local effect of the blastocyst on estrogen and progesterone receptors in the rat endometrium. *Science* **207**: 1083–1085.

LONGCHAMPT, J. and AXELROD, L. R. (1964) Contribution to steroid biosynthesis in human fetal adrenal. *Res. Steroids* **1**: 269–277.

LOPEZ BERNAL, A., ANDERSON, A. B. M., DEMERS, L. M. and TURNBULL, A. C. (1982) Glucocorticoid binding by human fetal membranes at term. *J. Clin. Endocr. Metab.* **55**: 862–865.

LOPEZ BERNAL, A., ANDERSON, A. B. M. and TURNBULL, A. C. (1984) The measurement of glucocorticoid receptors in human placental cytosol. *Placenta* **5**: 105–116.

LOWE, W. L. Jr., BOYD, F. T., CLARKE, D. W., RAIZADA, M. K., HART, C. and LeROITH, D. (1986) Development of brain insulin receptors: structural and functional studies of insulin receptors from whole brain and primary cell cultures. *Endocrinology* **119**: 25–35.

LUSTER, M. I., FAITH, R. E., McLACHLAN, J. A. and CLARK, G. C. (1979) Effect of "in utero" exposure to diethylstilbestrol on the immune response in mice. *Toxicol. Appl. Pharmacol.* **47**: 279–285.

LUSTER, M. I., BOORMAN, G. A., DEAN, J. H., LUEBKE, R. W. and LAWSON, L. D. (1980) The effect of adult exposure to diethylstilbestrol in the mouse: alterations in immunological functions. *J. Reticuloendothel. Soc.* **28**: 561–569.

LUZZANI, F. and SOFFIENTINI, A. (1980) Studies on cutosol progestin-binding components in the utero-placental unit of the pregnant hamster. *J. Steroid Biochem.* **13**: 697–701.

LYE, S. J. and CHALLIS, J. R. G. (1984) In vivo adrenocorticotropin (1-24)-induced accumulation of cyclic adenosine monophosphate by ovine fetal adrenal cells is inhibited by concomitant infusion of metopirone. *Endocrinology* **115**: 1584–1587.

LYONS, W. R. (1958) Hormonal synergism in mammary growth. *Proc. Royal Soc., Series B,* **149**: 303–325.

LYONS, W. R., LI, C. H. and JOHNSON, R. E. (1958) The hormonal control of mammary growth and lactation. *Rec. Prog. Horm. Res.* **14**: 219–254.

LYTTLE, C. R., GARAY, R. V. and DeSOMBRE, E. R. (1979) Ontogeny of the estrogen inducibility of uterine peroxidase. *J. Steroid Biochem.* **10**: 359–363.

MacLAUGHLIN, D. T. and RICHARDSON, G. S. (1976) Progesterone binding by normal and abnormal human endometrium. *J. Clin. Endocr. Metab.* **42**: 667–678.

MacLUSKY, N. J., LIEBERBURG, I. and McEWEN, B. S. (1979) The development of estrogen receptor systems in the rat brain: perinatal development. *Brain Res.* **178**: 129–142.

MADILL, D. and BASSETT, J. M. (1973) Corticosteroid release by adrenal tissue from foetal and newborn lambs in response to corticotrophin stimulation in a perfusion system in vitro. *J. Endocr.* **58**: 75–87.

MAGRE, S. and JOST, A. (1980) The initial phases of testicular organogenesis in the rat. An electron microscopy study. *Arch. Anat. Micros.* **69**: 297–318.

MARCAL, J. M., CHEW, N. J., SALOMON, D. S. and SHERMAN, M. I. (1975) Delta 5,3β-hydroxy-steroid dehydrogenase activities in rat trophoblast and ovary during pregnancy. *Endocrinology* **96**: 1270–1279.

MARSH, J. (1975) The role of cAMP in gonadal function. *Adv. Cyclic Nucleotide Res.* **6:** 137–199.

MARSHALL, R. N., UNDERWOOD, L. E., VOINA, S. J., FOUSHEE, D. B. and VAN WYK, J. J. (1974) Characterization of the insulin and somatomedin-C receptors in human placental cell membranes. *J. Clin. Endocr. Metab.* **39:** 283–291.

MARTEL, D. and PSYCHOYOS, A. (1976) Endometrial content of nuclear estrogen receptor and receptivity for ovoimplantation in the rat. *Endocrinology* **99:** 470–475.

MARTEL, D. and PSYCHOYOS, A. (1978) Progesterone-induced oestrogen receptors in the rat uterus. *J. Endocr.* **76:** 145–154.

MARTEL, D. and PSYCHOYOS, A. (1981) Estrogen receptors in the nidatory sites of the rat endometrium. *Science* **211:** 1454–1455.

MARTEL, D., MONIER, M-N., PSYCHOYOS, A. and DeFEO, V. J. (1984) Estrogen and progesterone receptors in the endometrium, myometrium, and metrial gland of the rat during the decidualization process. *Endocrinology* **114:** 1627–1634.

MARTIAL, J. A., BAXTER, J. D., GOODMAN, H. M. and SEEBURG, P. H. (1977) Regulation of growth hormone messenger RNA by thyroid and glucocorticoid hormones. *Proc. Natl Acad. Sci. USA* **74:** 1816–1820.

MARTIN, C. E., CAKE, M. H., HARTMANN, P. E. and COOK, I. F. (1977) Relationship between foetal corticosteroids, maternal progesterone and parturition in the rat. *Acta Endocr. (Copenh.)* **84:** 167–176.

MARTIN, L. and FINN, C. A. (1968) Hormonal regulation of cell division in epithelial and connective tissues of the mouse uterus. *J. Endocr.* **41:** 363–371.

MASHIACH, S., BARKAI, G., SACK, J., STERN, E., BRISH, M., GOLDMAN, B. and SERR, D. M. (1979) The effect of intra-amniotic thyroxine administration on fetal lung maturity in man. *J. Perinat. Med.* **7:** 161–170.

MAULÉON, P., BÉZARD, J. and TERQUI, M. (1977) Very early and transient secretion of oestradiol-17β by foetal sheep ovary in vitro. *Ann. Biol. Anim. Biochim. Biophys.* **17:** 399–401.

MAYEUX, P., BILLAT, C., FELIX, J. M. and JACQUOT, R. (1983) Evidence for glucocorticosteroid receptors in the erythroid cell line of fetal rat liver. *J. Endocr.* **96:** 311–319.

McCORMACK, S. A. and GLASSER, S. R. (1976) A high-affinity estrogen-binding protein in rat placental trophoblast. *Endocrinology* **99:** 701–712.

McCORMACK, S. A. and GLASSER, S. R. (1978) Ontogeny and regulation of a rat placental estrogen receptor. *Endocrinology* **102:** 273–280.

McCORMICK, P. D., RAZEL, A. J., SPELSBERG, T. C. and COULAM, C. B. (1981) Evidence for an androgen receptor in the human placenta. *Am. J. Obstet. Gynecol.* **140:** 8–13.

McDONNELL, D. P., MANGELSDORF, D. J., PIKE, J. W., HAUSSLER, M. R. and O'MALLEY, B. W. (1987) Molecular cloning of complementary DNA encoding the avian receptor for vitamin D. *Science* **235:** 1214–1217.

McEWEN, B. S. (1983) Gonadal steroid influences on brain development and sexual differentiation. In: *International Review of Physiology*, Vol. 27, Greep, R. O. (Ed.), University Park Press, Baltimore, pp. 99–145.

McEWEN, B. S., LIEBERBURG, I., MacLUSKY, N. and PLAPINGER, L. (1977) Do estrogen receptors play a role in the sexual differentiation of the rat brain? *J. Steroid Biochem.* **8:** 593–598.

McNEILLY, A. S. and FRIESEN, H. G. (1977) Binding of prolactin to the rabbit mammary gland during pregnancy. *J. Endocr.* **74:** 507–508.

MEANEY, M. J., SAPOLSKY, R. M., AITKEN, D. H. and McEWEN, B. S. (1985) [3H]-Dexamethasone binding in the limbic brain of the fetal rat. *Dev. Brain Res.* **23:** 297–300.

MEANS, A. R. and VAITUKAITIS, J. L. (1972) Peptide hormone "receptors": specific binding of [^{3}H]-FSH to testis. *Endocrinology* **90:** 39–46.

MEDLOCK, K. L., SHEEHAN, D. M. and BRANHAM, W. S. (1981) The postnatal ontogeny of the rat uterine estrogen receptor. *J. Steroid Biochem.* **15:** 285–288.

MENDELSON, C. R., BROWN, P. K., MacDONALD, P. C. and JOHNSTON, J. M. (1981)

Characterization of a cytosolic estrogen-binding protein in lung tissue of fetal rats. *Endocrinology* **109:** 210–217.

MENDELSON, C. R., CHEN, C., BOGGARAM, V., ZACHARIAS, C. and SNYDER, J. M. (1986) Regulation of the synthesis of the major surfactant apoprotein in fetal rabbit lung tissue. *J. Biol. Chem.* **263:** 2939–2947.

MENDELSON, C. R., SNYDER, J. M., GALLAPSY, S. E. and JOHNSTON, J. M. (1979) Development of human fetal lung in organ culture: effect of progesterone. *61st Ann. Meeting of the American Endocrine Soc.,* Abst. No. 966.

MENDELSON, C. R., MacDONALD, P. C. and JOHNSTON, J. M. (1980) Estrogen binding in human fetal lung tissue cytosol. *Endocrinology* **106:** 368–374.

MENDELSON, C. R., JOHNSTON, J. M., MacDONALD, P. C. and SNYDER, J. M. (1981) Multihormonal regulation of surfactant synthesis by human fetal lung in vitro. *J. Clin. Endocr. Metab.* **53:** 307–317.

MERCADO-SIMMEN, R. C., BRYANT-GREENWOOD, G. D. and GREENWOOD, F. C. (1980) Relaxin receptor in the rat myometrium: regulation by estrogen and relaxin. *Endocrinology* **110:** 220–226.

MERCADO-SIMMEN, R. C., BRYANT-GREENWOOD, G. D. and GREENWOOD, F. C. (1982) Characterization of the binding of ^{125}I-relaxin to rat uterus. *J. Biol. Chem.* **255:** 3617–3623.

MESTER, J., MARTEL, D., PSYCHOYOS, A. and BAULIEU, E. E. (1974) Hormonal control of estrogen receptor in uterus and receptivity for ovoimplantation in the rat. *Nature* **250:** 776–778.

MICHAEL, R. P., BONSALL, R. W. and REES, H. D. (1989) The uptake of [^{3}H]-testosterone and its metabolites by the brain and pituitary gland of the fetal macaque. *Endocrinology* **124:** 1319–1326.

MIDGLEY, A. R. (1973) Autoradiographic analysis of gonadotropin binding to rat ovarian tissue sections. *Adv. Exp. Med. Biol.* **36:** 365–378.

MIELE, L., CORDELLA-MIELE, E. and MUKHERJEE, A. B. (1987) Uteroglobin: structure, molecular biology, and new perspectives on its function as a phospholipase A2 inhibitor. *Endocr. Rev.* **8:** 474–490.

MILEWICH, L., GEORGE, F. W. and WILSON, J. D. (1977) Estrogen formation by the ovary of the rabbit embryo. *Endocrinology* **100:** 187–196.

MILGROM, E., ATGER, M., PERROT, M. and BAULIEU, E-E. (1972) Progesterone in uterus and plasma: VI. Uterine progesterone receptors during the estrus cycle and implantation in the guinea pig. *Endocrinology* **90:** 1071–1078.

MILLAN, M. A., CARVALLO, P., IZUMI, S.-I., ZEMEL, S., CATT, K. J. and AGUILERA, G. (1989) Novel sites of expression of functional angiotensin II receptors in the late gestation fetus. *Science* **244:** 1340–1342.

MILLER, H. C. and FUTRAKUL, P. (1968) Birthweight, gestational age and sex as determining factors in the incidence of respiratory distress syndrome of prematurely born infants. *J. Pediatrics* **72:** 628–635.

MILLER, K. G., MILLS, P. and BAINS, M. G. (1973) A study of the influence of pregnancy on the thymus gland of the mouse. *Am. J. Obstet. Gynecol.* **117:** 913–918.

MILLET, A. and PASQUALINI, J. R. (1978) Liaison spécifique de la ^{3}H-progesterone à une protéine du plasma du foetus de cobaye. *C. R. Acad. Sci. (Paris)* **287:** 1429–1432.

MILLS, E. S. and TOPPER, Y. J. (1969) Mammary alveolar epithelial cell: effect of hydrocortisone on ultrasturcture. *Science* **165:** 1127–1128.

MILLS, E. S. and TOPPER, Y. J. (1970) Some ultrastructural effects of insulin, hydrocortisone, and prolactin on mammary gland explants. *J. Cell Biol.* **44:** 310–328.

MOHLA, S., CLEM-JACKSON, N. and HUNTER, J. B. (1981) Estrogen receptors and estrogen-induced gene expression in the rat mammary glands and uteri during pregnancy and lactation: changes in progesterone receptor and RNA polymerase activity. *J. Steroid Biochem.* **14:** 501–508.

MOHRI, T., KITAGAWA, H. and RIGGS, T. R. (1974) Action of insulin on amino acid uptake by the immature rat uterus in vitro. *Biochim. Biophys. Acta* **363:** 249–260.

MOLSBERRY, R. L., CARR, B. R., MENDELSON, C. R. and SIMPSON, E. R. (1982) Human chorionic gonadotropin binding to human fetal testes as a function of gestational age. *J. Clin. Endocr. Metab.* **55:** 791–794.

MONDER, C. and COUFALIK, A. (1972) Separation of glycogen formation and aminotransferase activity induced by cortisol in fetal rat liver. *Endocrinology* **91:** 257–261.

MOOG, F. (1953) The functional differentiation of the small intestine. *J. Exp. Zool.* **124:** 329–346.

MORGAN, D. O. and ROTH, R. A. (1986) Mapping surface structure of the human insulin receptor with monoclonal antibodies. Localization of main immunogenic regions to the receptor kinase domain. *Biochemistry* **25:** 1364–1371.

MORISHIGE, W. K., PEPE, G. J. and ROTHCHILD, I. (1973) Serum luteinizing hormone, prolactin and progesterone levels during pregnancy in the rat. *Endocrinology* **92:** 1527–1530.

MORREALE DE ESCOBAR, G., PASTOR, R., OBREGON, M. J. and ESCOBAR DEL REY, F. (1985) Effects of maternal hypothyroidism on the weight and thyroid hormone content of rat embryonic tissues, before and after onset of fetal thyroid function. *Endocrinology* **117:** 1890–1900.

MORRISS, F. H. Jr., TUCHMAN, C., CRANDELL, S. S., RIDDLE, L. M., FITZGERALD, B. J. and WEST M. S. (1986) Ontogeny of ovine fetal liver and kidney plasma membrane insulin receptors and fetal growth. *Proc. Soc. Exp. Biol. Med.* **181:** 24–32.

MOSTELLO, D. J., HAMOSH, M. and HAMOSH, P. (1981) Effect of dexamethasone on lipoprotein lipase activity of fetal rat lung. *Biol. Neonate* **40:** 121–128.

MUECHLER, E. K., FLICKINGER, G. L. and MIKHAIL, G. (1974) Estradiol receptors in the oviduct and uterus of the rabbit. *Fertil. Steril.* **25:** 893–899.

MUELLER, G. C., HERRANEN, A. M. and JERVELL, K. (1958) Studies on the mechanism of action of estrogens. *Rec. Prog. Horm. Res.* **14:** 95–139.

MUELLER, P. L., GLUCKMAN, P. D., KAPLAN, S. L., RUDOLPH, A. M. and GRUMBACH, M. M. (1979) Hormone ontogeny in the ovine fetus. V. Circulating prolactin in mid- and late gestation and in the newborn. *Endocrinology* **105:** 129–134.

MUKHERJEE, A. B., LAKI, K. and AGARWAL, A. K. (1980) Possible mechanism of success of an allotransplantation in nature: mammalian pregnancy. *Med. Hypotheses* **6:** 1043–1055.

MULAY, S., GIANNOPOULOS, G. and SOLOMON, S. (1973) Corticosteroid levels in the mother and fetus of the rabit during gestation. *Endocrinology* **93:** 1342–1348.

MULAY, S., VARMA, D. R. and SOLOMON, S. (1982) Influence of protein deficiency in rats on hormonal status and cytoplasmic glucocorticoid receptors in maternal and fetal tissues. *J. Endocr.* **95:** 49–58.

MULAY, S., PHILIP, A. and SOLOMON, S. (1983) Influence of maternal diabetes on fetal rat development: alteration of insulin receptors in fetal liver and lung. *J. Endocr.* **98:** 401–410.

MULCHAHEY, J. J., DiBLASIO, A. M., MARTIN, M. C., BLUMENFELD, Z. and JAFFE, R. B. (1987) Hormone production and peptide regulation of the human fetal pituitary gland. *Endocr. Rev.* **8:** 406–425.

MULDOON, T. G. (1978) Characterization of mouse mammary tissue estrogen receptors under conditions of differing hormonal backgrounds. *J. Steroid Biochem.* **9:** 485–494.

MULDOON, T. G. (1979) Mouse mammary tissue estrogen receptors: ontogeny and molecular heterogeneity. In: *Ontogeny of Receptors and Reproductive Hormone Action*, Hamilton, T. H., Clark, J. H. and Sadler, W. A. (Eds), Raven Press, New York, pp. 225–247.

MULDOON, T. G. (1980) Regulation of steroid hormone receptor activity. *Endocr. Rev.* **1:** 339–364.

MULDOON, T. G. (1981) Interplay between estradiol and prolactin in the regulation of steroid hormone receptor levels, nature, and functionality in normal mouse mammary tissue. *Endocrinology* **109:** 1339–1346.

MUNCK, A. and BRINCK-JOHNSEN, T. (1968) Specific and non-specific physiochemical interactions of glucocorticoids and related steroids with rat thymus cells in vitro. *J. Biol. Chem.* **243:** 5556–5565.

MUNFORD, R. E. (1963) Changes in the mammary gland of rats and mice during pregnancy, lactation and involution. I. Histological structure. *J. Endocr.* **28:** 1–15.

MURPHY, B. E. P. (1979) Cortisol and cortisone in human fetal development. *J. Steroid Biochem.* **11:** 509–513.

MURR, S. M., BRADFORD, G. E. and GESCHWIND, I. I. (1974) Plasma luteinizing hormone, follicle-stimulating hormone and prolactin during pregnancy in the mouse. *Endocrinology* **94:** 112–116.

NANDI, S. (1958) Endocrine control of mammary gland development and function in the C3H/He Crgl mouse. *J. Natl Cancer Inst.* **21:** 1039–1063.

NARBAITZ, R., STUMPF, W. E. and STAR, M. (1980) Estrogen receptors in mammary gland primordia of fetal mouse. *Anat. Embryol.* **158:** 161–166.

NATHANIELSZ, P. W. (1975) Thyroid function in the fetus and newborn mammal. *Br. Med. Bull.* **31:** 51–56.

NATHANIELSZ, P. W., COMLINE, R. S., SILVER, M. and THOMAS, A. L. (1973) Thyroid function in the foetal lamb during the last third of gestation. *J. Endocr.* **58:** 535–546.

NELSON, W. O. and PFIFFNER, J. J. (1930) Experimental production of deciduomata in rat by extract of corpus luteum. *Proc. Soc. Exp. Biol. Med.* **27:** 863–866.

NEUFELD, N. D., CORBO, L. M. and KAPLAN, S. A. (1981) Plasma membrane insulin receptors in fetal rabbit lung. *Pediat. Res.* **15:** 1058–1062.

NEUMANN, F. and ELGER, W. (1966) The effect of the anti-androgen 1,2α-methylene-6-chloro-delta4,6-pregnadiene-17β-ol-3,20-dione-17alpha-acetate (cyproterone acetate) on the development of the mammary glands of male foetal rats. *J. Endocr.* **36:** 347–352.

NGUYEN, B. L., GIAMBIAGI, N., MAYRAND, C., LECERF, F. and PASQUALINI, J. R. (1986) Estrogen and progesterone receptors in the fetal and newborn vagina of guinea pig: biological, morphological and ultrastructural responses to tamoxifen and estradiol. *Endocrinology* **119:** 978–988.

NGUYEN B. L., HATIER R., JEANVOINE G., ROUX M., GRIGNON G. and PASQUALINI J. R. (1988) Effect of oestradiol on the progesterone receptor and on morphological ultrastructures in the foetal and newborn uterus and ovary of the rat. *Acta Endocr. (Copenh.)* **117:** 249–259.

NICHOLAS, T. E., JOHNSON, R. G., LUGG, M. A. and KIM, P. A. (1978) Pulmonary phospholipid biosynthesis and the ability of the fetal rabbit lung to reduce cortisone to cortisol during the final ten days of gestation. *Life Sci* **22:** 1517–1524.

NICOLL, C. A. and BERN, H. A. (1972) In: *Ciba Fdn Symp. Lactogenic Hormones*, Wolstenholme, G. E. W. and Knight, J. (Eds.), Churchill, London, pp. 299–317.

NIELSEN, H. C. (1985) Androgen receptors influence the production of pulmonary surfactant in the testicular feminization mouse fetus. *J. Clin. Invest.* **76:** 177–181.

NIELSEN, H. C. and TORDAY, J. S. (1981) Sex differences in fetal rabbit pulmonary surfactant production. *Pediat. Res.* **15:** 1245–1247.

NIELSEN, H. C., ZINMAN, H. M. and TORDAY, J. S. (1981) Dihydrotestosterone (DHT) inhibits fetal pulmonary surfactant production in vivo. *Pediat. Res.* **15:** 728A.

NISHIZUKA, Y. (1986) Studies and perspectives of protein kinase C. *Science* **233:** 305–312.

NISSENSON, R., FLOURET, G. and HECHTER, O. (1978) Opposing effects of estradiol and progesterone on oxytocin receptors in rabbit uterus. *Proc. Natl Acad. Sci. USA* **75:** 2044–2048.

NOLIN, J. M. and WITORSCH, R. J. (1976) Detection of endogenous immunoreactive prolactin in rat mammary epithelial cells during lactation. *Endocrinology* **99:** 949–958.

NOZU, K., DEHEJIA, A., ZAWISTOWICH, L., CATT, K. J. and DUFAU, M. L. (1981) Gonadotropin-induced receptor regulation and steroidogenic lesions in cultured Leydig cells. Induction of specific protein synthesis by chronic gonadotropin and estradiol. *J. Biol. Chem.* **258:** 12875–12882.

O'KEEFE, E. and CUATRECASAS, P. (1974) Insulin receptors in murine mammary cells: comparison in pregnant and non-pregnant animals. *Biochim. Biophys. Acta* **343:** 64–77.

ODOM, M. J., SNYDER, J. M., BOGGARAM, V. and MENDELSON, C. R. (1988) Glucocorticoid regulation of the major surfactant associated protein (SP-A) and its messenger ribonucleic acid and of morphological development of human fetal lung *in vitro*. *Endocrinology* **123:** 1712–1720.

OGASAWARA, Y., OKAMOTO, S., KITAMURA, Y. and MATSUMOTO, K. (1983) Proliferative pattern of uterine cells from birth to adulthood in intact, neonatally castrated, and/or adrenalectomized mice, assayed by incorporation of [^{125}I]iododeoxyuridine. *Endocrinology* **113:** 582–587.

OGLE, T. F. (1980) Characteristics of high affinity progesterone binding to rat placental cytosol. *Endocrinology* **106:** 1861–1868.

OGLE, T. F. (1981) Kinetic and physicochemical characteristics of an endogenous inhibitor to progesterone-receptor binding in rat placental cytosol. *Biochem. J.* **199:** 371–381.

OGLE, T. F. (1983a) Action of glycerol and sodium molybdate in stabilization of the progesterone receptor from rat trophoblast. *J. Biol. Chem.* **258:** 4982–4988.

OGLE, T. F. (1983b) Progesterone binding to the placental receptor in cytosol and nuclear compartments at various stages of pregnancy in the rat. *65th Ann. Meeting American Endocrine Soc.* San Antonio, 1983, Abst. 1027.

OGLE, T. F. (1986) Evidence for nuclear processing of progesterone receptors in rat placenta. *J. Steroid Biochem.* **25:** 183–190.

OGLE, T. F. (1987) Nuclear acceptor sites for progesterone-receptor complexes in rat placenta. *Endocrinology* **121:** 28–35.

OGLE, T. F. and BEYER, B. K. (1982) Steroid-binding specificity of the progesterone receptor from rat placenta. *J. Steroid Biochem.* **16:** 147–150.

OGLE, T. F. and MILLS, T. M. (1983) Estimation of molecular parameters of the endogenous inhibitor to progesterone-receptor binding in rat trophoblast. *J. Steroid Biochem.* **18:** 699–705.

OKA, T. and TOPPER, Y. J. (1971) Hormone-dependent accumulation of rough endoplasmic reticulum in mouse mammary epithelial cells in vitro. *J. Biol. Chem.* **246:** 7701–7707.

OKA, T., PERRY, J. W. and TOPPER, Y. T. (1974) Changes in insulin responsiveness during development of mammary epithelium. *J. Cell Biol.* **62:** 550–556.

OKULICZ, W. C., EVANS, B. W. and LEAVITT, W. W. (1981) Progesterone regulation of estrogen receptor in the rat uterus: a primary inhibitory influence on the nuclear fraction. *Steroids* **37:** 463–470.

OLIN, P., VECCHIO, G., EKHOLM, R. and ALMQVIST, S. (1970) Human fetal thyroglobulin: characterization and in vitro biosynthesis studies. *Endocrinology* **86:** 1041–1048.

OLIVER, C., ESKAY, R. L. and PORTER, J. C. (1980) Developmental changes in brain TRH and in plasma and pituitary TSH and prolactin levels in the rat. *Biol. Neonate* **37:** 145–152.

OLIVER, I. T., BLUMER, W. F. C. and WITHAM, I. J. (1963) Free ribosomes during maturation of rat liver. *Comp. Biochem. Physiol.* **10:** 33–38.

OLSON, M. E., SHEEHAN, D. M. and BRANHAM, W. S. (1983) The postnatal ontogeny of rat uterine ornithine decarboxylase: acquisition of a second peak of estrogen-induced enzyme activity. *Endocrinology* **113:** 1826–1831.

ORTH, J. M. (1982) Proliferation of Sertoli cells in fetal and postnatal rats: a quantitative autoradiographic study. *Anat. Rec.* **203:** 485–492.

ORTH, J. M. (1984) The role of follicle-stimulating hormone in controlling Sertoli cell proliferation in testes of fetal rats. *Endocrinology* **115:** 1248–1255.

PADAYACHI, T., PEGORARO, R. J., HOFMEYR, J., JOUBERT, S. M. and NORMAN, R. J. (1987) Decreased concentrations and affinities of oestrogen and progesterone receptors of intrauterine tissue in human pregnancy. *J. Steroid Biochem.* **26:** 473–479.

PAGANO, G., CASSADER, M., MASSABRIO, M., BOZZO, C., TROSSARELLI, G. F., MENATO, G. and LENTI, G. (1980) Insulin binding to human adipocytes during late pregnancy in healthy, obese, and diabetic state. *Horm. Metab. Res.* **12:** 177–181.

PASQUALINI, J. R. and COSQUER-CLAVREUL, C. (1978) Purification of the cytosol oestradiol-receptor complex from foetal guinea-pig uterus using electrofocusing on polyacrylamide plates. *Experientia* **34:** 268–269.

PASQUALINI, J. R. and NGUYEN, B. L. (1976) Mise en évidence des récepteurs cytosoliques et nucléaires de l'oestradiol dans l'utérus de foetus de cobaye. *C.R. Acad. Sci. Paris* **283:** 413–416.

PASQUALINI, J. R. and NGUYEN, B. L. (1979a) Uterine progesterone receptors in the guinea-pig foetus: changes with gestational age and induction by oestrogens. *J. Endocr.* **81:** 144P–145P.

PASQUALINI, J. R. and NGUYEN B. L. (1979b) Progesterone receptors in the foetal uterus of guinea-pig: its stimulation after oestradiol treatment. *Experientia* **35:** 1116–1117.

PASQUALINI, J. R. and NGUYEN, B. L. (1980) Progesterone receptors in the fetal uterus and ovary of guinea pig, evolution during fetal development and induction and stimulation in estradiol-primed animals. *Endocrinology* **106:** 1160–1165.

PASQUALINI, J. R. and PALMADA M. N. (1971) Estradiol-17-β (E2) receptors in guinea pig fetal brain. *Endocrinology* (Suppl.) **88**-A-242 53rd Meeting Endocrine Society.

PASQUALINI, J. R. and PALMADA, M. (1972) Etude du récepteur de l'oestradiol-17β dans le cerveau du foetus de cobaye. *C. R. Acad. Sci. Paris* **274:** 1218–1221.

PASQUALINI, J. R. and SUMIDA, C. (1971) Formation de récepteurs spécifiques aldostérone-macro-molécules au niveau du cytosol et du noyau du tissu rénal de foetus de cobaye. *C. R. Acad. Sci. Paris* **273:** 1061–1063.

PASQUALINI, J. R. and SUMIDA, C. (1977a) Mineralocorticoid receptors in target tissues. In: *Receptors and Mechanism of Action of Steroid Hormones, Part II, Modern Pharmacology-Toxicology*, Vol. 8, Pasqualini, J. R. (Ed.), Marcel Dekker, Inc., New York, pp. 399–511.

PASQUALINI, J. R. and SUMIDA, C. (1977b) Aldosterone and estradiol receptors in the fetal kidney of guinea pig. In: *Multiple Molecular Forms of Steroid Hormone Receptors*, Agarwal, M. K. (Ed.), Elsevier/North-Holland Biomedical Press, Amsterdam, pp. 199–214.

PASQUALINI, J. R. and SUMIDA, C. (1980) Ontogeny of steroid receptors in the guinea pig. In: *Development of Responsiveness to Steroid Hormones, Advances in the Biosciences*, Vol. 25, Kaye, A. M. and Kaye M. (Eds), Pergamon Press, Oxford, pp. 95–106.

PASQUALINI, J. R. and SUMIDA, C. (1986) Ontogeny of steroid receptors in the reproductive system. *Intl Rev. Cytology* **101:** 275–324.

PASQUALINI, J. R., WIQVIST, N. and DICZFALUSY, E. (1966) Biosynthesis of aldosterone by human foetuses perfused with corticosterone at mid-term. *Biochim. Biophys. Acta* **104:** 515–523.

PASQUALINI, J. R., NGUYEN, B. L., UHRICH, F., WIQVIST, N. and DICZFALUSY, E. (1970) Cortisol and cortisone metabolism in the human foeto-placental unit at midgestation. *J. Steroid Biochem.* **1:** 209–219.

PASQUALINI, J. R., SUMIDA, C. and GELLY, C. (1972) Mineralocorticosteroid receptors in the foetal compartment. *J. Steroid Biochem.* **3:** 543–556.

PASQUALINI, J. R., SUMIDA, C., GELLY, C. and NGUYEN, B. L. (1973) Formation de complexes ^{3}H-oestradiol-macromolécules dans les fractions cytosoliques et nucléaires du tissu rénal du foetus de cobaye. *C. R. Acad. Sci. Paris* **276:** 3359–3362.

PASQUALINI, J. R., SUMIDA, C., and GELLY, C. (1974a) Studies on the mechanism of formation of [^{3}H] aldosterone macromolecule complexes in the foetal guinea pig kidney. *Acta Endocr. (Copenh.)* **77:** 356–367.

PASQUALINI, J. R., SUMIDA, C. and GELLY, C. (1974b) Steroid hormone receptors in fetal guinea pig kidney. *J. Steroid Biochem.* **5:** 977–985.

PASQUALINI, J. R., BEDIN, M. and COGNEVILLE, A. M. (1976a) Transformation of [1,2-3H] aldosterone in the foetal and placental compartments of the guinea pig. *Acta Endocr. (Copenh.)* **82:** 831–841.

PASQUALINI, J. R., SUMIDA, C. and GELLY, C. (1976b) Cytosol and nuclear ^{3}H-oestradiol binding in the foetal tissues of guinea pig. *Acta Endocr. (Copenh.)* **83:** 811–828.

PASQUALINI, J. R., SUMIDA, C., GELLY C. and NGUYEN, B. L. (1976c) Specific ^{3}H-estradiol binding in the fetal uterus and testis of guinea pig. Quantitative evolution of ^{3}H-estradiol receptors in the different fetal tissues (kidney, lung, uterus and testis) during fetal development. *J. Steroid Biochem.* **7:** 1031–1038.

PASQUALINI, J. R., SUMIDA, C., GELLY, C., NGUYEN, B. L. and TARDY, J. (1978a) Specific binding of estrogens in different fetal tissues of guinea pig during fetal development. *Cancer Res.* **38:** 4246–4250.

PASQUALINI, J. R., SUMIDA, C., NGUYEN, B. L. and GELLY C. (1978b) Quantitative evaluation of cytosol and nuclear 3H-estradiol specific binding in the fetal brain of guinea pig during fetal ontogenesis. *J. Steroid Biochem.* **9:** 443–447.

PASQUALINI, J. R., GULINO, A, NGUYEN, G. L. and PORTOIS, M. C. (1980a) Receptor and biological response to estriol in the fetal uterus of guinea pig. *J. Receptor Res.* **1:** 261–275.

PASQUALINI, J. R., SUMIDA, C., NGUYEN B. L., TARDY, J. and GELLY, C. (1980b) Estrogen concentrations and effect of estradiol on progesterone receptors in the fetal and new-born guinea-pigs. *J. Steroid Biochem.* **12:** 65–72.

PASQUALINI, J. R., SUMIDA, C., NGUYEN, B. L., TARDY, J. and GELLY, C. (1980c) Estrogen concentrations and effect of estradiol on progesterone receptors in the fetal and new-born guinea-pigs. *J. Steroid Biochem.* **12:** 65–72.

PASQUALINI, J. R., COSQUER-CLAVREUL, C., VIDALI, G. and ALLFREY, V. G. (1981) Effects of estradiol on the acetylation of histones in the fetal uterus of the guinea pig. *Biol. Reprod.* **25:** 1035–1039.

PASQUALINI, J. R., LANZONE, A., TAHRI-JOUTEI, A. and NGUYEN, B. L. (1982) Effects of seven different oestrogen sulphates on uterine growth and on progesterone receptor in the foetal uterus of guinea pig after administration to the mother. *Acta Endocr.* (*Copenh.*) **101:** 630–635.

PASQUALINI, J. R., COSQUER-CLAVREUL, C. and GELLY, C. (1983a) Rapid modulation by progesterone and tamoxifen of estradiol effects on nuclear histone acetylation in the uterus of the fetal guinea pig. *Biochim. Biophys. Acta* **739:** 137–140.

PASQUALINI, J. R., SUMIDA, C. and GULINO, A. (1983b) Receptors and biological responses to ovarian steroid hormones in the fetal and perinatal periods. In: *Reproductive Physiology IV, International Review of Physiology*, Vol. 27, Greep, R. O. (Ed.), University Park Press, Baltimore, pp. 225–273.

PASQUALINI, J. R., GULINO, A., SUMIDA, C. and SCREPANTI, I. (1984) Antiestrogens in fetal and newborn target tissues. *J. Steroid Biochem.* **20:** 121–128.

PASQUALINI, J. R., STERNER, R., MERCAT, P. and ALLFREY, V. G. (1989) Estradiol enhanced acetylation of nuclear high mobility group proteins of the uterus of newborn guinea pigs. *Biochem. Biophys. Res. Commun.* **161:** 1260–1266.

PAYNE, D. W. and KATZENELLENBOGEN, J. A. (1980) Differential effects of estrogens in tissues: a comparison of estrogen receptor in rabbit uterus and vagina. *Endocrinology* **106:** 1345–1352.

PAYVAR, F., WRANGE, Ö., CARLSTEDT-DUKE, J., OKRET, S., GUSTAFSSON, J. A., and YAMAMOTO, K. R. (1981) Purified glucocorticoid receptors bind selectively in vitro to a cloned DNA fragment whose transcription is regulated by glucocorticoids in vivo. *Proc. Natl. Acad. Sci.* (*USA*) **78:** 6628–6632.

PEARCE, P. and FUNDER, J. W. (1986) Cytosol and nuclear levels of thymic progesterone receptors in pregnant, pseudopregnant and steroid-treated rats. *J. Steroid Biochem.* **25:** 65–69.

PEARLMUTTER, A. F. and SOLOFF, M. S. (1979) Characterization of the metal ion requirement for oxytocin-receptor interaction in rat mammary gland membranes. *J. Biol. Chem.* **254:** 3899–3906.

PELEG, S., de BOEVER, J. and KAYE, A. M. (1979) Replenishment and nuclear retention of oestradiol-17β receptors in rat uteri during postnatal development. *Biochim. Biophys. Acta* **587:** 67–74.

PEREZ-CASTILLO, A., BERNAL, J., FERREIRO, B. and PANS, T. (1985) The early ontogenesis of thyroid hormone receptor in rat fetus. *Endocrinology* **117:** 2457–2461.

PERROT, M. and MILGROM, E. (1978) Immunochemical studies of guinea-pig progesterone binding plasma protein. *Endocrinology* **103:** 1678–1685.

PERROT-APPLANAT, M., LOGEAT, F., GROYER-PICARD, M. T. and MILGROM, E. (1985) Immunocytochemical study of mammalian progesterone receptor using monoclonal antibodies. *Endocrinology* **116:** 1473–1484.

PERRY, J. S., HEAP, R. B. and AMOROSO, E. C. (1973) Steroid hormone production by pig blastocysts. *Nature* **245:** 45–47.

PHELPS, D. S., CHURCH, S., KOUREMBANAS, S., TAEUSCH, H. W. and FLOROS, J. (1987) Increases in the 35 kDa surfactant-associated protein and its mRNA following in vivo dexamethasone treatment of fetal and neonatal rats. *Electrophoresis* **8:** 235–238.

PHOENIX, C. H., GOY, R. W., GERALL, A. A. and YOUNG, W. C. (1959) Organizing action of prenatally administered testosterone propionate on the tissues mediating mating behavior in the female guinea pig. *Endocrinology* **65:** 369–382.

PICARD, D. and YAMAMOTO, K. R. (1987) Two signals mediate hormone-dependent nuclear localization of the glucocorticoid receptor. *EMBO J.* **6:** 3333–3340.

PLAPINGER, L., LANDAU, I. T., McEWEN, B. S. and FEDER, H. H. (1977) Characteristics of estradiol-binding macromolecules in fetal and adult guinea pig brain cytosols. *Biol. Reprod.* **16:** 586–599.

PLAS, C. and DUVAL, D. (1986) Dexamethasone binding sites and steroid-dependent stimulation of glycogenesis by insulin in cultured fetal hepatocytes. *Endocrinology* **118:** 587–594.

PLAS, C., CHAPEVILLE, F. and JACQUOT, R. (1973) Development of glycogen storage ability under cortisol control in primary cultures of rat fetal hepatocytes. *Devel. Biol.* **32:** 82–91.

POLK, D., CHEROMCHA, D., REVICZKY, A. and FISHER, D. A. (1989) Nuclear thyroid hormone receptors: ontogeny and thyroid hormone effects in sheep. *Am. J. Physiol.* **256:** E543–E549.

POMERANTZ, S. M., FOX, T. O., SHOLL, S. A., VITO, C. C. and GOY, R. W. (1985) Androgen and estrogen receptors in fetal rhesus monkey brain and anterior pituitary. *Endocrinology* **116:** 83–89.

POSNER, B. I. (1974) Insulin receptors in human and animal placental tissue. *Diabetes* **23:** 209–217.

POSNER, B. I. (1976) Characterization and modulation of growth hormone and prolactin binding in mouse liver. *Endocrinology* **98:** 645–654.

POSNER, B. I., KELLY, P. A., SHIU, R. P. C. and FRIESEN, H. G. (1974) Studies of insulin, growth hormone and prolactin binding: tissue distribution, species variation and characterization. *Endocrinology* **95:** 521–531.

POST, M. and SMITH, B. T. (1984) Effect of fibroblast-pneumonocyte factor in the synthesis of surfactant phospholipids in type II cells from fetal rat lung. *Biochim. Biophys. Acta* **793:** 297–299.

POST, M., FLOROS, J. and SMITH, B. T. (1984a) Inhibition of lung maturation by monoclonal antibodies against fibroblast-pneumonocyte factor. *Nature* **308:** 284–286.

POST, M., TORDAY, J. S. and SMITH, B. T. (1984b) Alveolar type II cells isolated from fetal rat lung organotypic cultures synthesize and secrete surfactant-associated phospholipids and respond to fibroblast-pneumonocyte factor. *Exp. Lung Res.* **7:** 53–65.

POST, M., BARSOUMIAN, A. and SMITH, B. T. (1986) The cellular mechanism of glucocorticoid acceleration of fetal lung maturation. *J. Biol. Chem.* **261:** 2179–2184.

POTAU, N., RIUDOR, E. and BALLABRIGA, A. (1984) Insulin receptors in human brain. Ontogenic study., *7th Int. Cong. Endocrinology, Excerpta Medica Int. Cong. Ser.* 652, Elsevier Science Publishers, Abst. No. 2015, p. 1268.

PRATT, W. B. (1987) Transformation of glucocorticoid and progesterone receptors to the DNA-binding state. *J. Cell. Biochem.* **35:** 51–68.

PSYCHOYOS, A. (1960) Nouvelle contribution à l'étude de la nidation de l'oeuf chez la ratte. *C.R. Acad. Sci. Paris* **251:** 3073–3075.

PSYCHOYOS, A. (1969) Hormonal requirements for egg implantation. In: *Advances in Bio-sciences IV. Mechanisms Involved in Conception*, Raspe, G. (Ed.), Pergamon Press, London, pp. 275–290.

PSYCHOYOS, A. (1973a) Endocrine control of egg-implantation. In: *Handbook of Physiology, Endocrinology*, Vol. 2, Part 2, Greep, R. O. and Astwood, E. B. (Eds.), Am. Physiological Society, Washington D. C., pp. 187–215.

PSYCHOYOS, A. (1973b) Hormonal control of ovoimplantation. *Vit. Horm.* **31:** 201–256.

PSYCHOYOS, A. (1976) Hormonal control of uterine receptivity for nidation. *J. Reprod. Fertil.* (Suppl.) **25:** 17–28.

PUCA, G. A. and BRESCIANI, F. (1969) Interactions of 6,7-^{3}H-17β-estradiol with mammary gland and other organs of the C3H mouse *in vivo*. *Endocrinology* **85:** 1–10.

PULKKINEN, M. O. and KERO, P. (1977) Effect of progesterone on initiation of respiration of the newborn. *Biol. Neonate* **32:** 218–221.

PURI, R. K. and ROY, S. K. (1981a) Estradiol binding in different parts of the rabbit oviduct during egg transport. *Endokrinologie* **78:** 12–20.

PURI, R. K. and ROY, S. K. (1981b) Estradiol receptors in embryonic and inter-embryonic segments of uterus of the rabbit during implantation. *Indian J. Exp. Biol.* **19:** 26–28.

QUIRK, S. J. and CURRIE, W. B. (1984) Uterine steroid receptor changes associated with progesterone withdrawal during pregnancy and pseudopregnancy in rabbits. *Endocrinology* **114:** 182–191.

QUIRK, S. J., GANNELL, J., FINDLAY, J. K. and FUNDER, J. W. (1982) Glucocorticoid receptors in epithelial cells isolated from the mammary glands of pregnant and lactating rats. *Mol. Cell. Endocr.* **25:** 227–241.

QUIRK, S. J., GANNELL, J. E. and FUNDER, J. W. (1983) Aldosterone-binding sites in pregnant and lactating rat mammary glands. *Endocrinology* **113:** 1812–1817.

QUIRK, S. J., GANNELL, J. E. and FUNDER, J. W. (1984) Oestrogen administration induces progesterone receptors in lactating rat mammary gland. *J. Steroid Biochem.* **20:** 803–806.

RABII, J. and GANONG, W. F. (1976) Responses of plasma estradiol and plasma LH to ovariectomy, ovariectomy plus adrenalectomy and estrogen injection at various ages. *Neuroendocrinology* I. **20:** 270–281.

RAESIDE, J. I. (1983) Gonadotrophic stimulation of androgen secretion by the early fetal pig ovary in organ culture. *Biol. Reprod.* **28:** 128–133.

RAJANIEMI, H. J., RÖNNBERG, L., KAUPPILA, A., YLÖSTALO, P., JALKANEN, M., SAASTAMOINEN, J., SELANDER, K., PYSTYNEN, P. and VIHKO, R. (1981) Luteinizing hormone receptors in human ovarian follicles and corpora lutea during menstrual cycle and pregnancy. *J. Clin. Endocr. Metab.* **108:** 307–313.

RAYNAUD, A. (1955) Observations sur les modifications provoquées par les hormones oestrogènes du mode de développement des mammelons des foetus de souris. *C. R. Acad. Sci. Paris* **240:** 674–676.

RAYNAUD, A. and DELOST, P. (1977) Inhibition du déveloooement des ébauches mammaires, chez les rongeurs, sous l'effet de la sécretion du testicule foetal et des hormones sexuelles. *Colloq. Int. C.N.R.S. sur les Mécanismes de la Rudimentation des Organes chez les Embryons de Vertébrés,* **266:** 71–84.

RAYNAUD, A. and FRILLEY, M. (1949) Le développement embryonaire de la glande mammaire de la souris, après destruction, au moyen des rayons X, des glandes génitales de l'embryon. *Bull. Soc. Zool. France* **74:** 156–159.

RAYNAUD, J. P. (1973) Influence of rat estradiol binding plasma protein (EBP) on uterotrophic activity. *Steroids* **21:** 249–258.

RAYNAUD, J. P., MOGUILEWSKY, M. and VANNIER, B. (1980) Influence of rat estradiol binding plasma protein (EBP) on estrogen binding to its receptor and on induced biological responses. In: *The Development of Responsiveness to Steroid Hormones. Advances in the Biosciences,* Vol. 25, Kaye A. M. and Kaye M. (Eds), Pergamon Press, Oxford, pp. 59–75.

REITER, E. O., GOLDBERG, R. L., VAITUKAITIS, J. L. and ROSS, G. T. (1972) A role for endogenous estrogen in normal ovarian development in the neonatal rat. *Endocrinology* **91:** 1537–1539.

REVESZ, C., CHAPPEL, C. I. and GAUDRY, R. (1960) Masculinization of female fetuses in the rat by progestational compounds. *Endocrinology* **66:** 140–144.

REYES, F. I., WINTER, J. S. D. and FAIMAN, C. (1973) Studies on human sexual development. I. Fetal gonadal and adrenal sex steroids. *J. Clin. Endocr. Metab.* **37:** 74–78.

REYES, F. I., BORODITSKY, R. S., WINTER, J. S. D. and FAIMAN, C. (1974) Studies on human sexual development. II. Fetal and maternal serum gonadotropin and sex steroid concentrations. *J. Clin. Endocr. Metab.* **38:** 612–621.

RICHARDS, J. E., SHYAMALA, G. and NANDI, S. (1974) Estrogen receptor in normal and neoplastic mouse mammary tissues. *Cancer Res.* **34:** 2764–2772.

RICHARDS, J. S. and KERSEY, K. A. (1979) Changes in theca and granulosa cell function in antral follicles developing during pregnancy in the rat gonadotropin receptors, cyclic AMP and estradiol-17beta. *Biol. Reprod.* **21**: 1185–1201.

RICHARDS, J. S., IRELAND, J. J., RAO, M. C., BERNATH, G. A., MIDGLEY, A. R. and REICHERT, L. E. (1976) Ovarian follicular development in the rat: hormone receptor regulation by estradiol, follicle stimulating hormone and luteinizing hormone. *Endocrinology* **99**: 1562–1570.

RICHARDS, S. R., MALARKEY, W. B., NICOL, S. J. and MATTHEWS, R. H. (1984) Assessment of mammary lactogenic receptor changes in pregnant rabbits. *Am. J. Obstet. Gynec.* **149**: 159–164.

RICKETTS, A. P., GALIL, A. K. A., ACKLAND, N., HEAP, R. B. and FLINT, A. P. F. (1980) Activation by corticosteroids of steroid metabolizing enzymes in ovine placental explants in vitro. *J. Endocr.* **85**: 457–469.

RIEMER, R. K., GOLDFIEN, A. C., GOLDFIEN, A. and ROBERTS, J. M. (1986) Rabbit uterine oxytocin receptors and in vitro contractile response: abrupt changes at term and the role of eicosanoids. *Endocrinology* **119**: 699–709.

RIEUTORT, M. (1974) Pituitary content and plasma levels of growth hormone in foetal and weanling rats. *J. Endocr.* **60**: 261–268.

ROBERT, M. F., NEFF, R. K., HUBBELL, J. P., TAEUSCH, H. W. and AVERY, M. E. (1976) Association between maternal diabetes and the respiratory distress syndrome in the newborn. *New Engl. J. Med.* **294**: 357–360.

ROBSON, J. M. (1937) The action of progesterone on the uterus of the rabbit and its antagonism by oestrone. *J. Physiol.* **88**: 100–111.

ROONEY, S. A. (1979) Biosynthesis of lung surfactant during fetal and early postnatal development. *Trends in Biochem. Sci.* (August): 189–191.

ROONEY, S. A., WAI-LEE, T. S., GOBRAN, L. and MOTOYAMA, E. K. (1976) Phospholipid content, composition and biosynthesis during fetal lung development in the rabbit. *Biochim. Biophys. Acta* **431**: 447–458.

ROONEY, S. A., GOBRAN, L. I., MARINO, P. A., MANISCALCO, W. M. and GROSS, I. (1979a) Effects of betamethasone on phospholipid content, composition and biosynthesis in fetal rabbit lung. *Biochim. Biophys. Acta* **572**: 64–76.

ROONEY, S. A., MARINO, P. A., GOBRAN, L. I., GROSS, I. and WARSHAW, J. B. (1979b) Thyrotropin-releasing hormone increases the amount of surfactant in lung lavage from fetal rabbits. *Pediatr. Res.* **13**: 623–625.

ROSE, J. C., KUTE, T. E. and WINKLER, L. (1985) Glucocorticoid receptors in sheep brain tissues during development. *Am. J. Physiol.* **249**: E345–E349.

ROSEMBLIT, N., ASCOLI, M. and SEGALOFF, D. L. (1988) Characterization of an antiserum to the rat luteal luteinizing hormone/chorionic gonadotropin receptor. *Endocrinology* **123**: 2284–2290.

ROSEN, J. M., O'NEAL, D. L., McHUGH, J. E. and COMSTOCK, J. P. (1978) Progesterone-mediated inhibition of casein mRNA and polysomal casein synthesis in the rat mammary gland during pregnancy. *Biochemistry* **17**: 290–297.

ROSEN, J. M., MATUSIK, R. J., RICHARDS, D. A., GUPTA, P. and RODGERS, J. D. (1980) Multihormonal regulation of casein gene expression at the transcriptional and post-transcriptional levels in the mammary gland. *Rec. Prog. Horm. Res* **36**: 157–193.

ROZENGURT, E. (1986) Early signals in the mitogenic response. *Science* **234**: 161–166.

RUIZ-BRAVO, N. and ERNEST, M. J. (1985) Multihormonal control of tyrosine aminotransferase activity in developing rat liver. *Endocrinology* **116**: 2489–2496.

SAEZ, J. M., MORERA, A. M., DAZORD, A. and BATAILLE, P. (1974) Interaction of ACTH with its adrenal receptors: specific binding of ACTH 1–24, its O-nitrophenyl sulfenyl derivative and ACTH 11–24. *J. Steroid Biochem.* **5**: 925–933.

SAIDAPUR, S. K. and GREENWALD, G. S. (1978) Peripheral blood and ovarian levels of sex steroids in the cyclic hamster. *Biol. Reprod.* **18**: 401–408.

SAKAI, S. and BANERJEE, M. R. (1979) Glucocorticoid modulation of prolactin receptors on mammary cells of lactating mice. *Biochim. Biophys. Acta* **582**: 79–88.

SAKAI, S., ENAMI, J., NANDI, S. and BANERJEE, M. R. (1978) Prolactin receptor on dissociated mammary epithelial cells at different stages of development. *Mol. Cell. Endocr.* **12**: 285–298.

SAKAI, S., BOWMAN, P. D., YANG, J., McCORMICK, K. and NANDI, S. (1979) Glucocorticoid regulation of prolactin receptors on mammary cells in culture. *Endocrinology* **104**: 1447–1449.

SAKAMOTO, H., LERANTH, C., MacLUSKY, N. J., SAITO, Y. and NAFTOLIN, F. (1987) Insulin specific binding sites in the myometrium of pregnant rats. *Endocrinology* **120**: 1951–1955.

SALA, N. L. and FREIRE, F. (1974) Relationship between ultrastructure and response to oxytocin of the mammary myoepithelium throughout pregnancy and lactation: effect of estrogen and progesterone. *Biol. Reprod.* **11**: 7–17.

SALISBURY, R. L., DUDLEY, S. D. and WEISZ, J. (1982) Effect of gonadotrophin-releasing hormone on circulating levels of immunoreactive luteinizing hormone in fetal rats. *Neuroendocrinology* **35**: 265–269.

SALOMON, D. S., ZUBAIRI, Y. and THOMPSON, E. B. (1978) Ontogeny and biochemical properties of glucocorticoid receptors in mid-gestation mouse embryos. *J. Steroid Biochem.* **9**: 95–107.

SANDERS, R. L., ENGLE, M. J. and DOUGLAS, W. H. J. (1981) Effect of dexamethasone upon surfactant phosphatidylcholine and phosphatidylglycerol synthesis in organotypic cultures of type II cells. *Biochem. Biophys. Acta* **664**: 380–388.

SAP, J., MUÑOZ, A., DAMM, K., GOLDBERG, Y., GHYSDAEL, J., LEUTZ, A., BEUG, H. and VENNSTRÖM, B. (1986) The c-erb-A protein is a high affinity receptor for thyroid hormone. *Nature* **324**: 635–640.

SAR, M. and STUMPF, W. E. (1976) Autoradiography of mammary glands and uteri of mice and rats after the injection of ³H-estradiol. *J. Steroid Biochem.* **7**: 391–394.

SCHEMESH, M. (1980) Estradiol-17β biosynthesis by the early bovine fetal ovary during the active and refractory phases. *Biol. Reprod.* **23**: 577–582.

SCHIRAR, A., CAPPONI, A. and CATT, K. J. (1980) Elevation of uterine angiotensin II receptors during early pregnancy in the rat. *Endocrinology* **106**: 1521–1527.

SCHNEIDER, W. and SHYAMALA, G. (1985) Glucocorticoid receptors in primary cultures of mouse mammary epithelial cells: characterization and modulation by prolactin and cortisol. *Endocrinology* **116**: 2656–2662.

SCHOFIELD, B. M. (1957) The hormonal control of myometrial function during pregnancy. *J. Physiol.* **138**: 1–10.

SCHOFIELD, B. M. (1960) Hormonal control of pregnancy by the ovary and placenta in the rabbit. *J. Physiol.* **151**: 578–590.

SCHULTZ, F. M. and WILSON, J. D. (1974) Virilization of the Wolffian duct in the rat fetus by various androgens. *Endocrinology* **94**: 979–986.

SCHWABE, C., STEINETZ, B. G., WEISS, G., SEGALOFF, A., McDONALD, J. K., O'BYRNE, E. M., HOCHMAN, J., CARRIERE, B. and GOLDSMITH, L. (1978) Relaxin. *Rec. Prog. Horm. Res.* **34**: 123–199.

SCREPANTI, I., GULINO, A. and PASQUALINI, J. R. (1982) The fetal thymus of guinea pig as an estrogen target organ. *Endocrinology* **111**: 1552–1561.

SEAMARK, R. F. and LUTWAK-MANN, C. (1972) Progestins in rabbit blastocysts *J. Reprod. Fertil.* **29**: 147–148.

SEDDIKI, T., DJIANE, J. and OLLIVIER-BOUSQUET, M. (1988) Localisation par immunofluorescence des récepteurs de la prolactine dans les cellules épithéliales mammaires de lapines en lactation à l'aide d'un anticorps monoclonal. *C.R. Acad. Sci. Paris* **307**: 427–432.

SENIOR, B. E. (1975) Cytoplasmic oestradiol-binding sites and their relationship to oestradiol content in the endometrium of cattle. *J. Reprod. Fertil.* **44**: 501–511.

SERENI, F., KENNEY, F. T. and KRETCHMER, N. (1959) Factors influencing the development of tyrosine-alpha-ketoglutarate transaminase activity in rat liver. *J. Biol. Chem.* **234**: 609–612.

SÉRON-FERRÉ, M., MONROE, S. E., HESS, D., PARER, J. T. and JAFFE, R. B. (1979) Prolactin concentrations in the monkey fetus during the last third of gestation. *Endocrinology* **104:** 1243–1246.

SHEEHAN, D. M., BRANHAM, W. S., MEDLOCK, K. L., OLSON, M. E. and ZEHR, D. R. (1981) Uterine responses to estradiol in the neonatal rat. *Endocrinology* **109:** 76–82.

SHEEHAN, D. M., BRANHAM, W. S., MEDLOCK, K. L. and ZEHR, D. R. (1982) Endogenous estrogen control of rat postnatal uterine development. *Teratology* **25:** 75A.

SHELLEY, S. A., BALIS, J. U., PACIGA, J. E., KNUPPEL, R. A., RUFFOLO, E. H. and BOUIS, P. J. Jr. (1982) Surfactant "apoproteins" in human amniotic fluid: an enzyme-linked immunosorbent assay for the prenatal assessment of lung maturity. *Am. J. Obstet. Gynecol.* **144:** 224–228.

SHERIDAN, P. J., BUCHANAN, J. M., ANSELMO, V. C. and MARTIN, P. M. (1979) Equilibrium: the intracellular distribution of steroid receptors. *Nature (London)* **282:** 579–582.

SHERMAN, M. R., CORVOL, P. L. and O'MALLEY, B. W. (1970) Progesterone-binding components of chick oviduct. I. Preliminary characterization of cytoplasmic components. *J. Biol. Chem.* **245:** 6085–6096.

SHERWOOD, O. D. (1988) Relaxin. In: *The Physiology of Reproduction*, Knobil, E. and Neill, J. (Eds), Raven Press, New York, pp. 585–673.

SHERWOOD, O. D., CRNEKOVIC, V. E., GORDON, W. L. and RUTHERFORD, J. E. (1980) Radioimmunoassay of relaxin throughout pregnancy and during parturition in the rat. *Endocrinology* **107:** 691–698.

SHIU, R. P. C. and FRIESEN, H. G. (1974a) Properties of a prolactin receptor from the rabbit mammary gland. *Biochem. J.* **140:** 301–311.

SHIU, R. P. C. and FRIESEN, H. G. (1974b) Solubilization and purification of a prolactin receptor from the rabbit mammary gland. *J. Biol. Chem.* **249:** 7902–7911.

SHIU, R. P. C. and FRIESEN, H. G. (1976) Blockade of prolactin action by an antiserum to its receptors. *Science* **192:** 259–261.

SHOLL, S. A. and GOY, R. W. (1978) Androgen and estrogen synthesis in the fetal guinea pig gonad. *Biol. Reprod.* **18:** 160–169.

SHOLL, S. A. and POMERANTZ, S. M. (1986) Androgen receptors in the cerebral cortex of fetal female rhesus monkeys. *Endocrinology* **119:** 1625–1631.

SHOREY, C. D. and HUGHES, R. L. (1973) Cyclical changes in the uterine endometrium and peripheral plasma concentrations of progesterone in the marsupial. *Trichosurus vulpecula. Austral. J. Zool.* **21:** 1–19.

SHORT, J. M., WYNSHAW-BORIS, A., SHORT, H. P. and HANSON, R. W. (1986) Characterization of the phosphoenolpyruvate carboxykinase (GTP) promoter-regulatory region. II. Identification of cAMP and glucocorticoid regulatory domains. *J. Biol. Chem.* **261:** 9721–9726.

SHUGHRUE, P. J., STUMPF, W. E. and SAR, M. (1988) The distribution of progesterone receptor in the 20-day-old fetal mouse; an autoradiographic study with [^{125}I]progestin. *Endocrinology* **123:** 2382–2389.

SHUGHRUE, P. J., STUMPF, W. E., SAR, M., ELGER, W. and SCHULZE, P.-E. (1989) Progestin receptors in brain and pituitary of 20-day-old fetal mice: an autoradiographic study using [^{125}I] progestin. *Endocrinology* **124:** 333–338.

SHYAMALA, G. (1973) Specific cytoplasmic glucocorticoid hormone receptors in lactating mammary glands. *Biochemistry* **12:** 3085–3090.

SHYAMALA, G. (1985) Regulation of mammary responsiveness to estrogen: an analysis of differences between mammary gland and the uterus. In: *Molecular Mechanism of Steroid Hormone Action*, Moudgil, V. K. (Ed.), Walter de Gruyter, Berlin, pp. 413–435.

SHYAMALA, G. and FERENCZY, A. (1982) The nonresponsiveness of lactating mammary gland to estradiol. *Endocrinology* **110:** 1249–1256.

SHYAMALA, G. and FERENCZY, A. (1984) Mammary fat pad may be a potential site for initiation of estrogen action in normal mouse mammary glands. *Endocrinology* **115:** 1078–1081.

SHYAMALA, G. and HASLAM, S. Z. (1980) Estrogen and progesterone receptors in normal mammary gland during different functional states. In: *Perspectives in Steroid Receptor Research*, Bresciani, F. (Ed.), Raven Press, New York, pp. 193–216.

SHYAMALA, G. and McBLAIN, W. A. (1979) Distinction between progestin- and glucocorticoid-binding sites in mammary glands. *Biochem. J.* **178**: 345–352.

SHYAMALA, G. and NANDI, S. (1972) Interactions of 6,7-³H-17β estradiol with the mouse lactating mammary tissue in vivo and in vitro. *Endocrinology* **91**: 861–867.

SHYAMALA, G., SINGH, R. K., RUH, M. F. and RUH, T. S. (1986) Relationships between mammary estrogen receptor and estrogenic sensitivity. II. Binding of cytoplasmic receptor to chromatin. *Endocrinology* **119**: 819–826.

SIEBERS, J. W., PETERS, F. and ENGEL, W. (1977a) Ovarian hCG-binding capacity during the oestrous cycle of the rat. *Acta Endocr. (Copenh.)* **85**: 850–854.

SIEBERS, J. W., PETERS, F., ZENZES, P. T., SCHMIDTKE, J. and ENGEL, W. (1977b) Binding of human chorionic gonadotrophin to rat ovary during development. *J. Endocr.* **73**: 491–496.

SIEBERS, J. W., WUTTKE, W. and ENGEL, W. (1977c) HCG-binding capacity of the rat ovary during pregnancy. *Acta Endocr. (Copenh.)* **86**: 173–179.

SIEGEL, T. W., GANGULY, S., JACOBS, S., ROSEN, O. M. and RUBIN, C. S. (1981) Purification and properties of the human placental insulin receptor. *J. Biol. Chem.* **256**: 9266–9273.

SIITERI, P. K., FEBRES, F., CLEMENS, L. E., CHANG, R. J., GONDOS, B. and STITES, D. (1977) Progesterone and maintenance of pregnancy. Is progesterone nature's immunosuppressant? *Ann. N. Y. Acad. Sci.* **286**: 384–397.

SILER-KHODR, T. M. and KHODR, G. S. (1978) Content of luteinizing hormone-releasing factor in the human placenta. *Am. J. Obstet. Gynec.* **130**: 216–219.

SILER-KHODR, T. M. and KHODR, G. S. (1981) Dose response analysis of GnRH stimulation of hCG release from human term placenta. *Biol. Reprod.* **25**: 353–358.

SIMPSON, A. A., SIMPSON, M. H. W., SINHA, Y. N. and SCHMIDT, G. H. (1973) Changes in concentration of prolactin and adrenal corticosteroids in rat plasma during pregnancy and lactation. *J. Endocr.* **58**: 675–676.

SINGH, M. M. and BOOTH, W. D. (1979) Origin of oestrogen in preimplantation rabbit blastocysts. *J. Steroid Biochem.* **11**: 723–728.

SKINNER, S. L., LUMBERS, E. R. and SYMONDS, E. M. (1968) Renin concentration in human fetal and maternal tissues. *Am. J. Obstet. Gynec.* **101**: 529–533.

SLOB, A. K., OOMS, M. P. and VREEBURG, J. T. M. (1980) Prenatal and early postnatal sex differences in plasma and gonadal testosterone and plasma luteinizing hormone in female and male rats. *J. Endocr.* **87**: 81–87.

SMITH, B. T. (1979) Lung maturation in the fetal rat acceleration by injection of fibroblast-pneumonocyte factor. *Science* **204**: 1094–1095.

SMITH, B. T. and SABRY, K. (1983) Glucocorticoid-thyroid synergism in lung maturation: a mechanism involving epithelial-mesenchymal interaction. *Proc. Natl Acad. Sci. USA* **80**: 1951–1954.

SMITH, D. E. and GORSKI, J. (1968) Estrogen control of uterine glucose metabolism. *J. Biol. Chem.* **243**: 4169–4174.

SOBHON, P. and JIRASATTHAM, C. (1974) Effect of sex hormones in the thymus and lymphoid tissue of ovariectomized rats. *Acta Anat.* **89**: 211–224.

SOLL, A. M., KAHN, C. R. and NEVILLE, D. M. (1975) Insulin binding to liver plasma membranes in the obese hyperglycemic (ob/ob) mouse, demonstration of a decreased number of functionally normal receptors. *J. Biol. Chem.* **250**: 7402–7407.

SOLOFF, M. S. (1975) Uterine receptor for oxytocin: effects of estrogen. *Biochem. Biophys. Res. Commun.* **65**: 205–212.

SOLOFF, M. S. and WIEDER, M. H. (1983) Oxytocin receptors in rat involuting mammary gland. *Can. J. Biochem. Cell Biol.* **61**: 631–635.

SOLOFF, M. S., ALEXANDROVA, M. and FERNSTRÖM, M. J. (1979) Oxytocin receptors: triggers for parturition and lactation? *Science* **204**: 1313–1315.

SOLOFF, M. S., FERNSTRÖM, M. A., PERIYASAMY, S., SOLOFF, S., BALDWIN, S. and WIEDER, M. (1983) Regulation of oxytocin receptor concentration in rat uterine explants by estrogen and progesterone. *Can. J. Biochem. Cell. Biol.* **61**: 625–630.

SOLOMON, S. and LEE, D. K. H. (1977) Binding of glucocorticoids in fetal tissues. *J. Steroid Biochemistry* **8**: 453–461.

SÖMJEN, D., SÖMJEN, G., KING, R. J. B., KAYE, A. M. and LINDNER, H. R. (1973) Nuclear binding of oestradiol-17β and induction of protein synthesis in the rat uterus during postnatal development. *Biochem. J.* **136**: 25–33.

SÖMJEN, G. J., KAYE, A. M. and LINDNER, H. R. (1974) Oestradiol-17β binding proteins in the rat uterus: changes during postnatal development. *Mol. Cell. Endocr.* **1**: 341–353.

SÖMJEN, G. J., KAYE, A. M. and LINDNER, H. R. (1976) Demonstration of 8S-cytoplasmic oestrogen receptor in rat Müllerian duct. *Biochim. Biophys. Acta* **428**: 787–791.

SOOS, M. A., SIDDLE, K., BARON, M. D., HEWARD, J. M., LUZIO, J. P., BELLATIN, J. and LENNOX, E. S. (1986) Monoclonal antibodies reacting with multiple epitopes on the human insulin receptor. *Biochem. J.* **235**: 199–208.

SPEEG, K. V., Jr. and HARRISON, R. W. (1979) The ontogeny of the human placental glucocorticoid receptor and inducibility of heat-stable alkaline phosphatase. *Endocrinology* **104**: 1364–1368.

SPELLACY, W. N. and GOETZ, F. C. (1963) Plasma insulin in normal late pregnancy. *New Engl. J. Med.* **268**: 988–991.

STACK, G. and GORSKI, J. (1983) The ontogeny of estrogen responsiveness reexamined: the differential effectiveness of diethylstilbestrol and estradiol on uterine deoxyribonucleic acid synthesis in neonatal rats. *Endocrinology* **112**: 2141–2146.

STANCHEV, P., RODRIGUEZ-MARTINEZ, H., EDQVIST, L. E. and ERIKSSON, H. (1985) Oestradiol and progesterone receptors in the pig oviduct during the oestrous cycle. *J. Steroid Biochem.* **22**: 115–120.

STEELE, P. A., FLINT, A. P. F. and TURNBULL, A. C. (1976) Activity of steroid C-17,20 lyase in the ovine placenta: effect of exposure to foetal glucocorticoid. *J. Endocr.* **69**: 239–246.

STERK, V. V. and KRETCHMER, N. (1964) Studies of small intestine during development. IV. Digestion of lactose as related to lactosuria in the rabbit. *Pediatrics* **34**: 609–614.

STRAIN, A. J., HILL, D. J., SWENNE, I. and MILNER, R. D. G. (1987) The regulation of DNA synthesis in human fetal hepatocytes by placental lactogen, growth hormone and insulin-like growth factor I/somatomedin-C. *J. Cell Physiol.* **132**: 33–40.

STROSSER, M. T. and MIALHE, P. (1975) Growth hormone secretion in the rat as a function of age. *Horm. Metab. Res.* **7**: 275–278.

STUMPF, W. E., NARBAITZ, R. and SAR, M. (1980) Estrogen receptors in the fetal mouse. *J. Steroid Biochem.* **12**: 55–64.

SUARD, Y. M. L., KRAEHENBUHL, J.-P. and AUBERT, M. L. (1979) Dispersed mammary epithelial cells. Receptors of lactogenic hormones in virgin, pregnant, and lactating rabbits. *J. Biol. Chem.* **254**: 10466–10475.

SUCHOWSKY, G. K. and JUNKMANN, K. (1961) A study of the virilizing effect of progestogens on the female rat fetus. *Endocrinology* **68**: 341–349.

SULTAN, C., MIGEON, B., ROTHWELL, S., ZERHOUNI, N., MAES, M. and MIGEON, C. J. (1980) Androgen receptors and metabolism in cultured human fetal fibroblasts. *Pediat. Res.* **13**: 67–69.

SULTAN, C., TERRAZA, A., DESCOMPS, B. and CRASTES DE PAULET, A. (1981) Récepteurs des androgènes chez le foetus de primate (*Macaca fascicularis*): résultats préliminaires. *C. R. Séances Soc. Biol.* **175**: 208–212.

SUMIDA, C. and PASQUALINI, J. R. (1979a) Determination of cytosol and nuclear estradiol-binding sites in fetal guinea pig uterus by ³H-estradiol exchange. *Endocrinology* **105**: 406–413.

SUMIDA, C. and PASQUALINI, J. R. (1979b) Relationship between cytosol and nuclear oestrogen receptors and oestrogen concentrations in the fetal compartment of guinea-pig. *J. Steroid Biochem.* **11:** 267–272.

SUMIDA, C. and PASQUALINI, J. R. (1980) Dynamic studies on estrogen response in fetal guinea pig uterus: effect of estradiol administration on estradiol receptor, progesterone receptor and uterine growth. *J. Receptor Res.* **1:** 439–457.

SUMIDA, C. and PASQUALINI, J. R. (1981) Stimulation of the incorporation of ^{3}H-leucine into proteins by oestradiol in the foetal uterus of the guinea pig. *Experientia* **37:** 782–783.

SUMIDA, C. and PASQUALINI, J. R. (1985) Receptors and biological responses of estrogens, antiestrogens and progesterone in the fetal and newborn uterus. In: *Molecular Mechanism of Steroid Hormone Action*, Moudgil, V. K. (Ed.), Walter de Gruyter, Berlin, pp. 471–504.

SUMIDA, C., GELLY, C. and PASQUALINI, J. R. (1978) DNA, protein and specific ^{3}H-estradiol binding in the nuclear fractions of fetal guinea pig kidney and lung during fetal development. *Biol. Reprod.* **19:** 338–345.

SUMIDA, C., GELLY, C. and PASQUALINI, J. R. (1980) Progesterone and oestradiol receptors in the uterus of oestradiol-primed fetal and newborn guinea-pigs. *J. Endocr.* **85:** 429–434.

SUMIDA, C., GELLY, C. and PASQUALINI, J. R. (1981) Progesterone antagonizes the effects of estradiol in the fetal uterus of guinea pig. *J. Receptor Res.* **2:** 221–232.

SUMIDA, C., GELLY, C. and PASQUALINI, J. R. (1982) Characteristics of the nuclear translocation of progesterone receptor in fetal guinea pig uterus "in vivo", "in vitro" and in organ culture. *Steroids* **39:** 431–444.

SUMIDA, C., GELLY, C. and PASQUALINI, J. R. (1983) De novo synthesis of progesterone receptor in the fetal uterus of guinea pig in organ culture and its control by progestins and triphenylethylene antiestrogens. *Biochim. Biophys. Acta* **755:** 488–496.

SUMIDA, C., LECERF, F. and PASQUALINI, J. R. (1988) Control of progesterone receptors in fetal uterine cells in culture: effects of estradiol, progestins, antiestrogens, and growth factors. *Endocrinology* **122:** 3–11.

SUTTER-DUB, M. T., SFAXI, A., LATRILLE, F., SODOYEZ-GOFFAUX, F. and SODOYEZ, J. C. (1984) Insulin binding and action in adipocytes of pregnant rats: evidence that insulin resistance is caused by post-receptor binding defects. *J. Endocr.* **102:** 209–214.

SZEGO, C. M. and ROBERTS, S. (1953) Steroid action and interaction in uterine metabolism. *Rec. Prog. Horm. Res.* **8:** 419–469.

TAKANO, K., HALL, K., FRYKLUND, L., HOLMGREN, A., SIEVERTSSON, H. and UTHNE, K. (1975) The binding of insulin and somatomedin A to human placental membrane. *Acta Endocr. (Copenh.)* **80:** 14–31.

TAKEDA, H., MIZUNO, T. and LASNITZKI, I. (1985) Autoradiographic studies of androgen-binding sites in the rat urogenital sinus and postnatal prostate. *J. Endocr.* **104:** 87–92.

TALWAR, G. P., SEGAL, S. J., EVANS, A. and DAVIDSON, O. W. (1964) The binding of estradiol in the uterus: a mechanism for depression of RNA synthesis. *Proc. Natl Acad. Sci. U.S.A.* **52:** 1059–1066.

TAN, J., JOSEPH, D. R., QUARMBY, V. E., LUBAHN, D. B., SAR, M., FRENCH, F. S. and WILSON, E. M. (1988) The rat androgen receptor: primary structure, autoregulation of its messenger ribonucleic acid, and immunocytochemical localization of the receptor protein. *Mol. Endocr.* **12:** 1276–1285.

TAPANAINEN, J., KELLOKUMPU-LEHTINEN, P., PELLINIEMI, L. and HUHTANIEMI, I. (1981) Age-related changes in endogenous steroids of human fetal testis during early and midpregnancy. *J. Clin. Endocr. Metab.* **52:** 98–102.

TARDY, J. and PASQUALINI, J. R. (1980) Autoradiographic studies on the fetal and newborn uteri of the guinea pig after injection of ^{3}H-progesterone into non-treated and into estradiol-primed animals. *Cell Tissue Res.* **213:** 213–220.

TARDY, J. and PASQUALINI, J. R. (1983) Localization of ^{3}H-estradiol and gonadotropin-releasing hormone (GnRH) in the hypothalamus of the fetal guinea pig. *Exp. Brain Res.* **49:** 77–83.

TARDY, J., NGUYEN, B. L. and PASQUALINI, J. R. (1983) Characterization of estradiol receptors, autoradiographic localization after ³H-estradiol administration and detection of gonadotrophin releasing hormone (GnRH) in the hypothalamus of the fetal guinea pig. In: *Neuropeptides, Neurotransmitters and Regulation of Endocrine Processes*, Endröczi H. et al. (Eds), Publishing House, Hungarian Acad. of Sci., pp. 145–152.

TAYLOR, H. C. Jr., WARNER, R. C. and WELSH, C. A. (1939) The relationship of the estrogens and other placental hormones to sodium and potassium balance at the end of pregnancy and in the puerperium. *Am. J. Obst. Gynec.* **38:** 748–777.

TAYLOR, M. J., JENKIN, G., ROBINSON, J. S., THORBURN, G. D., FRIESEN, H. and CHAN, J. S. D. (1980) Concentrations of placental lactogen in chronically catheterized ewes and fetuses in late pregnancy. *J. Endocr.* **85:** 27–34.

TERADA, N., KURODA, H., NAMIKI, M., KITAMURA, Y. and MATSUMOTO, K. (1984) Augmentation of aromatase activity by FSH in ovaries of fetal and neonatal mice in organ culture. *J. Steroid Biochem.* **20:** 741–745.

THORBURN, G. D. (1974) The role of the thyroid gland and the kidneys in fetal growth. *Ciba Fdn. Symp.* **27:** 185–214.

THORBURN, G. D. and HOPKINS, P. S. (1973) Thyroid function in the foetal lamb. In: *Foetal and Neonatal Physiology*, Proc. Sir Joseph Barcroft Centenary Symp., Comline, R. S., Cross, K. W., Dawes, G. S. and Nathanielsz, P. W. (Eds), Cambridge Univ. Press, Cambridge, pp. 488–507.

TOFT, D. and GORSKI, J. (1966) A receptor molecule for estrogens: isolation from the rat uterus and preliminary characterization. *Proc. Natl Acad. Sci. U.S.A.* **55:** 1574–1581.

TOPPER, Y. T. and FREEMAN, C. S. (1980) Multiple hormone interactions in the developmental biology of the mammary gland. *Physiol. Rev.* **60:** 1049–1106.

TORDAY, J. S. and NIELSEN, H. C. (1981) Surfactant phospholipid ontogeny in fetal rabbit lung lavage and amniotic fluid. *Biol. Neonate* **39:** 266–271.

TORDAY, J. S., SMITH, B. T. and GIROUD, C. J. P. (1975) The rabbit fetal lung as a glucocorticoid target tissue. *Endocrinology* **96:** 1462–1467.

TORDAY, J. S., OLSON, E. B. Jr. and FIRST, N. L. (1976) Production of cortisol from cortisone by the isolated, perfused fetal rabbit lung. *Steroids* **27:** 869–880.

TORDAY, J. S., NIELSEN, H. C., FENCL, M. and AVERY, M. E. (1981) Sex differences in fetal lung maturation. *Am. Rev. Resp. Dis.* **123:** 205–208.

TRAMS, G., ENGEL, B., LEHMANN, F. and MAASS, H. (1973) Specific binding of oestradiol in human uterine tissue. *Acta Endocr. (Copenh.)* **72:** 351–360.

TSAI-MORRIS, C-H., KNOX, G., LUNA, S. and DUFAU, M. L. (1986) Acquisition of estradiol-mediated regulatory mechanism of steroidogenesis in cultured fetal rat Leydig cells. *J. Biol. Chem.* **261:** 3471–3474.

TSAI-MORRIS, C-H., KNOX, G. F. and DUFAU, M. L. (1988) Gonadotropin induction of a regulatory mechanism of steroidogenesis in fetal Leydig cell cultures. *J. Steroid Biochem.* **29:** 285–291.

TSUTSUI, K. and KAWASHIMA, S. (1987) Properties of the binding of follicle-stimulating hormone to the fetal rat testis. *Endocr. Japon* **34:** 717–725.

TULCHINSKY, D., HOBEL, C. J., YEAGER, E. and MARSHALL, J. R. (1972) Plasma estrone, estradiol, estriol, progesterone and 17-hydroxyprogesterone in human pregnancy. I. Normal pregnancy. *Am. J. Obstet. Gynecol.* **112:** 1095–1100.

TWOMBLY, G. H. (1951) Tissue localization and excretion routes of radioactive diethylstilbestrol. *Acta Unionis Internationalis contra Cancerum* **7:** 882–888.

TWOMBLY, G. H. and SCHOENEWALDT, E. F. (1951) Tissue localization and excretion routes of radioactive diethylstilbestrol. *Cancer* **4:** 296–302.

TYDEN, O., BERNE, C. and ERIKSSON, U. (1980) Lung maturation in fetuses of diabetic rats. *Pediat. Res.* **14:** 1192–1195.

Van OBBERGHEN, E. and GAMMELTOFT, S. (1986) Insulin receptors: structure and function. *Experientia* **42:** 727–734.

VERHAGE, H. G., AKBAR, M. and JAFFE, R. C. (1980) Cyclic changes in cytosol progesterone receptor of human Fallopian tube. *J. Clin. Endocr. Metab.* **51**: 776–780.

VERHOEVEN, G. and WILSON, J. D. (1976) Cytosol androgen binding in submandibular gland and kidney of the normal mouse and the mouse with testicular feminization. *Endocrinology* **99**: 79–92.

VEYSSIÈRE, G., BERGER, M., JEAN-FAUCHER, C., DE TURCKHEIM, M. and JEAN, C. (1976) Levels of testosterone in the plasma, gonads, and adrenals during fetal development of the rabbit. *Endocrinology* **99**: 1263–1268.

VEYSSIÈRE, G., BERGER, M., JEAN-FAUCHER, C., DE TURCKHEIM, M. and JEAN, C. (1977) Effect of luteinizing hormone (LH) and LH-releasing hormone (LHRH) on testosterone production in vivo, in fetal rabbit testis in late gestation. *Biol. Neonate* **32**: 327–330.

VEYSIÈRE, G., BERGER, M., CORRE, M., JEAN-FAUCHER, C., DE TURCKHEIM, M. and JEAN, C. (1979) Percentage binding of testosterone and dihydrotestosterone and unbound testosterone and dihydrotestosterone in rabbit maternal and fetal plasma during sexual organogenesis. *Steroids* **34**: 305–317.

VEYSIÈRE, G., BERGER, M., JEAN-FAUCHER, C., DE TURCKHEIM, M. and JEAN, C. (1980) Ontogeny of pituitary gonadotrophin hormone activity and of testicular responsiveness to gonadotrophins in foetal rabbit. *Acta Endocr. (Copenh.)* **94**: 412–418.

VEYSIÈRE, G., BERGER, M., JEAN-FAUCHER, C., DE TURCKHEIM, M. and JEAN C. (1982) Pituitary and plasma levels of luteinizing hormone and follicle-stimulating hormone in male and female rabbit fetuses. *J. Endocr.* **92**: 381–387.

VINICOR, F. and KIEDROWSKI, L. (1982) Characterization of the hepatic receptor for insulin in the perinatal rat. *Endocrinology* **110**: 782–790.

VINICOR, F., HIGDON, G., CLARK, J. F. and CLARK, C. M. Jr. (1976) Development of glucagon sensitivity in neonatal rat liver. *J. Clin. Invest.* **58**: 571–578.

VITO, C. C. and FOX, T. O. (1979) Embryonic rodent brain contains estrogen receptors. *Science* **204**: 517–519.

VITO, C. C. and FOX, T. O. (1982) Androgen and estrogen receptors in embryonic and neonatal rat brain. *Dev. Brain Res.* **2**: 97–110.

VITO, C. C., WIELAND, S. J. and FOX, T. O. (1979) Androgen receptors exist throughout the 'critical period' of brain sexual differentiation. *Nature*, **282**: 308–310.

VU HAI, M. T., LOGEAT, F. and MILGROM, E. (1978) Progesterone receptors in the rat uterus: variations in cytosol and nuclei during the oestrous cycle and pregnancy. *J. Endocr.* **76**: 43–48.

WALTERS, M. R. and CLARK, J. H. (1977) Cytosol progesterone receptors of the rat uterus: assay and receptor characteristics. *J. Steroid Biochem.* **8**: 1137–1144.

WALTERS, M. R. and CLARK, J. H. (1979) Relationship between the quantity of progesterone receptor and the antagonism of estrogen-induced uterotrophic response. *Endocrinology* **105**: 382–386.

WANG, N. S., KOTAS, R. V., AVERY, M. E. and THURLBECK, W. M. (1971) Accelerated appearance of osmiophilic bodies in fetal lungs following steroid injection. *J. Appl. Physiol.* **30**: 362–365.

WANG, S.-L., RAIZADA, M. K. and SHIVERICK, K. T. (1987) Ontogeny of insulin receptors in the rat hemochorial placenta. *Dev. Biol.* **123**: 487–493.

WARREN, D. W., HALTMEYER, G. C. and EIK-NES, K. B. (1975) The effect of gonadotrophins on the fetal and neonatal rat testis. *Endocrinology* **96**: 1226–1229.

WARREN, D. W., DUFAU, M. L. and CATT, K. J. (1982) Hormonal regulation of gonadotropin receptors and steroidogenesis in cultured fetal rat testes. *Science* **218**: 375–377.

WARREN, D. W., HUHTANIEMI, I. T., TAPANAINEN, J., DUFAU, M. L. and CATT, K. J. (1984) Ontogeny of gonadotropin receptors in the fetal and neonatal rat testis. *Endocrinology* **114**: 470–476.

WARREN, D. W., HUHTANIEMI, I. T., DUFAU, M. L. and CATT, K. J. (1987) Regulation of LH receptors and steroidogenesis in the foetal rat testis in vivo. *Acta Endocr. (Copenh.)* **115**: 189–195.

WASNER, G., HENNERMANN, I. and KRATOCHWIL, K. (1983) Ontogeny of mesenchymal androgen receptors in the embryonic mouse mammary gland. *Endocrinology* **113**: 1771–1780.

WATANABE, Y. G. (1981) Immunohistochemical study of the responsiveness of LH cells of fetal rats to synthetic LHRH in vitro. *Cell Tissue Res.* **221:** 59–66.

WATERMAN, M., MURDOCH, G. H., EVANS, R. M. and ROSENFELD, M. G. (1985) Cyclic AMP regulation of eukaryotic gene transcription by two discrete molecular mechanisms. *Science* **229:** 267–269.

WATERS, M. J., LUSINS, S. and FRIESEN, H. G. (1984) Immunological and physicochemical evidence for tissue specific prolactin receptors in the rabbit. *Endocrinology* **114:** 1–10.

WATSON, J., ANDERSON, F. B., ALAM, M., O'GRADY, J. E. and HEALD, P. J. (1975) Plasma hormones and pituitary luteinizing hormone in the rat during the early stages of pregnancy and after post-coital treatment with tamoxifen (ICI 46,474). *J. endocr.* **65:** 7–17.

WEINBERGER, C., HOLLENBERG, S. M., ROSENFELD, M. G. and EVANS, R. M. (1985) Domain structure of human gluocorticoid receptor and its relationship to the v-erbA oncogene product. *Nature* **318:** 670–672.

WEINBERGER, C., THOMPSON, C. C., ONG, E. S., LEBO, R., GRUOL, D. J. and EVANS, R. M. (1986) The c-erb-A gene encodes a thyroid hormone receptor. *Nature* **324:** 641–646.

WEITLAUF, H. M. (1988) Biology of implantation. In: *The Physiology of Reproduction*, Knobil, E. and Neill, J. (Eds), Raven Press, New York, pp. 231–262.

WELSHONS, W. V., KRUMMEL, B. M. and GORSKI, J. (1985) Nuclear localization of unoccupied receptors for glucocorticoids, estrogens, and progesterone in GH3 cells. *Endocrinology* **117:** 2140–2147.

WENIGER, J. P., CHOURAQUI, J. and ZEIS, A. (1985) Steroid conversions by the 19-day old foetal rat ovary in organ culture. *Biol. Chem.* **366:** 555–559.

WEST, N. B., VERHAGE, H. G. and BRENNER, R. M. (1977) Changes in nuclear estradiol receptor and cell structure during estrous cycles and pregnancy in the oviduct and uterus of cats. *Biol. Reprod.* **17:** 138–143.

WEST, N. B., NORMAN, R. L., SANDOW, B. A. and BRENNER, R. M. (1978) Hormonal control of nuclear estradiol receptor content and the luminal epithelium in the uterus of the golden hamster. *Endocrinology* **103:** 1732–1741.

WHITSETT, J. A., JOHNSON, C. L. and HAWKINS, K. (1979) Differences in localization of insulin receptors and adenylate cyclase in the human placenta. *Am. J. Obstet. Gynec.* **133:** 204–207.

WHITSETT, J. A., WEAVER, T. E., LIEBERMAN, M. A., CLARK, J. C. and DAUGHERTY, C. (1987) Differential effects of epidermal growth factor and transforming growth factor-β on synthesis of Mr = 35,000 surfactant-associated protein in fetal lung. *J. Biol. Chem.* **262:** 7908–7913.

WIEGERINCK, M. A. H. M., POORTMAN, J., AGEMA, A. R. and THIJSSEN, J. H. H. (1980) Estrogen receptors in human vaginal tissue. *Maturitas* **2:** 59–67.

WIEST, W. G. (1970) Progesterone and 20-alpha-hydroxypregn-4-en-3-one in plasma, ovaries and uteri during pregnancy in the rat. *Endocrinology* **87:** 43–48.

WIKSTRÖM, A. C., BAKKE, O., OKRET, S., BRÖNNEGÅRD, M. and GUSTAFSSON, J-Å. (1987) Intracellular localization of the glucocorticoid receptor: evidence for cytoplasmic and nuclear localization. *Endocrinology* **120:** 1232–1242.

WILLIAMS, P. F. and TURTLE, J. R. (1979) Purification of the insulin receptor from human placental membranes. *Biochem. Biophys. Acta* **579:** 367–374.

WILLMAN, E. A. and COLLINS, W. P. (1978) The metabolism of prostaglandin E2 by tissues from the human uterus and foeto-placental unit. *Acta Endocr. (Copenh.)* **87:** 632–642.

WILSON, J. D. (1973) Testosterone uptake by the urogenital tract of the rabbit embryo. *Endocrinology* **92:** 1192–1199.

WILSON, J. D. and LASNITZKI, I. (1971) Dihydrotestosterone formation in fetal tissues of the rabbit and rat. *Endocrinology* **89:** 659–668.

WILSON, J. D. and SIITERI, P. K. (1973) The role of steroid hormones in sexual differentiation. *Proc. IVth In. Congr. Endocrinol. Excerpta Medica Int. Congr.* **273:** 1051–1056.

WILSON, M., MORGANTI, A. A., ZERVOUDAKIS, I., LETCHER, R. L., ROMNEY, B. M., VON

OEYON, P., PAPERA, S., SEALEY, J. E. and LARAGH, J. H. (1980) Blood pressure, the renin-angiotensin system and sex steroids throughout normal pregnancy. *Am. J. Med.* **68:** 97–104.

WINTERS, A. J., COLSTON, C., MacDONALD, P. C. and PORTER, J. C. (1975) Fetal plasma prolactin levels. *J. Clin. Endocr. Metab.* **41:** 626–629.

WINTERS, A. J., ESKAY, R. L. and PORTER, J. C. (1974) Concentration and distribution of TRH and LRH in the human fetal brain. *J. Clin. Endocr. Metab.* **39:** 960–963.

WINTOUR, E. M., BROWN, E. H., DENTON, D. A., HARDY, K. J., McDOUGALL, J. G., ODDIE, C. J. and WHIPP, G. T. (1975) The ontogeny and regulation of corticosteroid secretion by the ovine foetal adrenal. *Acta Endocr. (Copenh.)* **79:** 301–316.

WITTLIFF, J. L., GARDNER, G. G., BATTEMA, W. L. and GILBERT, P. J. (1972) Specific estrogen receptors in the neoplastic and lactating mammary gland of the rat. *Biochem. Biophys. Res. Comm.* **48:** 119–125.

WRIGHT, P. A., CREW, M. D. and SPINDLER, S. R. (1987) Discrete positive and negative thyroid hormone-responsive transcription regulatory elements of the rat growth hormone gene. *J. Biol. Chem.* **262:** 5659–5663.

WU, B., KIKKAWA, Y., ORZALESI, M. M., MOTOYAMA, E. K., KAIBARA, M., ZIGAS, C. J. and COOK, C. D. (1973) The effect of thyroxine on the maturation of fetal rabbit lungs. *Biol. Neonate* **22:** 161–168.

YANG, K. and CHALLIS, J. R. G. (1989) Fetal and adult sheep adrenal cortical cells contain glucocorticoid receptors. *Biochem. Biophys. Res. Commun.* **162:** 604–611.

YEOH, G. C. T., ARBUCKLE, T. and OLIVER, I. T. (1979) Tyrosine aminotransferase induction in hepatocytes cultured from rat fetuses treated with dexamethasone in vitro. *Biochem. J.* **180:** 545–549.

YMER, S. I. and HERINGTON, A. C. (1986) Binding and structural characteristics of a soluble lactogen-binding protein from rabbit mammary gland cytosol. *Biochem. J.* **237:** 813–820.

YMER, S. I., STEVENSON, J. L. and HERINGTON, A. C. (1989) Differences in the developmental patterns of somatotrophic and lactogenic receptors in rabbit liver cytosol. *Endocrinology* **125:** 516–523.

YOCHIM, J. M. and DeFEO, V. J. (1962) Control of decidual growth in the rat by steroid hormones of the ovary. *Endocrinology* **71:** 134–142.

YOCHIM, J. M. and DeFEO, V. J. (1963) Hormonal control of the onset, magnitude and duration of uterine sensitivity in the rat by steroid hormones of the ovary. *Endocrinology* **73:** 317–326.

YOSHINAGA, K., HAWKINS, R. A. and STOCKER, J. F. (1969) Estrogen secretion by the rat ovary in vivo during the estrous cycle and pregnancy. *Endocrinology* **85:** 103–112.

YOUNES, M. A., BESCH, N. F. and BESCH, P. K. (1981) Estradiol and progesterone binding in human term placental cytosol. *Am. J. Obst. Gynecol.* **141:** 170–174.

YOUNES, M. A., BESCH, N. F. and BESCH, P. K. (1982) Evidence for an adrogen binding component in human placental cytosol. *J. Steroid Biochem.* **16:** 311–315.

YU, W. C. Y. and LEUNG, B. S. (1982) Variation of cytoplasmic content of estrogen and progesterone receptors in the mammary gland and uterus of rats at time of parturition. *Biol. Reprod.* **27:** 658–664.

ZEILMAKER, G. H. (1963) Experimental studies on the effects of ovariectomy and hypophysectomy on blastocyst implantation in the rat. *Acta Endocr. (Copenh.)* **44:** 355–366.

ZELEZNIK, A. J., MIDGLEY, A. R. and REICHERT, L. E. (1974) Granulosa cell maturation in the rat: increased binding of human chorionic gonadotropin following treatment with follicle-stimulating hormone in vivo. *Endocrinology* **95:** 818–825.

ZEMEL, S., MILAN, M. A. and AGUILERA, G. (1989) Distribution of angiotensin II receptors and renin in the mouse fetus. *Endocrinology* **124:** 1774–1780.

3

Sex Differentiation and Fetal Endocrinology

Contents

Introduction

Sex separation took place relatively late during evolution. Unicellular organisms rarely exchange genetic material. Many nonvertebrate species are hermaphrodites (bisexual) or (chiefly insects) parthogenic; the female can reproduce without being fertilized by the male. In higher developed species chromosome exchange imparts definite evolutionary advantage and gender is not always firmly 'fixed'. In lower vertebrates (amphibians and fishes), exogenous estrogens change males into functional females and androgens produce the opposite effect. Many species of marine fishes are protogynous; adult females spontaneously reverse sex and become males when environmental conditions so demand. Exposure of bird embryos to sex hormones will impose the sex dictated by the hormone and mature individuals will reproduce albeit only temporarily. After some time the being will revert to gender dictated by the chromosomal make-up. To mammalian embryos exogenous steroids are teratogenic; exposure produces reorganization in internal and external genitalia but gonadal sex remains unchanged.

In birds the dominant sex is female and only the left ovary is functional. Estrogens from the developing ovary must be present for the development of sex organs. Otherwise, the organism will develop as a male. If the ovary is removed shortly after castration the rudimentary right gonad will develop into a small testis.

In mammals the role is reversed: the dominant sex is male. In the presence of androgens the individual will differentiate as male. If androgens are absent the entity will develop as a female. Yet, it would be wrong to consider females as the 'weaker' sex. In humans, male embryos have a higher incidence of abortions and miscarriages and

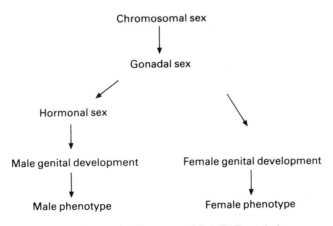

FIG 3.1. Sequential Processes of Sex Differentiation.

the frequency of death during the infant period is higher for boys. The ratio of males to females conceived is believed to be 115:100. By birth the ratio is 105:100 and is equal in the 30-year-old group; by the age of 65 years, 84 women but only 70 men remain alive. Most of male mortality is associated with cardiovascular diseases, the result of high androgen and low estrogen production; estrogen decreases low density lipoproteins, the main component of atherosclerotic plaques.

Sexual differentiation is a sequential process (Fig. 3.1). Chromosomal sex, established when the sperm and the ovum unite, determines the development of the gonads; the embryonic testes secrete two hormones which block the development of female organs, direct the formation of the internal and external genitalia, of mammary glands and (later in life) of secondary sex characteristics (phenotype).

1. Genetic Sex

The recognition that chromosomes determine sex in vertebrate (and invertebrate) species is less than 90 years old. Prior to the 1900s, it was believed that the sex of an individual is determined by environmental factors, such as maternal nutrition. Several groups (McClung, 1902; Stevens, 1905; Morgan, 1910) expanded Mendel's findings and deduced the importance of chromosomes in the determination of sex.

The sex-determining chromosomes can be either same (homogametic) or different (heterogametic). In lower vertebrates the difference is not fixed. In birds the female is heterogametic and lays two different kinds of eggs. In mammals the female is homogametic: she has two XX chromosomes, while the male is heterogametic; he has one X and one Y chromosome in all cells. The sex chromosomes are individual in most, but not all species. In the mongoose the Y chromosome has been translocated onto a chromosome not connected with sex determination (autosome). In some marsupials and bats the X chromosome has been fused to an autosome.

The Y chromosome does not determine maleness in all mammals: marsupials eliminate in extragonadal cells either the Y or the X chromosome to form an XO cell but the spermatogonia are always XY; the chromosomal make-up of the fertile female wood lemming is XY; the oregon vole (*Microtus oregoni*) eliminates the X chromosome from germ cells and produces YO sperm while the male vole (*Ellolius lutescens*) has no Y chromosomes and YO make-up in all cells.

In humans there are 22 paired autosomes plus the sex XY (male) and XX (female) chromosome (Painter, 1923). The X chromosome is larger than the Y chromosome and is essential for viability; it carries not only the sex-determining genes but also at least 60 others for characteristics such as vision, blood clotting, blood-group substance, sex-linked diseases (muscular dystrophy) and others. The Y chromosome carries mainly regulatory loci, located on the short arm, directing the formation of the testis.

In females, one of the X chromosomes becomes inactivated in most cells at an early stage of embryonic development but not in oocytes. Their development requires genetic activity from both chromosomes. In males the X chromosome is inactivated in primary spermatocytes. An active presence is usually associated with meiotic failure (see Lyon, 1972).

The presence of the Y chromosome predisposes the individual to become a male; in its absence a female develops but not always. In several species males develop having the XX chromosome code. Such individuals are sterile but of the male phenotype. The maleness is the result of retention of a fraction (0.2%) of the Y chromosome (Y_P material) which codes for testis development (Jacobs and Strong, 1959). In XX males the material is attached to one of the XX chromosomes; in XY females this fraction is missing (Evans *et al.*, 1979).

Almost one quarter of human pre-implantation embryos are chromosomally imbalanced and few of them survive full term. Most of the errors occur in the oocyte (Anon., 1988). The reason for the high incidence of such imbalance is unknown. Another agent which may change sex ratio is viral infection. Drew *et al.* (1978) reported more sons (a sex ratio of 3.4) in mothers infected with hepatitis B virus.

Abnormalities in chromosome make-up that result in hermaphroditism and sterility have also been traced in goats, cats, mice and cattle (see Gowen, 1961). In men, five separate genetic defects are known to cause inadequate testosterone production and incomplete virilization of the sex ducts (Wilson, 1978). Each defect involves one or several enzyme faults required for the conversion of cholesterol to testosterone (20,22 desmolase, 3β-hydroxysteroid dehydrogenase, 17-hydroxylase, 17,20-desmolase, 17β-hydroxysteroid dehydrogenase). The discussion of such deviations is beyond the scope of this chapter.

1.1. The Testis-Determining Gene

A sex-determining gene was identified by Page *et al.* in 1987. The investigators compared DNA sequence in a 230-kilobase (kb) segment in XX men and XY women to determine which base sequence codes for the testis-determining factor (TDF). TDF is located on the short arm of the Y chromosome and measures most likely 140 kb. The gene, now known as the zinc-finger Y gene (Page, 1988) codes for a cysteine- and histidine-rich protein which coordinates with zinc to form a tetrahedral complex. The complex has been recognized earlier in humans (Kadonaga *et al.*, 1987), frogs (Brown *et al.*, 1985; Miller *et al.*, 1985) and *Drosophila* (Rosenberg *et al.*, 1986; Tautz *et al.*, 1987). It is believed that the protein affects directly only those cells (germs and Sertoli) in which it is expressed, probably in a cell-autonomous fashion. However, further investigations are needed to establish if the zinc-finger Y is really the TDF (Erickson and Verga, 1989).

1.1.1. The H–Y antigen

Sex dimorphism exists with respect to skin transplantation. If two highly inbred strains are mated the F^1 generation rejects grafts when the donor is a male and the recipient a female (Eichwald and Silmer, 1955). It was suggested that the incompatibility resulted from an antigen determined by genes located on the 'nonpairing short segment' of the Y chromosome. The antigen was named the H–Y antigen and the gene which codes for the antigen (H–Y gene) was believed for many years to be the testis-determining instrument (see Ohno, 1976; Polani, 1979).

Recent evidence does not support this view. The H–Y antigen is present in many strains of mice, rats, rabbits, but not in hamsters and guinea-pigs; its presence in humans is uncertain. Serological testing indicates wide distribution of the protein in diverse tissues of mice such as sperm, heart, kidney, liver, lymph nodes, salivary glands, skin, thymus, bone marrow, pituitary, pancreas and skeletal muscle (see Wachtel, 1983).

Sertoli cells secrete the antigen (Zenzes *et al.*, 1978) and gonadal cells have specific H–Y receptors (Müller *et al.*, 1978). The two groups believe that H–Y is synthesized in large amounts in the undifferentiated embryonic gonad. Disseminated in Sertoli cell precursors of the heterogametic male, it may aid in the differentiation of the Sertoli and Leydig cells. This hypothesis remains to be validated. Vojtísková and Poláčková (1966, 1971) and Poláčková and Vojtísková (1968) claimed that the expression of the antigen becomes manifest at the time of sexual maturation (about day 30 in mice). They noted that syngeneic male grafts from young males, from neonatally castrated male donors, tend to survive for a long time, or even permanently. Whether the prolonged graft survival was the result of a lack of H–Y antigen, or the absence of testosterone production, has not been answered.

The absence of the H–Y antigen in women has been credited with a higher frequency of autoimmune diseases but definitive proof is lacking. In men, two genes may direct the synthesis of the antigenic determinant: one located in the paracentrometic region of the Y arm and one on the Xp region (Goodfellow *et al.*, 1983); possibly a third gene may be situated on an unidentified autosome. The protein is 15–18 kD mol wt, probably with a carbohydrate moiety bound to plasma membrane in nonspecific association with microglobulins (see Wachtel, 1983).

2. Gonadal Sex

The primordial germ sex cells carry the genetic information and contribute to the presumptive gonad. During early embryonic development the vertebrate embryo is bisexual—it carries both the male and female structures from which forms only one pair of sex ducts. The anlage which give rise to male structures are the Wolffian ducts. Müllerian ducts are transformed into the female reproductive apparatus.

2.1. The Origin of Germ Cells

Primordial germ cells (PGC) develop in the epithelium of the yolk sac near the developing allantois. The cells differentiate from primitive cells of an early embryo, develop larger than somatic cells and transform into spermatogonia, or oogonia. The time of appearance of germ cells is controversial. Kelly (1977) claims that during the early divisions, PGC do not segregate from somatic cells. Gardner (1977) reported that 4–5-day-old (post-coitum) blastocysts in mice can give rise to germ cells. Hertig *et al.* (1956) claimed that one of the eight cells comprising the inner cell mass of a $4\frac{1}{2}$-day-old human blastocyst might be a germ cell. Politzer (1933) found 49 PGC in a trilaminar presomite embryo with the chordomesodermal process. The numbers increased as the embryo developed: 37 in a four somite (segment) embryo, 30 in a seven-somite, 151 in an 18-somite and 586 in a 26-somite embryo. Jirásek (1962) detected germ cells using alkaline phosphatase stain in the allantois and the adjacent portion of the yolk sac of a bilaminar embryo with the secondary yolk sac (Fig. 3.2).

After segregating from somatic cells, PGCs multiply (by mitosis) and migrate from the hind gut through the mesentery to the medioventral area of the urogenital ridges, laterally to the radix of the mesentery (Fig. 3.3). The migration is an active process involving amoeba-like locomotion (Witschi, 1948; Blandau *et al.*, 1963). The cells may

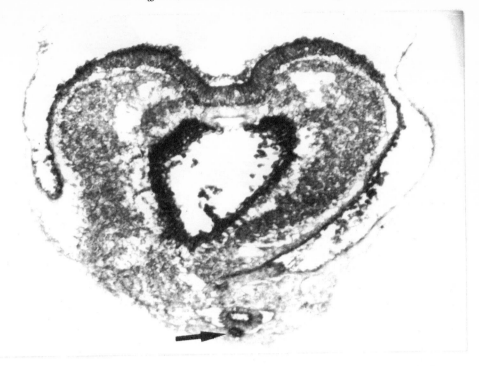

Fig 3.2. Primordial Germ Cells (arrow) Localized in the Allantois of an Early
Somite 26-day-old Human Embryo.
At this stage the endoderm of the gut still exhibits a high activity of alkaline
phosphatase. Distinguishing primordial germ cells located among endodermal cells of
the gut is difficult. (Magnification × 100.)

be attracted to the site where the gonads will form (gonadal ridges) by chemo-attraction. In birds and some mammals (cow, pig, sheep, goat) the cells may travel passively carried by the blood stream and 'home' on the gonadal ridges. The number of cells is believed to increase by mitosis during the passage from perhaps 100 to about 5000 in the fully developed undifferentiated gonad. The primordial germ cells develop into definitive germ cells towards the end of sex differentiation.

Not all primordial germ cells reach the gonadal anlage. Some are 'lost' during the migration while others may degenerate. Extragenital PGC are present in human embryos 6–35 mm long within the gut epithelium, in the mesentery, in the region of adrenals, near abdominal paraganglia and nerve cells, and along mesonephric and paramesonephric ducts. Dorsally PGC may be found in the region of the aorta and cranially to the anlage of the diaphragm. In fetuses longer than 30–35 mm these cells disappear (see Jirásek, 1977).

2.1.1. Definitive germ cells

Transformation of PGC into spermatogonia is related to the development of gonads. When the germ cells become incorporated into testicular cords they come into contact with Sertoli cells and change into spermatogonia. In the human the first spermatogonia

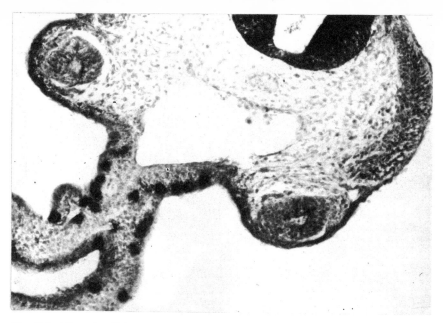

FIG 3.3. Migrating Primordial Germ Cells in the Epithelium of the Gut and in the
Mesentery of a 4.5-mm, 28-day-old Human Embryo.
Alkaline phosphatase strain. (Magnification × 100.)

appear in the 5-month-old embryo. The number may be determined by the number of
Sertoli cells produced during the embryonic stage (Orth *et al.*, 1988). During the
prenatal period, mitotic proliferation of spermatogonia is slow; spermatogonia which
are in contact with embryonal Sertoli cells do not enter meiosis. Active division with a
marked increase in numbers and meiosis begins only at puberty; meiotic division and
sperm formation proceeds during most of the adult life (Jirásek, 1988).

In contrast to males, the female is left with a finite number of oocytes; and post-natal
destruction in females is permanent and irreversible. In females all oogonia enter
meiotic prophase during fetal life. There are no special contacts to somatic cells before
meiosis begins. Oocyte number is highest before birth. In humans there are about seven
million in the 5-month-old embryo. Thereafter, the number decreases.

2.2. Development of the Gonads

The indifferent gonad arises from the condensation of three cellular components:
1. primordial germ cells; 2. mesoblastic cells from the surface (coelomic) epithelium
and 3. mesenchymal cells from the stroma of the urogenital (mesonephric) ridges
(Figs 3.4 and 3.5).

The primitive kidney (mesonephros) may be the source of, or may influence, the
formation of Leydig cells in the developing testis (Grinsted, 1982; Grinsted *et al.*, 1982).
In the embryonic female, mesonephros has the capacity to synthesize steroid hormones,
and to influence the steroidogenic capacity of the fetal ovary (Grinsted, 1982). In fetal
mice, the primitive kidney exerts a feminizing influence on the gonads. Gonads and

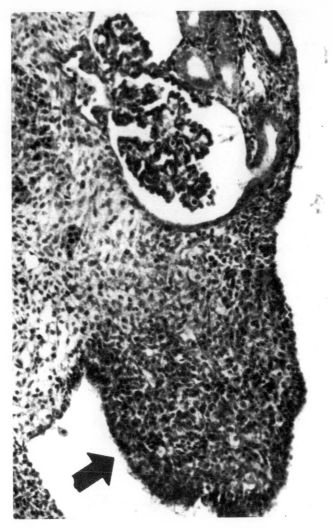

FIG 3.4. Indifferent Gonad (Genital Ridge) in a 9-mm, Approximately 36–38-day-
old Human Embryo.
The cellular tissue (arrow) located ventrally to the mesonephric nephrons is known
as the gonadal blastema. H- E- alcian blue. (Magnification × 100.)

ducts, cultured with mesonephros develop female characteristics regardless of sex
(Byskov and Grinsted, 1981).

2.3. Differentiation of the Genital Ducts

During the undifferentiated stage, two anlage for the development of male (Wolffian)
and female (Müllerian) ducts are present in the embryo. Masculinization of the male
genital apparatus will depend upon the presence of hormones originating in the male
gonad. In genetic females, or in castrated male embryos, the individual will form female

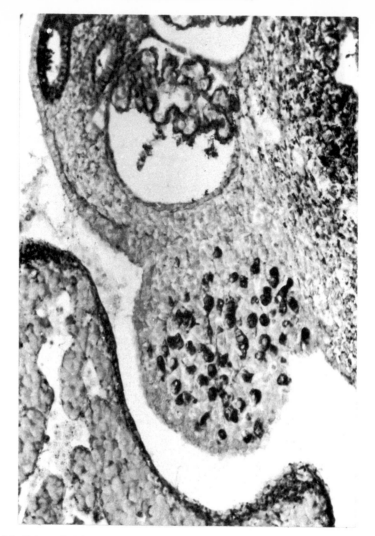

FIG 3.5. Primordial Germ Cells (dark) Concentrated Within the Gonadal Blastema. The mesonephric contribution can be demonstrated. The cells of the blastema, other than primordial germ cells, are mostly of coelomic origin. Human embryo 9 mm long, 36–38 days old. Alkaline phosphatase stain. (Magnification × 100.)

sexual organs. The timing of the process is of importance. Indifferent fetal mouse urogenital complex, grown *in vitro*, will differentiate into a male or female structure if explanted on day 11 of gestation. If the gonads are removed on day 10 they will remain undifferentiated (Taketo and Koide, 1981).

In males Wolffian ducts give rise to the epididymis, vas deferens and seminal vesicles; the urogenital sinus develops into the prostate, and the genital tubercle into the external genitalia. During the process of differentiation the Müllerian anlage regresses. In females the absence of testes causes involution of the Wolffian ducts and the Müllerian

Indifferent stage

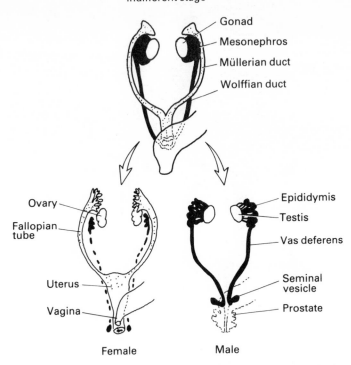

FIG 3.6. Internal Genital Tract Formation in Male and Female Embryos. Quoted from Wilson *et al.* (1981) with the permission of Academic Press.

TABLE 3.1. *Timing of Embryonic Gonadal Development in Several Mammalian Species*

Stage	Human (271–289)[a]	Rat (21–22)	Mouse (19)	Rabbit (30–32)
Germ cells				
identification	14–21	6–10	5–7	6–9
migration	21–42	10–13	8–11.5	6–13
Indifferent gonad	40–44	12–13.5	12.5	13–14
Testis				
embryonal	44–58	14–18	13–17	14–18
fetal	58–266 (birth)	18–21	17–19	19–33
Ovary				
embryonal	50–65	14–16.5	13–15.5	15–17
early fetal	64–115	17–20	15–18	18–22
late fetal	120–200	20–21	18–19	23–33

[a]Average length of pregnancy in days
Data courtesy of Dr J. Jirasek (Praha, Czechoslovakia).

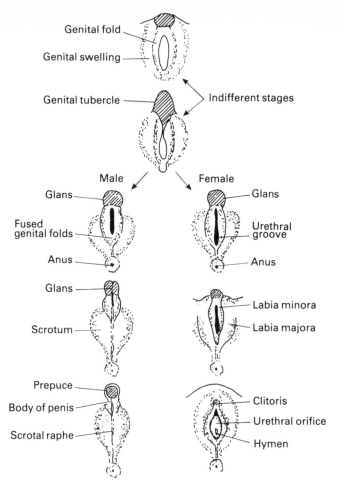

FIG 3.7. Formation of the External Genitalia in Male and Female Embryos.
Quoted from Wilson *et al.* (1981) with the permission of Academic Press.

ducts proliferate giving rise to the oviducts, uterus, cervix and a part of the vagina; the rest of the vagina is formed from the urogenital sinus.

The development of the external genitalia from the undifferentiated stage into the male structures also needs the presence of testosterone and the androgen receptor. In their absence the organization assumes a female character. Figures 3.6 and 3.7 show the formation of the internal genital tract and of the external genitalia in male and female embryos.

The time during which sexual differentiation takes place is remarkably similar in several mammals despite differences in the length of pregnancy (Table 3.1). The time of differentiation has been determined by dissecting fetuses of various ages, by evaluating the effect of testosterone on Wolffian duct differentiation *in vitro* (see Josso, 1970), and by transplanting female urogenital sinus into male recipients (Cunha, 1975).

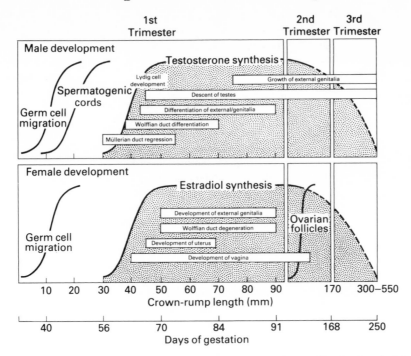

FIG 3.8. Sequences Between Gonadal Development, the Onset of Endocrine Activity
in the Gonads, and the Anatomical Differentiation of the Internal Genital Tract and
the External Genitalia in the Human Embryo.
Quoted from Wilson *et al.* (1981) with the permission of Academic Press.

Figure 3.8 gives the relationship between the development of the gonads, the onset of endocrine function of the gonads and the anatomical differentiation of the internal genital tract and the external genitalia in the human embryo (Wilson *et al.*, 1981).

In true hermaphrodites the sex ducts will differentiate depending upon the gonadal tissue in the ovotestis. In female mice the presence of 15% testicular tissue in ovaries is sufficient to decrease the proliferation of Müllerian ducts. If more than 85% of the tissue is testis, the Müllerian tissue atrophies and Wolffian ducts proliferate (Andersen *et al.*, 1983).

2.3.1. SEXUAL DIFFERENTIATION IN THE HUMAN

Morphological changes which accompany the differentiation of the gonads and the sex ducts were studied in detail in the human embryo. Table 3.2 shows the relationship between embryonic age, the length of the embryo, and development.

2.3.1.1. The Testes

(a) *Embryonic Testes*

Transformation of the indifferent genital ridge into embryonal testis begins in a 14–20 mm long embryo, 43–49 days old. During the change primordial germ cells

TABLE 3.2. *Timetable and Staging of Human Prenatal Development*

Periods	Age (days)	Length (mm)	External characteristics	Stage
Embyronal period				
Blastogenesis	0–2	0.2	Unicellular (fertilized oocyte)	1
	2–4	0.2	Blastomeric (16–20 blastomeres, morula)	2
	4–6	0.4	Blastodermic (blastocyst)	3
			Bilaminar embryo stage (round-shaped embryonic disk)	
	6–15	0.1	bilaminar plate	4–1
			primary yolk sac	4–2
		0.2–0.4	secondary yolk sac	4–3
			Trilaminar embryo stage (pear-shaped embryonic disk)	
	15–17	0.4–1.0	with primitive streak	5–1
	17–20	1.0–2.0	with notochordal process	5–2
Early organogenesis			Early somite stage (shoe-sole-shaped embryo)	
	20–21	1.5–2.0	completely open neural groove	6–1
	21–26	1.5–4.0	neural tube closing, both ends open	6–2
	26–30	3–5	one or both neuropores closed	6–3
			Stage or limb development (C-shaped embryo)	
	28–32	4–6	bud of proximal extremity	7–1
	31–35	5–8	buds of proximal and distal extremities	7–2
	35–38	7–10	proximal extremity, two segments	7–3
	37–42	8–12	proximal and distal extremity, two segments	7–4
	42–44	10–14	digital rays, foot plates	7–5
	44–51	13–21	digital tubercles	7–6
	51–53	19–24	digits, toe tubercles	7–7
			Late embryonal stage (embryo with differentiated extremities including fingers and toes)	
	52–56	22–25	Eyes open	8–1
	56–60	27–35	Fusing eyelids	8–2
Fetal period	60–182+	31–200	Fetus with fused eyelids	9
Perinatal period	170–266+	201–350	Third trimester fetus (newborn with open eyes)	10

After Jirasek (1983).

(PGC) become irregularly shaped and lose temporarily the ability to stain for alkaline phosphatase and glycogen. Contact with embryonic Sertoli cells induces cord formation. At the same time the amount of the mesenchymal interstitial connective tissue increases. The cords become distinct and separated from the surface epithelium by a primitive tunica albuginea. PGCs concentrate within the gonadal blastema, become embedded within testicular cords, regain rounded shape and stain again for alkaline phosphatase and glycogen.

There is no ingrowth of the cords from the surface epithelium. The testicular cords appear rapidly throughout the entire gonadal anlage (Fig. 3.9). Each testicular cord

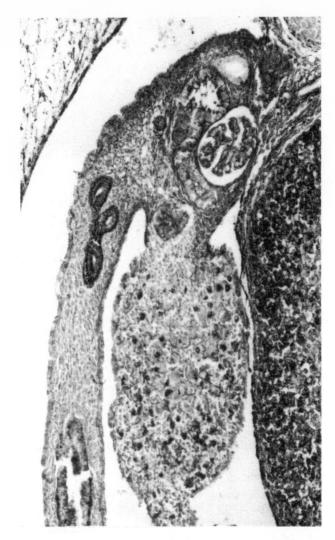

FIG 3.9. Differentiation of the Gonadal Blastema into the Embryonal Testis.
Basement membranes formed *in situ*, divide gonadal blastema into testicular cords.
Human embryo 16 mm long, 44 days old. Alkaline phosphatase stain. (Magnification × 100.)

forms a peripheral portion, contributing the primordium of the seminiferous tubule, and a central portion, which forms the rete cord. Rete cords interconnect and contact the epigenital mesonephric tubules to establish the urogenital junction (Fig. 3.10). Mesenchymal cells adjacent to the basement membranes of epithelial cells (surface epithelium, seminiferous cords, rete) differentiate into connective tissue of the propria of cords, the testicular mediastinum and the tunica albuginea. The spaces between the seminiferous cords contain a special mesenchyme rich in proteoglycans.

The connective tissue might be derived from the mesenchyme of the urogenital (mesonephric) ridges, whereas the 'special loose interstitial mesenchyme' separating the

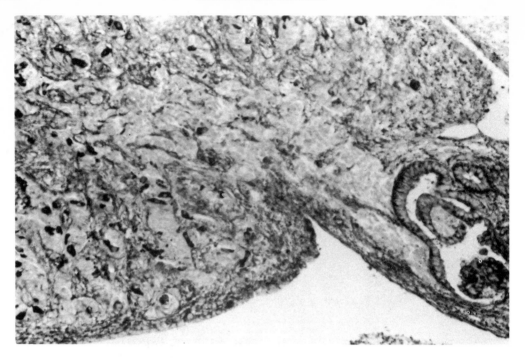

FIG 3.10. Embryonal Testis of a 19 mm, Approximately 48 Days Old Embryo.
Cords of rete testis originating from gonadal blastema contact epigenital mesonephric
nephrons. the urogenital junction (junction between testis and epididymis) becomes
established. Alcian blue: PAS.

cords (and later giving rise to the steroid-producing cells) might originate from coelomic cells of the blastema not incorporated into the cords. Wartenberg (1978; 1985) suggested that mesonephric cells participate in the histogenesis of testicular cords. The concept that Sertoli cells are mesonephric in origin is misleading. Embryonal testis does not contain any steroid-producing interstitial cells. A special proteoglycan present within the interstitium of the embryonal testis is considered to be related to the Müllerian-inhibiting factor produced by the mesenchymal cells within the testicular interstitium (Jirásek, 1977) and not by the embryonal Sertoli cells as suggested by Josso *et al.* (1977; 1985).

(b) *Fetal Testes*

Fetal testes are characterized by the presence of steroid-producing epithelioid interstitial cells (Fig. 3.11) originating from fibroblast-like mesenchymal cells (Jirásek, 1967). The interstitial (Leydig) cells are characterized by the presence of LH-hCG receptors at the cellular membranes and by the presence of cytoplasmic 3β-hydroxysteroid dehydrogenase. The production of fetal testicular androgens begins at week 9 post-conception (Jirásek, 1967; 1971) (see Vol I, Chapters 2 and 3). The amount of interstitial cells increases until the end of the third month, declining thereafter. The Sertoli cells of the fetal testis remain embryonal in character, and in spite of androgens present, do not

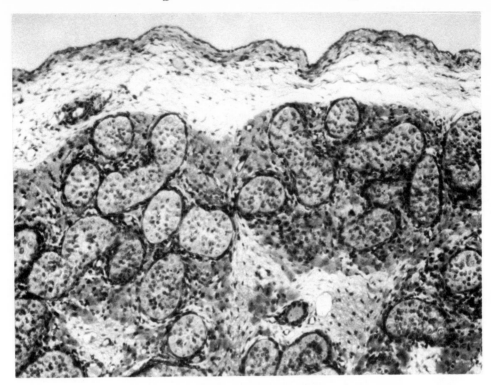

FIG 3.11. Fetal Testis with Interstitial Leydig Cells Located in the Spaces Between
Seminiferous Cords.
The propria of cords and the tunica albuginea are evident. Human fetus 75 mm CR
length. H- E- alcian blue. (Magnification × 100.)

further differentiate nor bind androgens. Fetal spermatogonia exhibit only a weak
mitotic activity and they do not differentiate prenatally into spermatocytes.

Within the first two post-natal months, the interstitial cells completely disappear. The
fetal testis changes into the prepubertal (quiescent) testis. Testicular cords remain
unlumenized lined with spermatogonia and immature Sertoli cells. With the beginning
of puberty, interstitial Leydig cells reappear, Sertoli cells become sensitive to androgens
and differentiate into 'adult-type' Sertoli cells and spermiogenesis begins. The presence
of lumen in the seminiferous tubules and spermiogenesis are characteristic features of
adult testes.

2.3.1.2. The Ovary

(a) *Embryonic Ovary*

The development of the human embryonic ovary is characterized by repeated mitotic
divisions of PGC within the gonadal blastema and proliferation of the coelomic and
mesenchymal cells. There is no ingrowth of medullary and cortical ovarian cords from
the surface. The medullary portion of the embryonal ovary results from differentiation
of the connective tissue within the gonadal blastema. Development of the cortical

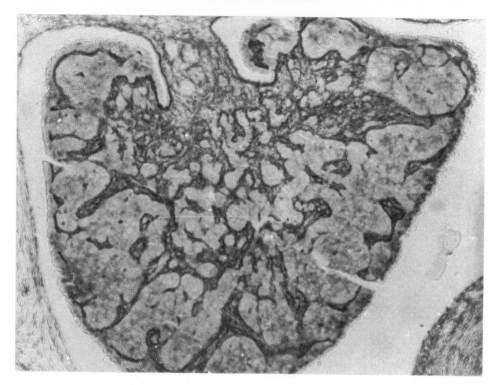

FIG 3.12. Differentiation of Connective Tissue Within the Embryonal Cord. Early
Fetal Ovaries Give Rise to the So-called medullary and Cortical Ovarian Cords.
Ovary of a 45-cm human fetus. Silver impregnation of reticulum. (Magnifica-
tion × 100.)

portion of the embryonal (and the later fetal) ovary results from mitotic proliferation
of PGC located mostly under surface epithelium (Fig. 3.12). The medullary cords
contain both embryonal granulosa cells and oogonia. The deepest portions of the
medullary cords form the ovarian rete, and connect with the epigenital mesonephric
nephrons. The so-called cortical cords result from mitotic proliferation of germ cells.
The proliferation of germ cells, which are in contact with the incompletely separated
surface epithelium, creates the so-called 'neogenic zone' of the embryonal ovary.
Reticular fibers differentiate within the connective tissue, sharply delineating ovarian
stroma from epithelial ovarian components (i.e. surface epithelium, cortical cords,
medullary cords and rete). The ovarian stroma contains mesenchymal cells of dual
origin: 1. cells from coelomic epithelium and 2. cells from mesenchyme of urogenital
ridges. Steroid-producing cells which demonstrate (histochemically) 3β-hydroxysteroid
dehydrogenase or meotic activity are absent.

(b) *Fetal Ovary*

Isogenic groups of meiotic oocytes develop in the deepest portions of cortical
medullary cords. Mitotic proliferation of oogonia begins under the surface epithelium.

Isolated primary follicles are not present. The first leptotene oocytes appear in the deepest layers of cortical cords and in medullary cords, in 35–40-mm fetuses (day 60–65 post-conception). Zygotene oocytes make their appearance around day 80, first diploene around day 50 (Baker, 1963; 1972). The groups of oocytes undergoing meiotic prophase are incompletely separated by granulosa cells. The connective tissue

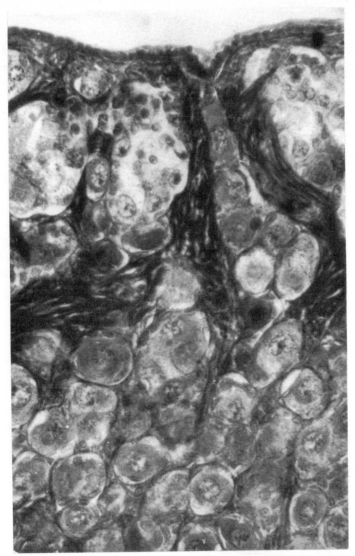

FIG 3.13. Cortical Portion of a Perinatal Ovary of a Newborn.
Underneath the surface epithelium there are still oocytes in groups. Similar groups represent the most advanced germinal structure in early fetal ovaries. Isolated primary follicles, similar to those found in late fetal ovaries are present in deeper areas of ovarian cortex. Growing follicles and vesicular follicles, characteristic for a perinatal ovary are present in the deepest portion of the cortex and in the medulla (not seen in the picture). Azan. (Magnification × 200.)

separating 'cords' of germinal tissue do not contain any epithelioid steroid-producing cells. In germinal cells the meiotic wave spreads from the deepest medullary cords towards the surface.

Primary follicles appear with a complete single layered granulosa cell, separated by connective tissue from the rest of cord, in the late fetal ovary. First primary follicles are derived from oocytes located within medullary cords and within the deepest portions of cortical cords. Differentiation of primary follicles spreads from the medullar towards the cortical surface. Under the surface epithelium mitotic proliferation of oogonia continues. During differentiation of the primary follicles, after the meiotic prophase has been completed, adjacent granulosa cells flatten and spread over the surface of the oocyte. The connective tissue invades from under the granulosa cells into the cords and separates individual primary follicles (Fig. 3.13). If the sheet of granulosa cells around the oocyte is incomplete, the connective tissue comes in direct contact with the oocyte which degenerates. Primitive granulosa cells, which do not participate in follicular differentiation, mix with the connective tissue and contribute to the mesenchyme of ovarian stroma. It has not been possible to demonstrate any ovarian cells containing 3β-hydroxysteroid dehydrogenase within the late fetal ovary by histochemical methods.

The total number of germ cells sharply decreases, as primary follicles are formed. The population of ovarian germ cells in the 18–22-week-old fetus may reach five to seven million in each ovary. At birth approximately two million germ cells remain; half of them may be degenerating (Baker, 1963). The ovaries of a 20-year-old woman contain only about 400 000 oocytes. Of these approximately 400 ovulate during the entire reproductive period.

(c) Perinatal Ovary

The perinatal ovary is characterized by the presence of growing preantral follicles filled by multilayered granulosa cells and by anthral follicles. Anthral follicles are located deep in the cortex or within the ovarian medullar. The stroma surrounding multilayered growing follicles becomes organized into a cellular theca interna and a fibrous theca externa. Epithelioid cells in the theca interna and interstitial cells in the medullary stroma exhibit 3β-hydroxysteroid dehydrogenase activity. The follicular anthrum becomes evident at the same time. The steroidogenic cells are mostly derived from thecal cells of atretic follicles.

2.3.1.3. The Wolffian (Mesonephric) Ducts

In humans Wolffian ducts originate as pronephric ducts dorsolateral to the segmented pronephric blastema. The cellular material of mesonephric ducts is derived from glycogen-rich ectodermal buds evaginating from surface epithelium to the glycogen-free pronephric blastema (Politzer, 1953; Jirásek, 1971). The mesonephric ducts grow caudally as solid cords into the area of the mesonephric blastema, contact laterally the primordia of mesonephric nephrons, become lumenized and in 27–28 somite embryos (4–5 mm long, 28–32 days old) enter the hind gut. The terminal portion of the hind gut develops into a cloaca (Streeter, 1951).

2.3.1.4. The Müllerian (Paramesonephric) Ducts

Primordia of Müllerian ducts invaginate from coelomic (mesodermal) epithelium on the lateral side of the epigenital portion of the mesonephric ridge. The invaginating epithelium represents extension of the surface epithelium of embryonal gonads (but does not contain any germ cells). The cellular cords of each paramesonephric duct grow caudally in contact with the mesonephric duct, cross the mesonephric duct ventrally and become lumenized. Caudally to the crossing, both paramesonephric ducts run parallel between the mesonephric ducts (Fig. 3.14). The tips of the paramesonephric

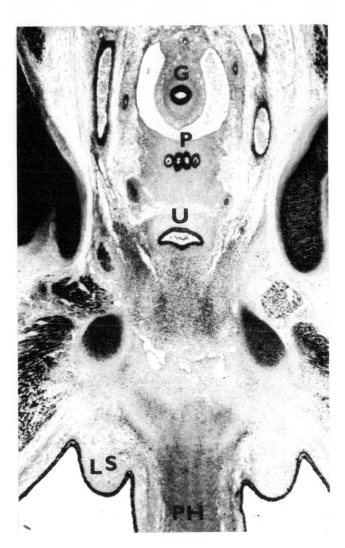

FIG 3.14. Transverse Section Through the Pelvis of a 26-mm Human Embryo. P: paramesonephric ducts located between mesonephric ducts; U: urogenital sinus; LS: labioscrotal swellings; PH: phallus; G: gut. Alcian blue: PAS. (Magnification × 40.)

ducts contact the endodermal epithelium of the urogenital sinus between the openings of the mesonephric ducts in 30–35 mm embryos (56–60 days of age) in the area known as the Müllerian tubercle. The parallel portions of the mesonephric ducts fuse into a single uterovaginal canal.

2.3.1.5. The Urogenital Sinus and the External Genitalia

In 7–10 mm long embryos (35–38 days old) the terminal portion of the hind gut, known as the cloaca, is closed by the cloacal membrane. The cloaca becomes divided by the urorectal septum into the dorsal portion (the anorectal canal) and the ventral portion (the primitive urogenital sinus). As the primary ureters (Wolffian ducts) enter the primitive urogenital sinus, the portion located above their openings is classified as the vesicourethral primordium, while the portion below the openings represents the definitive urogenital sinus. The vesicourethral canal gives rise to the lower portion of the urinary bladder, the whole female urethra, and the intramural and prostatic parts of the male urethra.

(a) *The Indifferent External Genitalia*

Primordia of the indifferent external genitalia appear around the cloacal membrane (Figs 3.15(a) and 3.15(b)). Two cutaneous elevations, known as the labioscrotal swellings, appear laterally from the genital tubercle (Fig. 3.16). Caudal ligaments of the urogenital ridge are anchored in these areas. As the urorectal septum reaches the cloacal membrane, contributing the primitive perineum, the cloacal membrane splits into the anal membrane closing the anus, and the urethral membrane (urethral plate) closing the urogenital sinus. The corporal portion of the urethral plate and later groove is delineated laterally by the urethral folds. The genital membrane disintegrates in embryos approximately 20 mm long, the anal membrane in embryos approximately 24 mm long. The derivative of the genital tubercle located above the external opening of the urogenital sinus is properly called the phallus.

(b) *Formation of the Genital Ducts and External Genitalia in the Male*

The canal ligament of the urogenital ridge (the gubernaculum) of each testis crosses the paramesonephric duct. The degeneration of the paramesonephric duct begins in the area of crossing exactly in the area where the duct is exposed to the Müllerian-inhibiting substance, MIS (see Section 3.2.2 below). In the exposed cells of the paramesonephric duct the activity of lysosomal acid hydrolases increases, the lysosomes rupture and the liberated enzymes destroy the cells. Regression of the paramesonephric ducts extend cranially as well as caudally, next reaching the terminal cranial and caudal ends of the ducts (Jirásek, 1977, 1983, 1985). In males, the closed cranial portion of each paramesonephric duct transforms into a cystic appendix testis, hydatid of Morgagni. The terminal caudal portions of former Müllerian ducts develop into the utriculus prostaticus.

The male development of the mesonephric derivatives, and of the external genitalia, is androgen-dependent (see Section 3.2 below). Growth of the epididymis and the vas deferens is testosterone-dependent; growth of the seminal vesicles, the prostate, the bulbourethral glands, as well as growth and differentiation of the external genitalia are dihydrotestosterone-dependent (Siiterii and Wilson, 1974). Five to twelve testosterone-stimulated epigenital mesonephric tubules connecting rete testis with the mesonephric duct become the ductuli efferentes of epididymis. The proximal portion of the mesonephric duct, incorporated within the mesonephric ridge, becomes the duct of

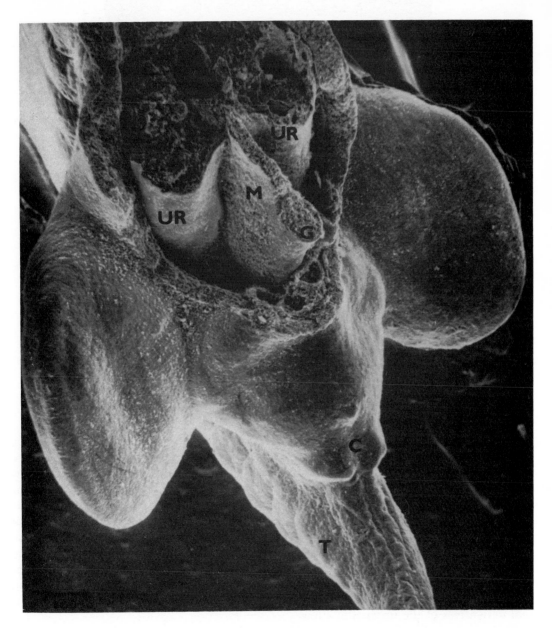

FIG 3.15(a). Transverse Dissection of an 8-mm Human Embryo.
UR: urogenital sinus; M: mesentery; G: gut; C: cloacal membrane; T: tail; SEM.

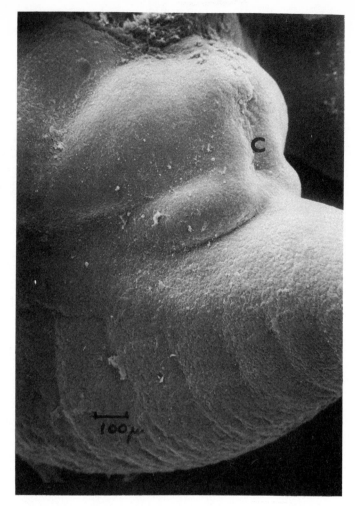

FIG 3.15(b). Genital Tubercle of a 10-mm Human Embryo.
C: cloacal membrane, SEM.

epididymis. The distal portion of the mesonephric duct, located between the mesonephric ridge and the urogenital sinus, transforms into the vas deferens. The terminal portion of the vas deferens located between the opening of the seminal vesicle and the urethra develops into the ejaculatory duct. Seminal vesicles originate as evaginations of mesonephric ducts. Under the influence of androgens, the urogenital sinus gives rise to the lower prostatic and membranous portions of the male urethra, whilst the formation of the cavernous urethra (penile and glandular) depends on the development of the urethral plate and groove, and is closely related to morphogenesis of the penis. The prostate and the bulbourethral glands are androgen-sensitive endodermal derivatives of the urogenital sinus.

External genitalia in normal males develop during the third month post-conception (Figs 3.17, 3.18 and 3.19). In 40–45-mm fetuses (week 9) the anogenital distance

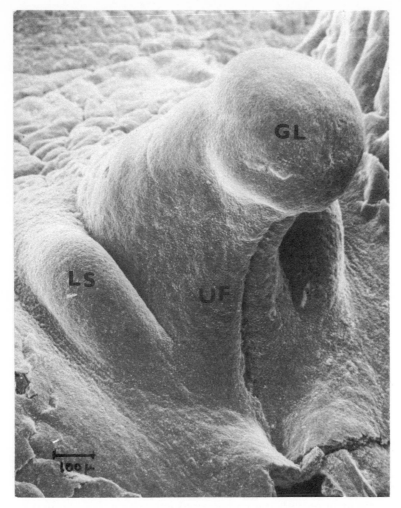

FIG 3.16. Indifferent External Genitalia of a 22-mm Human Embryo.
GL: glans of phallus; UF: urethral fold; LS: labioscrotal swelling; SEM.

lengthens, the labioscrotal swellings fuse in the mid-line, forming the scrotum and the rims of the urethral folds fuse postero-anteriorly closing the cavernous penile urethra.

(c) *Formation of the Genital Ducts and External Genitalia in the Female*

The superior (mesonephric) portions of paramesonephric (Müllerian) ducts contribute the uterine tubes. The tubes are included within a peritoneal fold (mesonephric ridge), known as the broad ligament. The tubes descend with the ovaries. The inferior portions of both paramesonephric ducts fuse into a single uterovaginal canal with an uterine and a vaginal segment. The vaginal segment becomes attached to the

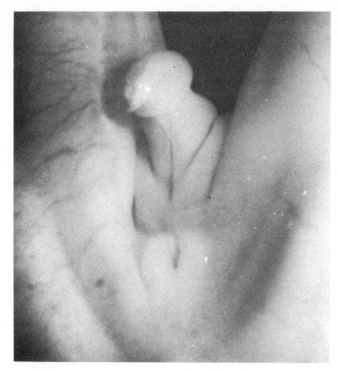

FIG 3.17. Masculinization of External Genitalia in a 35 mm Fetus. Lengthening of the anogenital distance. (Magnification × 20.)

urogenital sinus by a short endodermal vaginal bulb. In the uterine segment, the mesenchyme accompanying the paramesonephric ducts fuses with the mesenchyme of mesenephric ducts, increases in amount and forms the uterine wall. The epithelium of the vaginal segment fuses with the endodermal epithelium, contributed by the urogenital sinus and transforms into the vaginal plate. The vaginal plate is formed by multilayered squamous epithelium developing around the single layered cylindrical epithelium of paramesonephric origin. The vagina becomes lumenized by degeneration of the paramesonephric epithelium. The hymen develops as an incomplete septum between the endodermal portion of the vagina and the urogenital sinus in the area of the paramesonephric tubercle.

During the development of the external genitalia, and during the formation of the vagina, the urogenital sinus elongates sagitally and changes into the vaginal vestibule. During the process the anogenital distance (the perineum) does not increase, and neither do the labioscrotal swellings, nor the urethral folds (Fig. 3.20). The phallus bends caudally. Subsequently the derivative of the genital tubercle transforms into the clitoris, the rims of the urethral folds become the labia minora, and the labioscrotal swellings the labia majora (Fig. 3.21). The cavernous tissue associated with the urethral folds contributes the two vestibular bulbi. No hormones are required for female transformation of genital ducts and external genitalia (Jost, 1953).

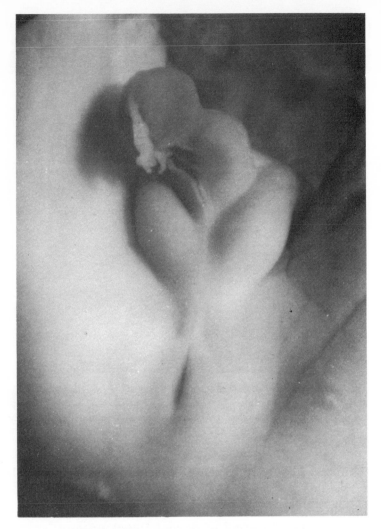

FIG 3.18. Masculinization of External Genitalia in a 50-mm Fetus.
Scrotal raphe has been formed, cavernous urethra is closing. Epithelial plug of the
glans originates from ectoderm of the cloacal membrane. (Magnification × 20.)

2.3.2. DEVELOPMENT OF THE MAMMARY GLANDS

The developing mammary anlage is sex hormone-dependent (Raynaud, 1947; 1949; Jean and Delost, 1964; Jean 1971a,b). In 16-day-old male mouse fetuses, mammary rudiments atrophy from the action of testosterone. The hormone acts directly on the mesenchyme which condenses around epithelial gland buds and causes their necrosis (Dürenberger and Kratochwill, 1980).

The female anlage is sensitive to pharmacological doses of androgens; their presence during the critical period of organogenesis abolishes the development. The anlage is

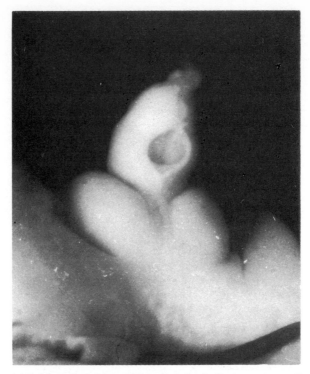

FIG 3.19. Masculinization of External Genitalia in a 52-mm Fetus.
Labioscrotal swellings are unified by the raphe scroti into the scrotum. Raphe of
penis closes the corporal portion of cavernous urethra. A physiologic hypospadia is
present at this stage. (Magnification × 20.)

about ten times more sensitive to exogenous testosterone than to dihydrotestosterone
(Goldman *et al.*, 1976).

3. The Control of Sexual Development

The critical role played by the embryonic testis in the control of differentiation of sex
ducts has been mainly elucidated by Jost in rabbits (Jost, 1947; 1953) and in rats (Jost,
1972a,b; Jost *et al.*, 1973). Jost developed a theory which states that the testes of the
developing male fetus superimpose masculinity on a basically female state; in the
absence of testes the organism develops into a female. Experimental evidence which
support the concept is:

1.   Müllerian ducts do not develop in males but are present in castrated male fetuses.
The observation suggests that fetal testes must *actively inhibit* the growth of Müllerian
ducts.
2.   If testis tissue is implanted, on one side, into castrated male fetuses, normal male sex
ducts develop, but on that side only. Both Müllerian and Wolffian ducts remain on the
other side. The observation suggests that testes *actively stimulate* the growth of Wolffian
ducts.

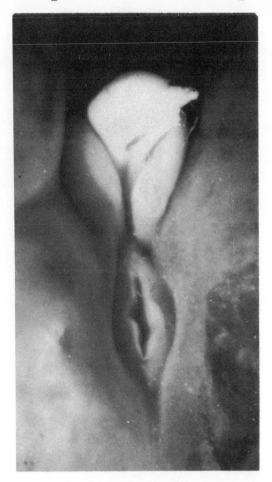

FIG 3.20. Feminization of External Genitalia in a 40-mm Human Fetus.
The labioscrotal swellings do not fuse, the phallus bends ventrally. (Magnification × 25.)

Exogenous androgens, or estrogens, are teratogenic in both sexes. In females androgens suppress proliferation of regional parts (vaginal segments), the vagina does not form, the prostate buds are stimulated to a male-like form, and the rest of genitalia develop into a male-like form. Estrogens precipitate precocious development in females. In males estrogens cause abnormalities to a varying degree depending upon the status of the duct, the dose and the species. A vaginal cord may develop, the growth of the prostate is suppressed, and the external genitalia may become female-like (see Section 5 below).

3.1. Hormonal Influences Prior to Implantation

The pre-implantation embryo (PIE), the morula or the blastocyst, was believed to be capable of synthesizing steroid hormones, a function essential for maintenance of early

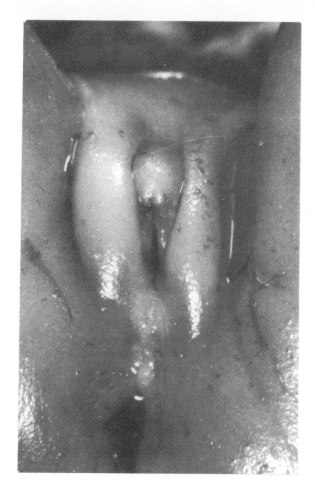

FIG 3.21. Female External Genitalia in a 120-mm Human Fetus.
Labioscrotal swellings give rise to the labia majora, the urethral folds become the
labia minora, the phallus transforms into the clitoris. (Magnification × 10.)

pregnancy. Dickmann and Dey (1974a) and Dickmann *et al.* (1976) studied the
appearance of 3β-hydroxysteroid dehydrogenase in rats, mice, hamsters, rabbits and
pigs and reported that enzyme activity began at the early morula stage, peaked at the
blastocyst stage and then declined and disappeared shortly after implantation. The
pattern of activity of 17β-hydroxysteroid dehydrogenase (*estradiol* was the substrate in
the incubation medium) was confined to similar developmental stages. Huff and
Eik-ness (1966) described a 6-day-old rabbit blastocyst able to convert acetate into
cholesterol and pregnenolone.

A tropic (LH-, or HG-like) activity using a radioreceptor assay has been demonstrated by Haour and Saxena (1974) in a 6-day-old rabbit blastocyst. Fishell *et al.*
(1984) detected the formation of hCG in the medium of two cultured human embryos.

Based on these results Dickmann *et al.* (1976) proposed that steroid hormones (estradiol), originating in the blastocyst, play a vital role in inducing implantation. Since 3β-hydroxysteroid dehydrogenase activity was found in PIE of hypophysec-tomized mother rats (Dickmann and Dey, 1974b), the conclusion was drawn that the activity in the glastocyst was autonomous.

Later investigation does not suppport this view. Angle and Mead (1979) were unable to observe (*in vivo* and *in vitro*) any significant conversion of pregnenolone to proges-terone but noted a significant uptake of progesterone and its conversion to unidentified metabolites. The group proposed that pre-implantation rabbit blastocysts are not capable of *de novo* synthesis but are able to sequester progesterone from the surrounding medium, and metabolize the hormone.

Evans and Kennedy (1980) demonstrated that, in hamsters, the signal which induces implantation (most likely prostaglandin E) originates in the blastocyst. The process is independent of maternal, or blastocyst, steroidogenesis.

3.2. The Role of the Embryonic Gonads

Testosterone is not the hormone which inhibits the growth of Müllerian ducts. In castrated male fetuses the hormone stimulates the development of Wolffian ducts into a normal male reproductive tract; in addition the animal will have a set of female reproductive organs. The observation demonstrates that testosterone does not inhibit the growth of female sex tissue. Exposure of intact embryos to anti-androgens results in underdeveloped genitalia in both sexes. Males do not develop internal genitalia while the external genitalia become feminized and a vaginal opening forms. In females, the genitalia also do not develop since the testes continue to secrete MIF (Neumann and Steinbeck, 1974). See also Section 5.1, below.

Fetal biosynthesis of steroid hormones, and the concentrations of various hormones (polypetide, glycoproteins and steroid) in the maternal, placental and fetal compart-ments have been described in Volume I, Chapters 2 and 3.

3.2.1. ANDROGENS

The presence of androgens sways the development of the female embryo in the male direction. Female embryos become virilized (cattle: Keller and Tandler, 1916; Lillie, 1916; 1917; swine: Hughes, 1929; sheep, and goats: Andersson, 1956) when the fetus becomes exposed to a male hormonal milieu by sharing a common placental circulation (freemartin). Females develop normally if blood circulation does not anastomose.

In mice a female fetus developing between two male embryos may become influenced by the proximity. The androgenic influence becomes expressed in adults by an increase in the average cycle length by $1\frac{1}{2}$ days (vom Saal and Bronson, 1980); the behavior of the females resembles in some respects male responses (Hauser and Gandelman, 1983).

Testosterone secretion by the embryonic testes induces transformation of Wolffian ducts into epididymis, vas deferens and seminal vesicles, of the urogenital sinus into the prostate and the formation of male external genitalia from the indifferent apparatus.

The production of testosterone by fetal testis has been demonstrated in sheep by **Pomerantz and Nalbandov** (1975); in monkeys by Resko *et al.* (1973); in rats by Warren *et al.* (1973) and Picon (1976); in mice by vom Saal and Bronson (1980); in rabbits by Catt *et al.* (1975), Veyssiere *et al.* (1976) and George *et al.* (1979); in guinea-pigs by Buhl *et al.* (1979); in pigs by Raeside and Middleton (1979) and in man by Huhtaniemi *et al.* (1970) and Siiterii and Wilson (1974). The concentration of testosterone is usually higher in male fetuses in cattle (Kim *et al.*, 1972; Challis *et al.*, 1974), humans (Abramovich and Rowe, 1973), rabbits (Veyssiere *et al.*, 1976), guinea-pigs (Buhl *et al.*, 1979), and rats (Weisz and Ward, 1980). In 23-day-old rabbit embryos, testosterone values in male plasma range from 48 to 269 pg/ml and in females between 29 and 113 pg/ml (Veyssiere *et al.*, 1976). The concentration varies from species to species and the time of gestation. Buhl *et al.* (1979) found in guinea-pigs (male differentiation takes place between day 20 and 24) average 3.04 ng testosterone/ both testes in 20-day-old fetuses and 3.94 ng/both testes on day 26. In pigs (differenti-ation takes place between days 25 and 27 in 1.6–2.2-mm long embryos), the testes produce during this time 20 ± 2.7 ng/24 h ($\pm$SD) of testosterone; the production increases to 181 ± 64.8 ng/24 h in 2.7-mm long embryos (Raeside and Middleton, 1979). In rat embryo, testes form between day 13.5 to 14.5. Steroidogenesis appears on day 15.50; the activity increases and reaches a plateau between days 19.5 and 20.5 of gestation (Ikonen and Niemi, 1966). Picon (1976) found 1.01 ng/testes of testosterone on day 14.5, and 9.12 ng/testes on day 18.5. The onset of the biosynthetic activity coincides with the period of sensitivity (day 16.5) of Wolffian ducts to androgens (Stinnakre, 1975).

However, the concentration of androgens in systemic circulation is of less importance in the differentiation of sex ducts; female embryos also produce testosterone. Veyssiere *et al.* (1976) found in 23-day-old rabbit male embryos, 48–269 pg/ml in blood and 29–113 pg/ml in female fetuses. Weisz and Ward (1980) reported 450–2800 pg/ml in male rat fetuses and 350–3850 in females. This shows that it is the local concentration in the tissue, the evolution of steroid hormone receptors (Catt *et al.*, 1975), metabolic clearance rate, the production rate and conversion rate of testosterone to 5α-dihy-drotestosterone (Pelardy and Delost, 1978), and the percentage of the two free steroids in maternal and fetal plasma which provide the dominant influence. This is fully discussed in Chapter 2. Adequate testosterone production is essential. Reduction of the amounts that circulate in plasma (such as by immunizing the mothers by serum against testosterone) leads to failure of proper formation of genitalia in males (Veyssiere *et al.*, 1979). Agents which block androgenic effects (anti-androgens) also prevent the proper development of the genital apparatus (see Section 5.1 below).

3.2.1.1. The Role of 5α-Dihydrotestosterone

Testosterone influences the development of internal genitalia whilst 5α-dihydrotestos-terone (5α-DHT) controls the development of external structures in rats and rabbits (Wilson and Lasnitzky, 1971; Wilson, 1973; Veyssiere *et al.*, 1982a), guinea-pigs (Rigaudiere, 1981) and humans (Wilson *et al.*, 1981). 5α-Dihydrogenase activity can be demonstrated only in the urogenital sinus and urogenital tubercle and only after virilization is well advanced.

Veyssiere *et al.* (1982a) compared the concentration of testosterone and dihy-drotestosterone in plasma, sex ducts and genital tubercle in rabbit fetuses of both sexes. In males, testosterone appeared successively in testis (day 19), mesonephros (day 20) and Wolffian ducts (day 22). In sexual ducts the concentration increased from day 20

TABLE 3.3. *Testosterone (T) and 5α-Dihydrotestosterone (5α-DHT) Concentrations in 25-day-old Rabbit Fetuses*

	Males				Females		
	Testes	Plasma	Sexual ducts	Genital tubercle	Plasma	Sexual ducts	Genital tubercle
T	2715 ± 224	171 ± 52	49.6 ± 16.5	ND	66 ± 14	ND	6.2
5α-DHT	63 ± 11	36 ± 7	22.2 ± 16.9	33.4 ± 9.8	17 ± 2	ND	10.6

Values: testes, pg/2 testes; plasma, pg/ml; sexual ducts, pg/both ducts; genital tubercle, pg $\pm$ SEM; ND, not detectable

Quoted from Veyssière *et al.* (1982a).

to 25 and then became stable until birth. Dihydrotestosterone appeared only on day 24. In female fetuses both testosterone and dihydrotestosterone were undetectable in sexual ducts: 5α-DHT was present in genital tubercle but the concentrations were lower than in males (Table 3.3). It should be noted that the variations (SE) were extremely large.

Reduction of testosterone to dihydrotestosterone takes place also in other tissues (abdominal skin, placenta, brain, kidney, intestines, lungs, etc) albeit to a much lower degree than in urogenital tubercle and sinus (Wilson and Lasnitzki, 1971).

3.2.1.2. The Biosynthesis of Steroid Hormones

The ability of fetal testes to convert C-21 precursors into C-19 androgenic steroids has been demonstrated in *in vitro* studies by various groups (for details see Volume I, Chapter 2). The appearance of different enzymes (17-hydroxylases, 17,20-desmolases, 17β-hydroxysteroid dehydrogenases), involved in the transformation of the precursors to the active hormone, is age-dependent and varies in different species. The activity of

TABLE 3.4. *3β-Hydroxysteroid Dehydrogenase, 5-ene → 4-ene Isomerase Activities in Mammalian Fetal Gonads*

Species	Positive reaction at stages given		Reference
	Testis	Ovary	
Rat	15–21 days		Niemi and Ikonen (1962)
Mouse	15.5 days		Hitzeman (1962)
	11–20 days		Baillie (1965)
	11–20 days	12–21	Baillie *et al.* (1966)
Guinea-pig	29–50 days	days	Price *et al.* (1964)
Human	9.5 cm		Bloch *et al.* (1962)
	18–23 days		Baillie *et al.* (1965)

the key enzymes in the synthesis of steroid hormones (3β-hydroxysteroid dehydrogenase and 5-ene $\rightarrow$ 4-ene isomerase) appears in the gonads at the time of sex differentiation (Table 3.4). In testes, the activity is localized in the inter-tubular spaces (Leydig cells). The enzyme also appears in the ovaries but the activity is minimal. Both the testes and ovaries contain the capacity for *de novo* synthesis of steroid hormones from cholesterol (George *et al.*, 1979).

Fetal testes produce androgens *in vitro* (Pointis and Mahoudeau, 1977) and *in vivo* (Kiser *et al.*, 1975). The ability of fetal testis to respond to hCG or LH, to produce androgens *in vitro* has been shown in humans (Abramovich *et al.*, 1974; Ahluwalia *et al.*, 1974; Huhtaniemi *et al.*, 1977), rats (Warren *et al.*, 1975; Weniger and Zeis, 1974; 1975; Sanyal and Villee, 1977; Feldman and Bloch, 1978; Paz *et al.*, 1980), mice (Weniger and Zeis, 1974; Pointis and Mahoudeau, 1975), rabbits (Catt *et al.*, 1975; George *et al.*, 1978a), guinea-pigs (Brinkmann, 1977), domestic pig (Raeside and Middleton, 1979), and cattle (Shemesh *et al.*, 1978). Table 3.5 shows the age at which the conversion of progesterone to testosterone takes place and Table 3.6 indicates the appearance of androgen-forming enzymes in testes of different species.

TABLE 3.5. *Conversion of Progesterone into Testosterone by Fetal Testes*

Species	Stage studied[a]	Reference
Human	5.5–8 cm; 9.5–11.5 cm	Bloch (1964)
	13 cm	Bloch *et al.* (1962)
	9–14.5 cm;	Ikonen and Niemi (1966)
	11 and 28 cm	Acevedo *et al.* (1963)
Rat	13.5–21.5 days[b]	Noumura *et al.* (1966)
	19.5 days	Bloch (1967)
Guinea-pig	3–4, 10 and 12 cm	Bloch (1967)
Rabbit embryo[b]	15–28 days	Lipsett and Tullner (1965)
Armadillo	10–11 cm	Bloch (1967)

[a]Indicates fetal length (crown–rump); [b]gestation age

TABLE 3.6. *Appearance of Androgen-forming Enzymes in Testes of Different Species, Based on Conversion of Pregnenolone or Progesterone to Testosterone or 4-Androstene-3,17-dione*

Species	Age	Reference
Human	3–7.5 months	Acevedo *et al.* (1961; 1963)
		Bloch *et al.* (1962)
Dog	Late gestation	Bloch (1966)
Mouse	14.5 days	Bloch *et al.* (1971; 1974)
Rat	13.5 days	Noumura *et al.* (1966)
	19.5 days	Bloch *et al.* (1974)
Rabbit	18 days	Lipsett and Tullner (1965)
Guinea-pig	Mid-gestation	Bloch (1966)
Armadillo	Late gestation	Bloch and Benirschke (1965)

TABLE 3.7. *Endogenous Neutral Steroids in Fetal Human Testes*

Steriod	Concentration (μg/100 g wet tissue)
3β-Hydroxy-5-pregnen-20-one	180
3β-Hydroxy-5-pregnen-20-one sulfate	24
5-Pregnene-3β,20α-diol (monosulfate)	22
Testosterone	170
4-Androstene-3,17-dione	18
3β-Hydroxy-5-androsten-17-one sulfate	45
3β,16α-Dihydroxy-5-androstene-17-one sulfate	66

After Huhtaniemi *et al.* (1970)

The onset of androgen secretion in the fetus is accompanied by alteration in the configuration and amount of cytoplasmic membranes which occur in sex-dependent tissues (Flickinger, 1974). Testicular tissue contains, in addition to testosterone, other C-21 and C-19 steroids. Huhtaniemi *et al.* (1970) and Huhtaniemi (1977) studied the endogenous hormone concentration in human fetal testes (12–24 weeks gestational age) and found testosterone, pregnenolone and other compounds (Table 3.7; see also Volume I, Chapter 2).

Androgen biosynthesis is altered in gonads of intersex individuals and freemartins (Bottiglioni *et al.*, 1971; Shore and Shemesh, 1981; Hunter *et al.*, 1982).

The pituitary provides the stimulus in most mammals (see Section 3.3 below). In the human, fetal kidneys also have the ability to synthesize chorionic gonadotropin (CG) in appreciable amounts (about one-half the amount of the placenta) (McGregor *et al.*, 1983). The sex of the fetus has no influence on the amount of CG produced by the placenta (Wide and Hobson, 1974; Hobson and Wide, 1975).

3.2.2. MÜLLERIAN-INHIBITING SUBSTANCE (MIS)

The presence of a substance which induces regression of the Müllerian ducts in male fetuses has been postulated by Jost (Jost, 1947; 1953). The substance has been named also anti-Müllerian hormone, Müllerian inhibitor, Jost's factor X and Müllerian-inhibiting factor. An assay to measure the activity of the substance based on *in vitro* organ culture was described by Donahoe *et al.* (1977) and Koike and Jost (1982). Vigier *et al.* (1982) developed a radioimmunoassay (RIA) and Necklaws *et al.* (1986) reported a solid phase sandwich RIA. A purification procedure based on the affinity of the glycoprotein to lectins was described by Picard and Josso (1980). The presence of MIS has been also reported in birds (Hutson *et al.*, 1981; Hutson and Donahoe, 1983).

MIS is a polypeptide, produced both by testes and ovaries during fetal life, and also post-natally. In rat testis MIS persists for 20 days after birth (Donahoe *et al.*, 1976) and in humans approximately two years after birth (Donahoe *et al.*, 1982). The peptide is not species-specific. Josso (1971; 1972) induced regression of fetal rat Müllerian tissue by MIS of human origin.

MIS is synthesized by seminiferous tubules (Josso, 1973) and Sertoli cells (Blanchard and Josso, 1974; Donahoe *et al.*, 1977; Picard *et al.*, 1978; Tran and Josso, 1982; Hayashi *et al.*, 1984). Germ cells do not make the hormone; MIS is present in human fetal testicular tissue deprived of germ cells by irradiation (Josso, 1974). The prenatal ovary lacks the ability to synthesize the substance but acquires the ability post-natally (Ueno *et al.*, 1989).

The concentration of MIS in bovine fetal serum was reported by Vigier *et al.* (1982). The group found the highest concentration between days 100 and 120 of fetal life, 30–35 mU/ml. The concentration declined to about 10 mU at birth (day 280). One unit was defined as the amount released by 1 g of fetal bovine testicular tissue incubated under standard conditions.

The hormone is a glycoprotein (Picard *et al.*, 1978). The sugar content is 8.3%; mannose represents 0.7%, galactose 1.3% and amino sugars the rest (glucosamine 2.8%, galactosamine 0.9%, and *N*-acetylneuraminic acid 2.6%). Budzik *et al.* (1982) speculated that the hormone may exert its activity by depleting Müllerian cells of zinc.

The inhibitor acts by blocking phosphorylation of tyrosine on membrane proteins, specifically the autophosphorylation of the epidermal growth factor (Donahoe *et al.*, 1987).

3.2.2.1. Control of MIS Secretion

Gonadotropin releasing factor injected into pregnant rats increases MIS production, whereas FSH injected postnatally lowers the biosynthesis. Follicle stimulating hormone controls indirectly the production of MIS in fetal rats (Bercu *et al.*, 1979) and guinea pigs (Zaaijer *et al.*, 1985) by stimulating the activity of Sertoli cells.

3.2.3. ESTROGENS

During the normal course of sexual development estrogens do not play any significant role. The ovary has the enzymatic capacity to produce estrogens from radiolabeled androgens *in vitro* (Milewich *et al.*, 1977) and *de novo* from cholesterol (George *et al.*, 1979). The lack of production is due to the absence of LH/hCG receptors (George *et al.*, 1979). See also Chapter 2. Given in pharmacological amounts estrogens provoke teratological changes (Section 5 below).

3.3. The Hypothalamus–Pituitary Axis

Throughout gestation the placenta is impermeable to most hormones (Josimovich, 1974; see Volume I, Chapter 4). The fetus is endocrinologically independent of the maternal environment and fetal hormones regulate the function of fetal endocrine glands and influence the endocrine milieu of the mother. The hormones secreted by the fetoplacental unit into maternal circulation control the physiological changes which take place during pregnancy. Only in diseases does the maternal endocrine system influence the fetus (see Volume I, Chapter 1, p. 56).

Fetal secretion of tropic hormones is governed by the embryonic hypothalamus but not in all cases. There is evidence to show that thyrotropin secretion is independent of both fetal and maternal brain function (Tanooka and Greer, 1978; see Section 4.2 below).

From the limited information available, it would appear that the capacity of the fetal brain to produce gonadotropin-releasing hormone develops prior to the capacity of the pituitary gland to respond, but many basic questions still remain unanswered. What cell types are responsible for the synthesis of hypophysiotropic hormones? What other types of input do they have in terms of control of hormone synthesis and release? To answer these questions is almost beyond the scope of present-day techniques; adequate micromethods must be developed to distinguish the peptide hormones which are present in minute quantities in a milieu that contains a large number of amino acids and peptides. The role of metals, such as calcium, in hormone release and intracellular transport and storage mechanisms in the fetus is only poorly understood.

If hormones and neurotransmitters are present in nonphysiological concentrations during fetal life, or shortly thereafter, they can act as teratogens leading to permanent functional disturbances of reproduction or metabolism (see Section 5 below).

For a full discussion of hormone concentrations in the maternal, placental and fetal compartments see Volume I, Chapter 3.

3.3.1. NEUROENDOCRINE FUNCTIONS

Adequate fetal neuroendocrine function is essential to stimulate the biosynthesis of androgens by the fetal testes and to induce (in some species) parturition by stimulating adrenal function (see Section 4.1 below).

The critical role of an intact hypothalamo–pituitary relationship was shown by Jost in 1947 who demonstrated that the removal of the pituitary gland, or fetal decapitation, in rabbits, led invariably to the formation of the female genitalia. Jost related the development to the lack of androgen production by fetal testis. Others confirmed the findings in different species, including primates. For example, removal of the maternal pituitary of pregnant rhesus monkeys has only a marginal effect on fetal organ weights (adrenals, thyroid, gonads) in males whereas ablation of the fetal gland results in marked decrease in weight of these organs (Gulyas *et al.*, 1977; Jaffe *et al.*, 1981).

3.3.1.1. Gonadotropin-Releasing Hormone

Gonadotropin-releasing hormone is produced both by the fetal brain and the placenta (Khodr and Siler-Khodr, 1980). An excessive production (or exogenous source) may lead to a down-regulation of GnRH receptors in Leydig cells (Dufau *et al.*, 1984). See Chapter 2 for a full discussion.

In the human fetus immunoreactive neurons to GnRH appear in the hypothalamic area at the age of 13 weeks scattered in the mediobasal, premamillary and anterior hypothalamus areas. The ending of the fibers lies close to the mantelplexus vessels, the only vessels present at this period (Bugnon *et al.*, 1977). The hypothalamus-vascular system is present in fetuses 11.5–17 weeks old (Thiveris and Currie, 1980). Similar observations on the development of the hypothalamic neurons have been made in other primate species (Barry, 1976).

In humans the hypothalamus produces GnRH early in life. Winters and co-workers (1974a) were able to detect immunoreactive GnRH in 4.5-week-old embryos while Aksel and Tyrey (1977) failed to detect GnRH in hypothalamic and corticol tissue in 5-week-old fetuses; immunoreactive hormone was present at 6 weeks. As the age of the fetus progressed from 16 to 20 weeks GnRH concentration in the hypothalamus increased from 1.2 to 29.3 pg/mg of wet tissue. No sex differences were detected. Aksel and Tyrey (1977) found no immunoreactive GnRH in the hypothalamus and thalamus at 5 weeks; the hormone was detectable in 6-week-old fetuses in the whole brain. The concentration in the hypothalamus rose with age; it was only 1.2 pg/mg at 16 weeks but 29 pg/mg 4 weeks later. Significant amounts were present in the thalamus $(8.5 \pm 0.19 \text{ pg/mg})$ and trace amounts in the cerebrum at 20 weeks. Clements *et al.* (1980) found an average of 280 pg in the whole hypothalamus of female, and 400 pg in male fetuses at 8–10 weeks. The difference was not statistically significant. The concentration was 4700 ± 640 pg ($\pm$ SD) in both sexes at 14–17 weeks.

In sheep fetus, GnRH is detectable 55 days post-coitum; there is no difference between males and females (Foster *et al.*, 1972a,b).

In the guinea-pig, GnRH appears first in 28-day-old embryos (but not earlier) and coincides with the appearance of LH in the pituitary (Schwanzel-Fukuda *et al.*, 1981).

In rats, GnRH can be detected as early as day 15, several days before gonadotropins become measurable (Chiappa and Fink, 1977).

3.3.1.2. Pituitary Gonadotropins

The pituitary forms early. In the human evaginated pituitary primordium appears in 4-week-old embryos and the telenephalon and diencephalon at 5 weeks. The cells proliferate, capillaries begin to form, and by week 9 the median eminence becomes distinguishable (Hyyppa, 1972). A fully developed hypothalamic vascular system is found in fetuses 11.5–16 weeks old (Pierson *et al.*, 1973; Thiveris and Currie, 1980).

In some rodents (mouse, rat) a mature system develops only post-natally (Table 3.8).

The identification of peptide-secreting cells (Pearse and Takor, 1976) suggests that the progenitors of hormone-secreting cells originate in the ventral neural ridges of the primitive neural tube, which gives rise also to the diencephalon. In their view, the whole gland originates from neural tissue, a deviation from the classical view which holds that the anterior pituitary results from the epithelial evagination of Rathke's pouch.

TABLE 3.8. *Development of the Hypothalamic-Hypophyseal Portal Vascular System in Several Species*

Species	Gestation length, days	Age at which developed[a]		
		Primary Plexus[b]	Portal vessels	Mature system
Mouse	19–20	1–5 pn[c]	16	28 pn
Rat	21–22	5 pn	21–22	40 pn
Rabbit	30–32	70–22	21	
Guinea-pig	65–70	40	40	50
Man	*c.* 280		Functional system by day	80

[a]Gestation days at which observed; [b]invasion of capillary loops into the median eminence; [c]pn, post-natal day
Adapted from Gluckman *et al.* (1981).

Release of gonadotropins from fetal pituitary cell cultured *in vitro* in response to stimulatory effects of the releasing hormone has been demonstrated by several groups (Groom *et al.*, 1971; Siler *et al.*, 1972; Siler-Khodr *et al.*, 1974; Groom and Boyns, 1973; Tamura *et al.*, 1973; Pasteels *et al.*, 1974; 1977; Goodyer *et al.* (1977). Gitlin and Biasucci (1969a,b) and Chowdhury and Steinberger (1975) noted incorporation of ^{14}C-labeled amino acids into both FSH and LH. The literature prior to 1975 has been reviewed by Kaplan *et al.* (1976a). An accurate assessment of gonadotropin secretion *in vitro* is difficult because of the large production of free α-subunits by cultured gonadotropins (Franchimont and Pasteels, 1972). The ability of human fetal pituitaries (in organ or in monolayer cultures) to respond to a GnRH stimulus has been also reported by Goodyer *et al.* (1977) who noted that the capacity increased with gestational age.

Cell cultures, originating from 5-week-old human embryos (Siler-Khodr *et al.*, 1979) or 12-day-old rat fetuses (Begeot *et al.*, 1979), grown only in the presence of fetal serum, have the ability to release stimulatory hormones (ACTH, GH, LH, PRL, TSH) into the medium. The observation may suggest that the pituitary possesses a partial potential for differentiation and secretion in the absence of hypothalamic influence.

It is not clear at present whether the gland can respond to the stimulation also *in vivo*. The catheterization of the stalk vessel in young fetuses is difficult, and measurements do not provide information on whether the release is pulsatile, or not. In later pregnancy, after sexual differentiation, the patterns are easier to establish. In the sheep the release of both hormones is pulsatile (Clark *et al.*, 1984).

In the adult, other major regulators of gonadotropin synthesis and secretion include catecholamines, α- and β-adrenergic agents and opioids. The contribution of these agents to the regulation of fetal hypothalamic-pituitary function is not known.

(a) *Humans*

The gland develops the capability to elaborate the various hormones at different times. In the human fetus the first cells which appear at 7 weeks are probably corticotrophin-containing cells. Gonadotropins become distinguishable about three weeks later (Baker and Jaffe, 1975). Scattered LH and FSH immunoreactive gonadotropins appear already in 8-week-old embryos but only α-subunits of the two hormones can be identified (Pasteels *et al.*, 1974; Dubois and Dubois, 1974; Bugnon *et al.*, 1977). β-Subunits (imparting biological activity) appear from week 15 onwards. Hagen and McNeilly (1975) failed to detect any β-subunits prior to week 16. Kaplan *et al.* (1976b) detected higher concentrations of α-LH and intact LH, in the pituitary of female fetuses than in males. The ratio α/β subunit reached the adult ratio at term. In contrast the pituitary of an anencephalic fetus contained predominantly only the α-subunits (Hagen and McNeilly, 1977). Consequently, the hypothalamus is needed for the secretion of both subunits; in the anencephalic fetus the pituitary secretes only the α-chain.

The same gonadotropins bind an immune serum specific for LH, and for FSH indicating that both hormones are secreted by the same cells but FSH secretion may precede LH secretion by several weeks. In 20-week-old human fetuses there is a sudden increase in both LH and FSH pituitary content (Levina, 1968; Reyes *et al.*, 1974).

Both chorionic gonadotropin and fetal LH may control fetal Leydig cell function. Clements *et al.* (1976) found CG concentrations much higher during weeks 11–17 (when testosterone concentrations are high during sexual differentiation) than the concentrations of LH. Levina (1972) and Siler-Khodr and Khodr (1980) believe that pituitary LH (and FSH) provide the main stimulation.

Peak production in male embryos of both gonadotropins coincides with the production of testosterone but the concentrations of FSH are lower than in females (Winter, 1982).

(b) *Other Species*

The emergence of pituitary function—appearance of LH and FSH in fetal circulation—has been measured in rhesus monkeys (Ellinwood and Resko, 1980); sheep (Foster *et al.*, 1972a,b; Sklar *et al.*, 1981); pigs (Elsaesser *et al.*, 1976; Colenbrander *et al.*, 1977; 1982); rats (Slob *et al.*, 1980; Picon and Habert, 1981) and mice (Pointis and Mahoudeau, 1976). The pituitary of ovine (Folster *et al.*, 1972a), bovine (Kiser *et al.*, 1975) and monkey (Tseng, 1977) fetuses will respond to an infusion of GnRH by releasing LH into blood. The technical problems during fetal studies are considerable; this is often reflected in high variations (SE often approaching the means).

(i) RHESUS MONKEY (GESTATION ABOUT 175 DAYS)

The pituitary of fetuses near term (150–159 days) responds to an infusion of synthetic GnRH (80 μg) by depletion of the secretory granules (Tseng, 1977), increase of blood LH (and testosterone in males) concentration, but not of estradiol (Norman and Spies, 1979).

(ii) PIGS (GESTATION 110–115 DAYS)

The pituitary begins to respond during the last third of fetal life (around day 80). Electrochemical stimulation of the hypothalamus is equally effective (Bruhn *et al.*, 1983). Colenbrander *et al.* (1977) detected LH (1.4–1.7 ng/ml plasma) 110 days post-coitum.

(iii) SHEEP (GESTATION ABOUT 148 DAYS)

The pituitary begins to respond to GnRH stimulation about day 80 of fetal life. The response increases with gestational age and is greatest between days 115–132 (Mueller *et al.*, 1981), Sklar *et al.* (1981) reported endogenous LH and FSH detectable in 59–64-day-old fetuses, highest between days 71–90 and low near term. Higher amounts of LH are found in females (3.2 $\pm$ 1.2 ng/ml before day 90) than in males (0.6 $\pm$ 0.1 ng/ml).

LH is released in pulsatile pattern. The impulse interval is about 2.4 h with a peak amplitude ranging from 1.2 to 11.5 ng/ml (Clark *et al.*, 1984).

(iv) RATS (GESTATION 21–22 DAYS)

In rats, the epithelial cells of Rathke's pouch in culture begin to differentiate in the presence of brain extracts, on days 11–13 (Ishikawa *et al.*, 1977). Magre and Dupouy (1973) and Dupouy and Magre (1973) performed detailed cytochemical evaluation of pituitaries obtained from 20-day-old fetuses. Sétaló and Nakane (1976) and Begeot *et al.* (1981) agreed that LH synthesis appears on day 17. Daikoku *et al.* (1980) used encephalectomy and immunohistochemical staining with an anti-GnRH serum from day 17.5 onwards and established that the hypothalamus begins to influence the pituitary gland only near term on day 20.5.

Between days 17–19, the pituitary functions autonomously. After this period hypothalamic control is essential for the development (Cohen *et al.*, 1971). Fetal decapitation causes a significant retardation in the increase of Leydig cell volume (Eguchi *et al.*, 1975). Ishikawa *et al.* (1977) observed that epithelial cells derived from Rathke's pouch of 11–13-day-old fetuses needed the presence of a brain factor to differentiate.

Orth (1984) demonstrated that FSH is needed to stimulate the expansion of Sertoli cells.

(v) MICE (GESTATION 19–20 DAYS)

Plasma concentrations of LH remain below detection levels until day 16 of gestation. The hormone can be detected in the pituitary gland as early as day 14 when testosterone is present in blood in measurable quantities (Pointis *et al.*, 1980).

(vi) GUINEA-PIG (GESTATION LENGTH 65–70 DAYS)

LH-producing cells can be detected in 29-day-old embryos; FSH cells appear earlier on day 24. Androgen secretion begins several days earlier, possibly independently of gonadotropic stimulation (Zaaijer *et al.*, 1985). Testis cell culture, obtained from 30-day-old fetuses, can be stimulated to produce androgens. Cells obtained from younger fetuses (25–29 days) do not respond (Brinkmann and van Straalen, 1979).

(vii) RABBIT (GESTATION LENGTH 30–32 DAYS)

Pituitaries obtained from 19- or 20-day-old (but not 18-day-old) male or female fetuses are capable of stimulating testosterone (and 5α-dihydrotestosterone) synthesis *in vitro* (Veyssière *et al.*, 1980a). The period is prior to the beginning of male sexual differentiation.

Immunoreactive LH can be detected in the pituitary on day 19, and in plasma one day later. FSH appears in the blood of females on day 27, and is absent in the plasma of males during gestation (Veyssière *et al.*, 1982b).

3.3.1.3. Prolactin

In adult humans, prolactin release is controlled by an inhibiting factor of the hypothalamus and blood concentration may increase under stress (Jaffe *et al.*, 1973; Euker *et al.*, 1975).

In primates (human, rhesus monkey) and sheep the pattern of PRL secretion during fetal life is similar. The concentration rises in late pregnancy in all three species. In humans, the hormone can be detected in several fetal tissues (pituitary and plasma); the highest concentration is in the amniotic fluid (see Volume I, Chapter 3). In the human fetus the hypothalamus exerts an inhibitory influence on prolactin release after 16 weeks (McNeilly *et al.*, 1977) but the full control of prolactin release is not understood.

In rodents prolactin appears first on the last day of gestation, or during the first day of post-natal life but the concentration remains low until the third week of life (see Volume I, Chapter 3).

In humans, and possibly other species, the hormone regulates water permeability across the amnion (Tyson and Pinto, 1978; Leontic *et al.*, 1979).

(a) *Human*

Human fetal pituitary begins to secrete PRI (*in vitro*) at the age of 12 weeks (Pasteels *et al.*, 1963). Minute amounts of the hormone can be found in some embryos by the age of 10 weeks; at term the concentration reaches 2000 ng/gland (Kaplan *et al.*, 1976a). There is no sex difference in the amounts present (Aubert *et al.*, 1975a,b). The concentration in fetal blood rises from about 5 ng/ml (week 10), to around 20 ng/ml in 20-week-old fetuses and 200 ng/ml in 34-week-old fetus and reaches almost 300 ng/ml at term. Thus the rise begins during the last 40% of fetal development (see Volume I, Chapter 3 for references).

(b) *Sheep*

In sheep, PRI concentration in fetal blood is low during most of gestation (Mueller *et al.*, 1979). It begins to rise only during the last 20% of gestational age. The synthesis of the hormone precedes the appearance in blood by several weeks (Leisti *et al.*, 1982).

The release is inhibited by dopaminergic nervous pathways (Gluckman *et al.*, 1979b; 1980a,b). In late gestation (day 105) the response is modulated by estrogens; infusion of estradiol into fetal circulation is followed by a rise of PRI in peripheral blood (Gluckman *et al.*, 1979a; 1983).

(c) *Rat*

In rats the hormone becomes detectable two to three days before parturition but the concentrations are very low (Amendomori *et al.*, 1970; Bast and Melampy, 1972; see also Volume I, Chapter 3). The development of prolactin-secreting cells takes place independently of hypothalamic control (Chatelain *et al.*, 1977). The pituitary is poorly sensitive to dopamine but more sensitive to TRH which helps to maintain hormone production (Khorram *et al.*, 1984). During the neonatal period, brain opioids may provide additional modulatory influence (Limonta *et al.*, 1989).

3.3.2. THE FEEDBACK MECHANISM

The pituitary of male fetuses responds to a negative feedback by steroid hormones; the female pituitary is insensitive in this respect. Gonadectomy of male rhesus fetuses near mid-gestation leads to an increase in LH concentration in peripheral blood, from 4.2 ± 1.0 ($\pm$SEM) to $46.3 \pm 7.9 \, \mu g/ml$. In female fetuses the intervention has no apparent effect; the LH concentration was 19.0 ± 2.8 and 22.9 ± 4.0, respectively (Ellinwood *et al.*, 1982).

Addition of estradiol ($0.1 \, \mu g/ml$) to a culture of human pituitary cells inhibited FSH and LH production while prolactin production was increased (Pasteels *et al.*, 1974). Since present-day information pertaining to estrogen concentration in human fetal brain (and the fetuses of other species as well) is poor, the significance of findings from *in vitro* studies can provide at best information of only speculative nature.

In male sheep, a 6-day infusion of estradiol towards the end of gestation (beginning days 105–106) caused a suppression of plasma LH (from $1.2 \pm 0.1 \, ng/ml$ to $0.1 \, ng/ml$) and of FSH from 5.6 to $3.3 \, ng/ml$ (Gluckman *et al.*, 1983). Endogenous opioids may modulate the feedback control in fetal sheep (Cuttler *et al.*, 1985), and rat (Limonta *et al.*, 1989).

Parvizi (1986) states that a catechol estrogen, 2-hydroxyestradiol ($5 \, \mu g$), infused into 105–108-day-old pig fetuses, lowered the concentration of LH in fetal plasma rapidly from 0.82 ± 0.21 (SEM) to $0.21 \pm 0.05 \, \mu g/l$. The concentration of LH in maternal plasma was not affected. The author speculated that the catechol estradiol acted by modifying catecholamine metabolism or neurotransmission.

It has been already stressed that the placenta is almost impermeable to maternal pituitary hormones, and chorionic gonadotropins (Volume I, Chapter 4); it must be assumed that the signals which stimulate gonadal steroidogenesis in the developing fetus arrive from its own hypothalmo-pituitary hormones. We have no knowledge at the present time whether the secretion of brain neurohormones is a function of the developing brain, or whether it is due to change in internal and/or external environment.

4.3.3. METABOLISM OF GONADAL HORMONES IN THE BRAIN

Adult brain is biochemically an active endocrine gland. Enzymes, located in the white matter, are capable of cleaving cholesterol and synthesizing pregnenolone, dehydroepiandrosterone and estrogens. Testosterone and estradiol stimulate and inhibit the release of GnRH, modulate electrical activity of hypothalamic neurons, affect cerebral blood flow, brain oxygen and glucose consumption, and phosphorus, protein and lipid metabolism (see Woodbury and Vernadakis, 1966). In the fetal brain androgens (Matsumoto and Arai, 1981) and estradiol (Uchibori and Kawashima, 1985) modulate the growth of axodendritic shaft and spine synapsis in the hypothalamus.

The *de novo* synthesis of estrogens in fetal brain has been thought by some to be of singular importance in the control of sex functions. To account for the obvious differences between adult male and female sex function it has been proposed that conversion of testosterone into estradiol 'masculinizes' male fetal brain. Reddy *et al.* (1974) stated '... the androgen effect on brain differentiation is via estrogenic metabolites formed at the site in the brain...'. McEwen *et al.* (1977) and Parsons *et al.* (1982) concurred and implicated the ventromedial nucleus as the site of action.

The correctness of the hypothesis is based mainly on the observation of the effect of androgens given shortly after birth to female rats; behavior responses were the end-point used in most studies. Reliance solely on behavior studies can be misleading. The observation by Shapiro *et al.* (1980) is illustrative: this group evaluated the behavior reaction of testicular feminized rats (Tfm) to either testosterone or estradiol. Testicular feminization is a hereditary defect found in humans, cattle, mice, and rats. The Tfm animals have XY cariotype, small undeveloped inguinal testes that secrete suboptimal amounts of testosterone but develop female genotype. The development is due to the absence of androgen receptor molecules in target organs. The authors concluded solely on the basis of injected sex hormones that in Tfm rats '... the testes are a source of testosterone that is subsequently aromatized to estrogens in the brain...'. Another argument against depending solely on behavior observations are the studies by Ciaccio who showed that untreated, castrated male rodents (hamsters) will respond as male or females, depending upon the manner in which testosterone, or estradiol, is supplied. (See Kincl, 1989 for a more complete discussion of this problem.)

The aromatization hypothesis explains some, but not all, of the experimental evidence. The evidence in favor is:

1. only androgens which can aromatize (i.e. those possessing 4-ene-3-keto moiety) are capable of inducing masculine behavior in females;
2. dihydrotestosterone (and derivatives) are not active this respect.

Unexplained by the hypothesis remain the following observations:

a. not all aromatizable androgens provoke the same response;
b. androstenedione permits somatic and genital development of males but does not block the evolution of feminine behavioral traits;
c. estrogens of maternal origin persist in newborn rats for several days without affecting behavioral development (Friend, 1977);
d. the metabolic yield of estrogens from androgens in the brain is low (less than 1%) (Naftolin *et al.*, 1972). Testosterone is present both in male and female rat fetuses. Maximal concentration in males reaches 2200 pg/ml and in females 1300 pg/ml (Weisz and Ward, 1980). Conversion of the difference (900 pg) would therefore provide an additional 9–10 pg of estrogen in the CNS of male embryos. It has not been established whether this difference would influence brain 'differentiation' towards 'maleness'.

Aromatase activity in fetal rat brain has been studied by George and Ojeda (1982). The authors found peak activity in hypothalamic tissue between days 18–20 of fetal life but apparently there was no contrast between sexes. Further, in 1-day-old rats, androstenedione concentration in blood was similar in males (0.24 ng/ml) and females (0.18 ng/ml) whereas there was significant disparity in the concentration of testosterone (1.08 ng/ml, and 0.06 ng/ml, respectively). The authors speculated that estradiol '... must be the major estrogen formed in the brain...' but provided no evidence to support the claim.

Formation of 5α-dihydrotestosterone in human fetal brain was described by Jenkins and Hall (1977) and Saitoh *et al.* (1982).

4. The Role of Other Endocrine Glands

The development of other endocrine systems is essential for the growth and maturation of the fetus (Hurley *et al.*, 1977). This section describes changes and development of other endocrine systems only insofar as such systems may have bearing on the development of reproductive functions. The time at which different tropic hormones appear in the human fetus is shown in Table 3.9. Their development varies from species to species and they are the overall function of growth (Table 3.10).

A detailed discussion of glucose, mineral and water metabolism is beyond the scope of this monograph.

TABLE 3.9. *Appearance of Various Hormones in the Pituitary and Blood of Human Fetuses*

	First detectable (weeks of fetal life)	
Hormone	Pituitary cells	Blood
ACTH	7	–
β-Lipotropin	8	–
β-Endorphin	8	–
GH	10.5	11
FSH	10	11–12
LH	10.5	11–12
PRL	10	10
TSH	12–13	–
MSH	14	–

Compiled from references cited in text.

TABLE 3.10. *Functional Development of Different Endocrine Systems in the Human, Sheep and Rat Fetuses. (The Time of Gestation at which an Endocrine Function First Appears has been Indicated as a Ratio of Total Gestation)*

	Time of first appearance		
Endocrine system	Human	Sheep	Rat
Hypothalamo-pituitary axis			
Growth hormone	0.25	0.6	–
ACTH	–	0.39	–
TSH	0.36	–	0.86
Thyroid	0.36	0.47	0.82
Adrenals	0.25	0.27	0.73

Compiled from references cited in text.

4.1. The Pituitary–Adrenal Axis

Adequate adrenal function in the fetus is of paramount importance. Glucocorticoids secreted by embryonic adrenals affect the maturation of a variety of enzyme systems including the liver (and thus influence the metabolism of sex hormones), the pancreas and the gastrointestinal tract; they influence the maturation of surfactants in lungs, and in several species (sheep, rats) fetal adrenals are involved in the initiation of parturition.

Placental transfer of cortical hormones and the interconversion of cortisol and cortisone, an important step in the control of fetal glucocorticoid activity, were discussed in Volume I, Chapter 4.

4.1.1. NEUROHORMONES

In rats, removal of the hypothalamus in 19-day-old fetuses leads to adrenal atrophy (Jost, 1966). The hypothalamus of 20-day-old fetuses contains corticotrophin-releasing factor (CRF) activity; the pituitary is responsive to its stimulating influence (Dupouy, 1975). Cortisol inhibits ACTH release induced by CRF (Dupouy, 1971; Dupouy, 1976).

4.1.2. ACTH AND RELATED PEPTIDES

Adrenocorticotropic hormone (ACTH) and melanocyte stimulating hormone (MSH) are the two principal hormone regulating fetal adrenal functions. Studies in human (anencephalic) and rat (decapitated) fetuses have shown that MSH also contributes to the control of fetal growth (Swaab et al., 1977).

4.1.2.1. Humans

The development of pituitary–adrenal systems takes place early in the human. Corticotrophin-containing cells appear at 7 weeks, melanotrophs at 14 weeks, gonadotrophs at 11, and thyrotrophs at 13 weeks (Baker and Jaffe, 1975). Substances exhibiting ACTH and MSH-like activity in human fetal pituitary are found from week 12 onwards; the same substances also appear in human blood and urine during pregnancy (Sulman, 1956).

Brubaker et al. (1982) separated ACTH, αMSH, and a third corticotrophic factor, not identical either to ACTH, MSH, or β-endorphin. All three hormones stimulated the synthesis of dehydroepiandrosterone and cortisol in adrenal cells obtained from 15–19-week-old fetuses. The maturation of the hypothalamo–pituitary axis at about week 20 of age is reflected in increased ACTH pituitary content (Pavlova et al., 1968).

Silman et al. (1977) studied human fetal pituitary content from weeks 12 to 38 of gestation and found αMSH (the designation α- and β- signifies hormones of different molecular weight; see the Appendix in Volume I for further information), and a corticotrophin-like intermediate lobe peptide (CLIP) rather than ACTH. The group advanced the hypothesis that these two peptides are the tropic hormones for the fetal zone of the adrenal gland. Winters et al. (1974b) detected about 250 pg/ml of ACTH in plasma of human fetuses at the end of the first trimester and about 120 pg/ml at term (see Volume I, Chapter 3 for more data).

4.1.2.2. Rodents

In rodents (rats) adrenal growth becomes pituitary-dependent late in gestation (days 17–20 of fetal life). Decapitation of the fetus *in utero* or ACTH administration prior to this time exerts no effect on adrenal histology, lipid distribution or ascorbic acid content of the glands (Cohen, 1963).

Cytodifferentiation of the corticotroph and melanotroph cells in the pituitary occurs independently of the influence of the hypothalamus (Chatelain *et al.*, 1976, 1979). The first ACTH cells appear in 17-day-old fetuses in the pars distalis. βMSH cells have been detected on day 15 in the anterior pituitary, and on day 17 in the intermediate lobe; αMSH appears on day 18 in the intermediate lobe (Dupouy and Dubois, 1975).

Shaha *et al.* (1984) investigated the appearance of immunoreactive β-endorphin cells (physicochemically similar to propiomelanocortin) in Leydig cells of fetal mice and hamsters.

4.1.2.3. Sheep

In sheep, adequate adrenal function is essential to initiate parturition (see Section 4.1.3 below). Both ACTH and αMSH are capable of stimulating the synthesis of adrenocortical hormones Llanos *et al.* (1979). However, Silman *et al.* (1979) were unable to detect the presence of any αMSH in fetal sheep pituitary near term.

4.1.3. ADRENOCORTICAL HORMONES

The capacity of fetal adrenals to synthesize corticoids (and other steroids) has been shown in *in vitro* experiments; human adrenal slices are able to utilize acetate and other precursors to form cortisol (Bloch and Benirschke, 1959; Villee *et al.*, 1959). Adrenals of other species (sheep) are likewise capable of corticoid biosynthesis *in vitro* (Davies and Ryan, 1973; Madill and Bassett, 1973).

The fetus acquires early in life the potential of corticosteroid biosynthesis but the sensitivity of the adrenals to ACTH needs to mature. Since the placenta is not permeable to ACTH (Genazzani *et al.*, 1975) the signal must originate in the fetus and indeed fetal hypophysectomy results in a decrease in cortisol production (Challis *et al.*, 1977a; 1985).

4.1.3.1. Humans

Huhtaniemi (1977) assayed adrenals obtained from 12–20-week-old human fetuses and detected 17α-hydroxylated C-21 steroids (and also C-19 steroids) but not cortisol. Most of the *de novo* synthesis of cholesterol takes place in the fetal zone (Carr *et al.*, 1982). The zone occupies about 80% of the adrenals in the fetus and atrophies after birth. The synthesis of other steroid hormones develops between weeks 25–32 of pregnancy (see Volume I, Chapter 2).

Near term the primate (rhesus monkey) fetal adrenals have steroidogenic capacity to produce cortisol, progesterone, estradiol and estrone in sufficient quantities to maintain fetal, as well as maternal, plasma concentrations (see Volume I, Chapter 3). In rhesus monkeys, ACTH, but not PRL, HG, or αMSH is an important regulator of adrenal function (Walsh *et al.*, 1979).

4.1.3.2. Rodents

Adrenal activity of rat adrenals is low prior to parturition (see above) and diurnal activity is absent during fetal life (Dupouy and Cohen, 1975). The function of the pituitary, and of the hypothalamus, is blocked by pharmacological doses of cortical hormones (Dupouy, 1974). The increase in maternal corticosterone (the main adrenal steroid in rats) production also depresses fetal ACTH production (D'Angelo *et al.*, 1973). The temporary unresponsiveness may protect the neonate adrenal against stress associated with parturition.

In rabbits the production of adrenocortical hormones is highest after birth (Hirose, 1977).

4.1.3.3. Sheep

In fetal sheep, the secretion of corticoids (Wintour *et al.*, 1975) in response to a fixed amount of ACTH increases with gestational age indicating a 'maturation' of 11β-, and 17α-hydroxylase activity (Anderson *et al.*, 1972). The change parallels the increase in fetal adrenal weight and corticosteroid concentration in fetal plasma (Bassett and Thorburn, 1973). ACTH stimulates steroid production in adrenal glands of 40-day-old fetuses (Wintour *et al.*, 1975). Adrenal cells isolated from 120-day-old fetus, stimulated by ACTH, possess the capacity to synthesize a variety of 11-, 17-, and 21-oxygenated pregnane derivatives (Durand *et al.*, 1982).

Most significant changes take place near term. There is a gradual rise in plasma corticoid concentration (see Volume I, Chapter 3) and the fetal adrenal weight doubles (Comline and Silver, 1961). The increase in cortisol production appears to result from maturational changes in the fetal adrenals and from an increase in pituitary stimulation (Challis *et al.*, 1976, 1977b). In addition to the ACTH, other stimuli may provoke an increase in adrenal output. Close to term prostaglandins (PGE) provoke a rapid three-fold increase in fetal cortisol plasma levels (Challis *et al.*, 1977b).

4.2. The Thyroid Gland

Adequate levels of thyroid hormones in mammalian fetuses are important for the development, differentiation and function of the nervous system (Bakke and Lawrence, 1966; Bakke *et al.*, 1970). Early in gestation thyroid hormones are probably not needed for fetal growth; thyroidectomy of rabbit fetuses does not immediately impair further fetal growth (Geloso *et al.*, 1968). Later during fetal life thyroid fetal deficiency in rodents and monkeys (Pickering, 1968), sheep (Erenberg *et al.*, 1974), man and other species (Geloso, 1961; Brassel and Boyd, 1975) results in a marked retardation of body growth, bone maturation and inhibits cell size growth in heart, lung and brain and delays myelination in the central nervous system. The rise in TSH concentrations in fetal serum and the pituitary gland correlates with the appearance of electrical activity in the brain and the formation of the portal system (Fig. 3.22).

The development of the various endocrine functions varies from species to species and is the function of overall growth (see Table 3.10). The development of the mammalian thyroid was reviewed by Fisher and Dussault (1979).

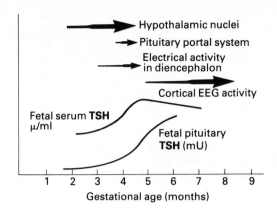

FIG 3.22. Correlation Between Development of the Hypothalamus, the Pituitary
Portal System, Vascular Higher Nervous System Electrical Activity, and Fetal
Pituitary and Fetal Serum TSH Concentrations in the Human Fetus.
As the pituitary portal system develops and the hypothalamus matures histologically
at about 20 weeks of gestation, there is a marked increase in pituitary TSH
concentration and an abrupt increase in serum TSH levels. After Fisher, 1974.

4.2.1. THE CONTROL OF THYROID FUNCTION

As with other hormones, the transport of TRH and TSH from the maternal to the
fetal compartment is severely limited by the placental barrier (see Volume I, Chapter
4) except possibly late in pregnancy; Kajihara *et al.* (1972) noted that rat placenta
becomes quite permeable to TRH (but not to TSH) near term (day 20 of gestation),
yet provided no information pertaining to the secretion of TRH. Transport of thyroid
hormones across the placenta in late pregnancy has also been shown in guinea-pigs,
rabbits, dogs, sheep, monkey and man (see Volume I, Chapter 4).

The autonomy of fetal thyroid function has been demonstrated in many experiments
in sheep (Wallace *et al.*, 1979). Hypophysectomy results in a fall of fetal TSH in plasma
but not on the maternal side (Thorburn and Hopkins, 1973). Administration of TRH
to ewes in doses which result in increases of TSH does not affect the concentration of
the hormone in the fetus (Thomas *et al.*, 1975). Similarly, injection of TRH into the
fetus does not influence maternal TSH plasma levels. Similarly, in rhesus monkeys,
injection of T_3 to the mother does not influence the pituitary response of the fetal
hypophysis to TSH (Melmed *et al.*, 1979). Administration of TRH caused a large
response of TSH in the fetal plasma (Azukizawa *et al.*, 1976).

In humans pituitary thyrotrophs become detectable by week 13 (Baker and Jaffe,
1975) and the thyroid begins to concentrate iodine. The ability increases more than
three-fold at the age of 22 weeks (Table 3.11). At this time the placenta is permeable
to iodine (Evans *et al.*, 1967). The fetal pituitary is capable of responding to TRH
stimulation; a monolayer culture grown from human pituitaries obtained from 10–14-
week-old embryos will respond to TRH (10^{-8} M concentration) by secreting more TSH
into the incubation medium. The effect is specific; TRH has no influence on the release
of PRL, GH, LH or FSH (Goodyer *et al.*, 1977). Immunoassayable TSH in serum
appears at about week 18 (Fisher *et al.*, 1970; Greenberg *et al.*, 1970).

TABLE 3.11. *^{131}I Uptake by the Human Fetal Thyroid Gland.
The Uptake was Studied 18–24 h after Maternal Injection*

Fetal age (weeks)	Mean thyroid weight (mg)	Mean ^{131}I thyroid concentration (% g)
13–15	21	1.6
17–21	109	1.4
22	203	4.6

After Evans *et al.* (1967).

Serum TSH increases rapidly between weeks 18 and 22, and remains stable until term; these changes are independent of changes in maternal thyroid function. The increase in concentration of iodinated thyronines in fetal plasma, serum TSH and the general maturation of the hypothalamo pituitary axis is paralleled by increases in thyroid-binding globulin (TBG) noticeably from about week 15 of pregnancy onwards (Greenberg *et al.*, 1970). The increase is probably influenced by augmented hepatic synthesis of TBG stimulated by enlarged concentrations of estrogens (Engström and Engström, 1959).

It is generally accepted that the thyroid function becomes fully operational by weeks 18–20 of pregnancy, at the time of brain maturation (Fig. 3.22).

In fetal rats encephalectomy on day 18 does not affect the pituitary–thyroid function (Tanooka and Greer, 1978); by day 19 TRH and TSH are present (Conklin *et al.*, 1973). Between this time and parturition there is a 10-fold increase in fetal pituitary TSH content (Florsheim *et al.*, 1966; D'Angelo and Wall, 1971). Administration of relatively high doses (12 μg) to a 21-day-old rat fetus results in histological evidence of thyroid activation (D'Angelo and Wall, 1972).

The metabolism of fetal thyroid is distinct from that of the adult metabolism by the presence of reverse T_3 (3′,5′-tri-iodothyronine) which circulates in high concentration. Probably decreased 5′-iodothyronine, and enhanced 5-iodothyronine deiodinase activities are responsible for elevated serum rT_3 and subnormal T_3 in fetal blood (see Volume I, Chapter 3).

4.3. Other Peptide Hormones

Proper balance of growth hormone, insulin function, water and mineral metabolism is indispensable for fetal growth and hence for the differentiation of sexual apparatus. This section provides an overview of the various hormones. Additional information pertaining to the concentrations can be found in Volume I, Chapter 3.

4.3.1. GROWTH HORMONE

In the adult, a rise in GH secretion may be induced by somatomedins, by infusion of amino acid or by insulin-induced hypoglycemia, and inhibited by glucocorticoids, catecholamines and somatostatin. Infusion of cortical hormones has been shown to inhibit GH secretion in several species (Reichlin, 1974). It may be that similar regulatory mechanisms are also operating in the fetus but the evidence is incomplete.

Human fetal pituitary content of GH reaches mg quantities (Matsukaki *et al.*, 1971), almost 1000 times higher than the concentration of PRL, FSH or LH and fetal plasma concentration is higher than in neonate. The concentration in blood reaches a peak at the end of the second trimester and then declines despite increasing concentrations in the pituitary. Increasing concentration is associated with the development of cerebral activity and hypothalamic secretion and the appearance of functional pituitary portal system (Begeot *et al.*, 1977; 1978a,b) (Fig. 3.23). This suggests a relationship between the inhibitory activity of the brain and falling fetal plasma levels of GH (Grumbach and Kaplan, 1973).

Inhibition of GH function in cell monolayer culture of human fetal pituitary cells by somatostatin (10^{-6}–10^{-9} M) has been reported by Goodyer *et al.* (1977) but the possible role of placental lactogen in respect to growth promotion in the fetus remains obscure.

Destruction of the pituitary in the rhesus monkey results in the disappearance of GH from fetal plasma (Chez *et al.*, 1970a) but hypoglycemia or arginine infusion did not result in an increase of GH plasma levels in nonhypophysectomized fetuses (Mintz *et al.*, 1969).

Growth hormone-dependent tropic substance, stimulating fetal brain proliferation, has been demonstrated in serum of rats (Sara *et al.*, 1976). The nondialyzable, heat-stable material is different from prolactin, placental lactogen, insulin and nerve growth factor.

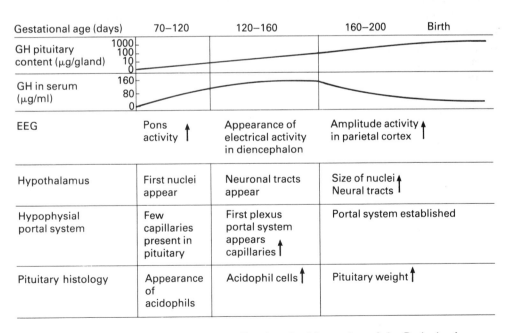

FIG 3.23. Schematic Representation Showing the Maturation of the Brain in the Human Fetus Compared to the Development of Growth Hormone (GH) Secretion Adapted from Grumbach and Kaplan (1973).

Somatostatin receptors are present in the pituitary of ovine fetuses at mid-gestation; its infusion lowers GH concentrations in plasma (Gluckman *et al.*, 1979b).

4.3.3. HORMONES OF THE NEUROHYPOPHYSIS, WATER AND ELECTROLYTE METABOLISM

When interpreting experiments designed to study water and electrolyte balance it must be borne in mind that data from one species cannot be readily applied to another. For example fluid movement in ungulates (sheep) is different from that of primates (human). In sheep, fetal urine gains access to the allantoic sac via the urachus and to the amnion via the urethra. There is no fluid compartment comparable to the allantoic sac in the human. Fetal renal blood flow and glomerular filtration rate are low compared to the adult (Barnes, 1976) but this has been determined in only a few species. Vasopressin will act on fetal kidney (Buddingh *et al.*, 1971) but its action will be the function of the glomerular filtration rate. The renin-angiotensin-aldosterone system may operate in the fetus. From the studies on fetal lamb it appears that all the components of the system are present (see Lee, 1974).

Oxytocin and vasopressin are closely related octapeptides sharing several physiological functions. In terms of fetal physiology the most important appears to be concerned with response to blood loss. In the adult, oxytocin-release stimuli arise in the peripheral areas of the nervous system (vagina, cervix, nipple) and from higher levels of the central nervous system.

Fetal oxytocin plasma concentration in the sheep rises sharply within hours preceding parturition and reaches a peak at delivery. The stimulatory mechanism has as yet to be identified. The rise is unlikely due to hypoxia since during delivery in sheep blood gas tensions fall only during the very terminal phases (Comline and Silver, 1972). The relationship between oxytocin release and adrenal function or prostaglandin release remains to be elucidated. In the human there is no large increase in oxytocin output at the time of delivery (Volume I, Chapter 5). These findings would indicate that '... oxytocin release (in the fetus) may play only a supportive role' (Chard, 1972).

Vasopressin (arginine vasopressin) is rapidly released from fetal lamb pituitary in response to oxygen decrease in the ewe (Alexander *et al.*, 1972) and in response to blood loss (Alexander *et al.*, 1974). Increases in plasma levels are accompanied by renin release (Broughton *et al.*, 1974).

The role of the third important hormone involved in fluid control, aldosterone, remains yet to be elucidated. In the rat increased aldosterone production is associated with depleted sodium stores (increased potassium) in plasma. Similar mechanisms may be a factor in fetal aldosterone production (Schneider and Mulrow, 1973).

4.4. Glucose Metabolism

After birth glucose metabolism is directed by the interrelationship between insulin and glucagon. Growth hormone (GH) acting via intermediates (somatomedins) and adrenal hormones provides additional homeostatic balance. The response of fetal GH to hypoglycemia has been tested by Bassett and Madill (1974) who reported that infusion of glucose into fetus led to lowered plasma GH concentration. Somatostatin, an inhibitor of GH and insulin has been identified immunochemically in the pancreas of

12-week-old human fetuses (Dubois *et al.*, 1975) but no information is available in respect of concentration.

Insulin is the main fetal growth hormone. While the absence of thyroxine, growth hormone, corticoids and sex steroids has little effect on somatic growth (but for disturbances noted above), abnormal insulin production during pregnancy may result in growth alterations. Increased body weight results from hyperinsulinemia (islet tumors), while pancreatic agenesis leads to poor muscle and adipose tissue development (Hill, 1976).

4.4.1. HUMANS

The placenta is probably impermeable to insulin (Volume I, Chapter 4) suggesting an independent fetal homeostasis. Insulin is present in 8–10-week-old human fetal pancreas (Adesanya *et al.*, 1966; Thorell, 1970) and plasma (Adam *et al.*, 1969). Maternal hyperglycemia leads to fetal hyperinsulinism (Obenshain *et al.*, 1969); infants born to diabetic mothers tend to be overweight (Hill, 1976). Injections of glucagon, cyclic AMP and amino acid mixture result in insulin release from beta cells (Adam *et al.*, 1969; King *et al.*, 1971; Milner *et al.*, 1972).

At term, elevated maternal glucose concentration leads to elevated blood glucose (Obenshain *et al.*, 1969).

4.4.2. MONKEYS

In monkeys, direct fetal insulin injection results in hypoglycemia (Chez *et al.*, 1970a). Administration of glucagon results in enhancement of insulin levels (Chez *et al.*, 1970b).

The monkey fetus will respond to injection of glucagon and amino acids by releasing insulin (Mintz *et al.*, 1969).

4.4.3. SHEEP

Infusion of glucose (i.v.) to fetal sheep *in utero* will result in elevation of fetal plasma glucose and insulin concentrations (Alexander *et al.*, 1968, 1969, 1970; Fiser *et al.*, 1974). Insulin response appears correlated with maternal plasma glucose levels and is not potentiated by glucagon (Bassett and Thorburn, 1971) indicating that in this species the cAMP-dependent part of the insulin secretory mechanism is not fully developed.

The concentrations of basic somatomedins (insulin-like growth factors) during gestation were reported by van Vliet *et al.* (1983).

4.4.4. RODENTS

The concentration of insulin begins to increase in fetal rats on about day 15 of gestation. At birth the rise is about 1000-fold greater (Rall *et al.*, 1979). The pancreas responds to an infusion of glucose only close to parturition (21.5 days) but not before (Kervran and Girard, 1974). The development of insulin-, glucagon- and somatostatin-positive cells during the development interval from day 16 post-coitum to 10 days of post-natal life was described by McEvoy and Madson (1980).

4.5. Mineral Metabolism

Almost nothing is known about the function of the parathyroid glands, the concentrations of parathyroid hormone and calcitonin in blood and other tissues and the possible controlling mechanism. Appropriate mineral balance, especially of calcium, is of utmost importance not only for bone calcification, but also muscular and nervous function. The placenta is apparently impermeable to parathyroid hormone and thyrocalcitonin (Wezeman and Reynolds, 1971) which suggests autonomous fetal development independent of maternal milieu. Hopefully with the advent of sensitive assay methods to study tissue concentrations and availability of cell membrane binding sites, these questions will be answered.

5. Teratologic Effects of Steroid Hormones

Exposure of the developing fetus to pharmacological amounts of steroid hormones may bring on fetal death (estrogens), malformations of the genitalia and mammary glands (androgens and estrogens), reduction in body growth, bone formation and the growth of internal organs (adrenocortical hormones) and lead to the development of cancer (estrogens, especially triphenylethylene derivatives). Table 3.12 summarizes the effects.

The literature devoted to the subject is voluminous and a full coverage is outside the scope of this chapter. We only highlight the most important effects on the developing gonads to provide an overview of this important subject. A more detailed review will be found in Kincl (1989) and in Pasqualini and Ojasoo (1991).

TABLE 3.12. *Teratological Effects of Steroid Hormones on the Developing Human Fetus Exposed During the First Trimester*

Hormone	Induced defects
Androgens	Virilization of female fetus
Estrogens	Cardiovascular, termination of pregnancy
Diethylstilbestrol (DES)	Carcinogenesis, uterine and vaginal lesions

5.1. Males

5.1.1. ANDROGENS

Exposure of fish and amphibian larvae to androgens changes all offspring into functional males; estradiol will produce females. In birds treatment of fertile eggs with gonadal hormones induces like changes but only temporarily. After some time, inverted animals will revert to their genetic sex. In mammals, genetic sex determines gonadal sex and exposure of embryos to sex hormones will change only somatic and behavioral sex.

During the undifferentiated stage, two anlage for the development of male (Wolffian) and female (Müllerian) ducts are present in the fetus.

Androgens cause proliferation of the duct in both sexes. Estrogens may cause a partial involution but in general the anlage is insensitive to estrogens (Raynaud, 1942).

The influence of sex hormones on the formation of genital organs was studied in the late 1930s. Mme. Dantchakoff working in Bratislava, and later in Paris, published between 1936 and 1939 a series of observations pertaining to the consequence of exposing guinea-pig fetuses to steroid hormones. A French physiologist, Raynaud (1939a,b; 1942), studied the influence of androgens and estrogens on the organization of sex organs in mice. Deanesly (1939) evaluated the reaction of rabbit embryos to both androgens and estrogens.

During pregnancy estrogens are biosynthesized in ever increasing amounts. The presence of high concentrations of α-fetoprotein may 'protect' the fetus from the deleterious consequences of estrogens circulating in the mother (Vannier and Raynaud, 1975; Payne and Katzenellenbogen, 1979). α-Fetoprotein most likely does not play a major role in other species. The protein is present mainly in rodents (rats) while in many species estradiol does reach the fetus but only as a conjugate, either a glucuronide or a sulfate (see Volume I, Chapters 2 and 3).

In the genetic male rat, Wolffian ducts display a transitory increase in lumen size and diameter when the embryo is 16.5 days old. In females the ducts begin to involute 24 h later. In females, androgens will maintain the ducts if injected before this time and will produce inconsistent changes if injected after involution has begun. The portion still present on day 18 is insensitive to androgens. The presence of androgens on day 15.5 has no effect on the development of the ducts (Stinnakre, 1975). The sensitivity of Wolffian ducts to hormonal influence varies from species to species.

A rapid and reliable method for assessing the effect of steroid hormones in rodents is the measurement of the distance between the anus and the urinary papilla (anogenital distance); the interval is shorter in females and longer in males. Androgenic hormones cause an increase in the distance in females (virilization) whereas estrogens have the opposite effect (feminization). Microscopic examination of the internal genital apparatus is necessary to reveal more significant malformations.

Androgens produce permanent hyperplasia of accessory sex organs. Dantchakoff (1938a) studied the influence of sex hormones in fetal guinea-pigs. She began injecting gravid animals (day 18) with 0.5–1 mg of testosterone propionate (TP), increased the dose to 2 mg five days later and implanted in the newborn 2 mg of the crystalline substance. She found in adolescent animals (31 days old) active spermatogenesis and hypertrophy of the epididymis, seminal vesicles and penis. Slob *et al.* (1973) found marginally increased body growth in male guinea-pigs born to mothers injected daily (from day 24 to 41) with 5 mg of TP. The weight increase was transitory and disappeared during post-natal growth. Brown-Grant and Sherwood (1971) found no aftermath in guinea-pigs born to mothers treated with 12.5 mg TP on days 33, 35 and 37 of gestation. In contrast, females became virilized (see section 2.6.1 above).

Kincl (1989) injected gravid rats daily (day 17–21) with 0.5 mg of TP. At the age of 80 days the males were lighter and sex organs were smaller but there was no evidence of spermatogenesis inhibition. Swanson and van der Werff ten Bosch (1964; 1965) also reported active spermatogenesis in adults exposed *in utero* to androgens.

5.1.2. ANTI-ANDROGENS

In males, compounds which compete with the action of androgens block the development of external genitalia and allow a partial development of the Müllerian ducts but do not prevent the development of Wolffian ducts or the differentiation of the gonads (Jost, 1972a,b). A German group led by Neumann (Neumann and Steinbeck, 1974) explored in rats the action of an anti-androgen (cyproterone acetate). The steroid, injected daily during days 17–20 of gestation, caused in genetic male offspring a shortening of the anogenital distance (the length was similar to that in females), and prevented the development of seminal vesicles and of the penis. The urethra was feminine and the urogenital sinus formed as a female vagina. Wolffian ducts regressed only partially. The development of the vagina in rats is incomplete at birth. To induce full feminine formation, the group treated newborn male offspring, in addition to *in utero* exposure, during the first 10–14 days after birth. Cyproterone acetate also induces in males female-like differentiation of mammary glands.

Goldman *et al.* (1972) generated in rabbits an antibody to testosterone conjugated at C-3 to bovine serum albumin via 3-carboxymethyloxime. Injected into pregnant rats (days 13–20) the antibody blocked in part the effect of testosterone. In genetic males the anogenital distance was shorter and testes were atrophied.

5.1.3. ESTROGENS

Estrogens induce paradoxically virilizing changes. Greene *et al.* (1939c,d; 1940; 1941) found in the male offspring at puberty cryptorchidism, atrophied testes and retained Müllerian ducts. Moore (1939) reported stimulation of Wolffian ducts by estrogens in the opossum of both sexes. Falconi and Rossi (1965) reported inhibition of sex organ formation by estrogens and noted that doses which induced the changes were close to embryotoxic doses. Stinnakre (1972) confirmed the paradoxical retention of Wolffian ducts in animals exposed to high estrogen doses.

A synthetic compound, diethylstilbestrol (DES), is highly toxic. Newbold *et al.* (1982) reported persistence of Müllerian ducts in male offspring born to mothers exposed to DES (100 μg/kg of body weight) between days 9 and 11.

Yasuda *et al.* (1977; 1985) described gonadal dysgenesis in male offspring born to mice dosed orally with ethynyl estradiol (0.01 mg/kg body weight) from days 11 to 17 of gestation. The 3 methyl ester (MEE) causes virilization in rats (Table 3.13).

Vannier and Raynaud (1975; 1980) used graded doses of estradiol (50, 250 and 1250 μg daily, days 16–20) in rats and reported that fetal wastage was dose-related: 66% of embryos died in animals injected with 1250 μg; the loss was 41% in the low dose group. A dose of 50 μg was sufficient to induce a decrease in the anogenital distance. Higher amounts led to greater teratogenic effects. Microscopic examination of fetuses (50 and 250 μg dose) revealed underdevelopment of seminal vesicles and coagulating glands, inhibition of ventral and dorsal prostate buds and epithelial proliferation of urethral walls. Males exposed to the high dose were sterile. In all males prostates were atrophic, penile development depressed (hypospadia) and testes were cryptorchidic.

Raynaud (1942) described in mice the feminization of the genital apparatus and atrophy of gubernacula (Raynaud, 1957; 1958). Injection on day 13 of gestation with 62 or 94 μg of estradiol dipropionate was enough to cause the atrophy.

TABLE 3.13. *Influence of Testosterone Propionate and 17-Ethynyl Estradiol 3-Methyl Ether (MEE) Injected to Female Rats from Day 17 to Day 21 of Pregnancy on the Development of Female Offspring*

Treatment	Daily dose (μg)	Total	With CL	Virilized	Virilization grade (number)	Prostate (mg $\pm$ SE)
0	0	35	24	0	0	0.0 $\pm$ 0.0
Testosterone propionate	500	14	6	13	1(13)[a]	8.8 $\pm$ 1.1
					2(8)[b]	15.0 $\pm$ 3.0
MEE	10	10	6	9	1(6)[a]	0.0 $\pm$ 0.0
					3(1)[b]	0.0 $\pm$ 0.0

[a]Autopsy at 45 days of age; [b]autopsy at 80 days of age; for the description of virilization grade see Table 3.15

Quoted from Kincl, 1989.

The differentiation of the epididymis, arrested by estrogens, can be reversed by concomitant administration of human chorionic gonadotropin (Hadziselimovic and Guggenheim, 1980).

5.2. Females

5.2.1. TESTOSTERONE

In genetic females (rodents, ungulates and primates) androgens prevent the regression of Wolffian ducts (virilization). The animals become sterile if the hormone is injected directly into the fetus to bypass metabolite formation in the mother.

A typical finding in virilized females is an increase in the anogenital distance, the presence of a prostate and more severe morphological changes.

Androgenization of female fetuses was reported in pigs (Elsaesser *et al.*, 1978), dogs (Beach and Kuehn, 1970; Beach 1975), and monkeys (Goy and Phoenix, 1971). In most studies changes in behavior were the end-point used to assess virilization changes. In a later study, Young *et al.* (1964) described the development of a hermaphrodite monkey (a female with well developed phallus). The daily testosterone propionate dose was 25 mg from post-coital day 40, 20 mg from day 51 to 70 and 10 mg from day 71 to 90.

5.2.1.1. Guinea-pigs

Dantchakoff (1936; 1937a,b) injected 0.05 mg directly into 20–23-day-old fetuses and gave a second injection (3 mg) 6–10 days later. The results were severe. Female embryos (45 days old) had, in addition to ovaries, two sets of secretory ducts (oviducts and sperm duct) located in a mid-point between the kidneys and the bladder (as in males), prostate, seminal vesicles and a rudimentary penis. The ovaries of adult

6-week-old females were cystic and contained some maturing follicles with degenerating ova; corpora lutea (CL) were absent (Dantchakoff, 1938a,b).

Phoenix *et al.* (1959), Goy *et al.* (1964) and Young *et al.* (1964) reconfirmed Dantchakoff's result. The reports state that sex organs were masculinized and CL did not form in the ovaries but no details were given. Brown-Grant and Sherwood (1971) used 12.5 mg of TP injected on days 29, 31 and 33 of embryonic life. The treatment induced gross malformations of lower genitalia in female offspring; the urethra opening was at the end of an enlarged phallus and the vaginal opening was absent. Fertility was not influenced. The ovaries appeared normal with old and new CL present.

Slob *et al.* (1973) found no changes in post-natal body growth of females born to does injected with TP (5 mg daily) between days 24 and 41 of gravidity.

5.2.1.2. Rats

Cagnoni *et al.* (1964) injected TP (10 mg) on day 16 and evaluated the effects in 120-day-old offspring. All females (only four survived) became virilized. Kincl (1989) injected graded doses of TP daily between days 15–19 and measured the anogenital distance on day 1, again on day 24 of life, and autopsied the animals when they were 60–80 days old. The degree of virilization was dose-related. A daily dose of 250 μg was sufficient to increase the anogenital distance in the genetic females and to produce more severe malformations. The function of the ovaries was not influenced (Table 3.14).

TABLE 3.14. *Influence of Testosterone Propionate Injected from Day 15 to Day 19 of Gestation on the Development of Female Offspring*

Treatment	Daily dose (μg)	Final body weight (g ± SE)	Anogenital distance mm ± SE		Total no. of pups	No. of abnormal pups[a]	Ventral prostate (mg ± SE)
			Day 1	Day 24			
0	0	63.4 ± 1.4	1.3 ± 0.1	9.75 ± 0.52	16	0	0.0 ± 0.0
Testosterone propionate	250	52.3 ± 2.8	2.7 ± 0.1	10.9 ± 0.4	18	18(1); 13(2); 1(3); 2(4)	9.4 ± 1.4
	750	46.6 ± 5.6	2.5 ± 0.0	14.6 ± 1.0	5	5(2); 5(3)	12.4 ± 1.2
	2250	52.5 ± 6.5	3.0 ± 0.2	14.3 ± 0.9	4	4(3); 4(4)	21.8 ± 4.1

[a]The numbers in parentheses indicate virilization grade found on visual inspection. An individual animal could exhibit one, or several malformations at the same time.
Virilization grades: 1. Vaginal opening at base of urinary papilla; 2. prostate present; 3. common vaginal-urinary opening; 4. blind vagina; autopsied at the age of 24 days.
Quoted from Kincl, 1989.

5.2.1.3. Mice

TP (25 μg and 250 μg) injected into 17-day-old fetuses caused virilization in adults (examined at 5–10 months) of the genitalia, absence of vaginal orifice and irreversible proliferation of the vaginal epithelium. There was no effect on the reproductive capacity. Injection of TP at birth did not masculinize the genitalia but blocked the reproductive capacity. The ovaries of 13/18 animals contained only cystic follicles and no CL (Taguchi *et al.*, 1977).

5.2.1.4. Sheep

Clarke *et al.* (1976; 1977) demonstrated that in sheep genitalia differentiate between days 40 and 50 of fetal life. Implantation of 1 g bolus of testosterone between days 30 and 80 (releasing about 7 mg daily) caused masculinization of the external genitalia. The ewes were born with a penis and an empty scrotal sac. A vaginal opening absent at birth developed slowly. In 10-month-old animals, a small opening became visible in addition to the one present at the tip of the fused labia. Small seminal vesicles and bulbourethral glands were also present. Exposure between days 50 and 100 caused only hypertrophy of the clitoris and restricted vaginal opening. Virilization was less severe in fetuses subjected to the same testosterone dose between days 70–120.

5.2.1.5. Hamsters

In female hamsters the development of the urogenital apparatus is complete after birth. The endodermal sinovaginal cord regresses, a vaginal introitus and a pair of vaginal pouches form during the first few days of post-natal life. Injection of 1 mg or less of testosterone propionate on day 9 of gestation speeds up the development of female sex organs. Injection of TP (5 mg or more) between days 10 and 12 inhibits the down-growth of the vagina which remains short and opens into the urogenital sinus— '... almost complete male type differentiation of the organs derived from urogenital sinus ...' (Brunner and Witschi, 1946). The females remain sterile and no corpora lutea form.

5.2.2. OTHER ANDROGENS

Dihydrotestosterone, the 'active' androgenic hormone in the male (Volume I, Chapter 2), causes virilization. The hormone forms from testosterone in the urogenital sinus and tubercle before sex differentiation (rabbits and rats) and in the Wolffian and Müllerian ducts after the sex has become established. Possibly the former tissues have an inherent enzymatic capacity for the reduction while the sex cords need to be exposed to testosterone before they become capable of a response (Wilson and Lasnitzki, 1971).

Both 5α-DHT and 5α-androstane-3α,17β-diol (5 mg) injected into pregnant guinea-pigs (days 28–36) or 1 mg (days 37–57), are potent enough to virilize female fetuses as the same dose of TP (van der Werff ten Bosch and Goldfoot, 1975). Goldman and Baker (1971) used two doses, 10 mg/kg and 50 mg/kg maternal body weight (or about 2 and 10 mg per pregnant rat), delivered the fetuses by Cesarean section on day 22 and measured the anogenital distance. Androstenedione was an active substance; in genetic females the average distance increased from 1.26 ± 0.10 mm (controls) to 1.70 ± 0.19 mm (low-dose group) and 2.71 ± 0.12 mm (high-dose group). Schultz and Wilson (1974) could not confirm the virilizing properties of androstenedione. DHT was androgenic at a dose of 4 mg; a daily dose of 1 mg produced no effect. Three other steroids (5α-androstane-3α,17β-diol, 17α-methyl testosterone and 17α-methyl DHT) were active (Table 3.15). Elger *et al.* (1970) confirmed the virilizing property of methyl

TABLE 3.15. *Virilizing Potency of Various Androgens (Female Fetuses) when Injected into the Gravid Rat*

Steroid studied	Daily dose (mg)	Injection period[a]	Estimated potency[b]	Reference
5α-DHT	4	14–21		1
	1,10/kg	13–20	~1.2	2
4α-A-3α	4	14–21		1
17β-diol	1,5,10/kg	13–20	1	2
A-dione	10,50/kg	13–20	0.4	2
5α-A-3β	1,10/kg	13–20	~0.2	2
17β-diol				
Androsterone	10/kg	13–20	0.1	2
17-MeT	4	14–21		1
	1,3,10	15–21		3
17-MeDHT	4	14–21		1

[a]Injection period during gestation (days); [b]testosterone = 1; ref. 1, Schultz and Wilson (1974), end-point based on gross examination of sex organs; ref. 2, Goldman and Baker (1971), end-point based on microscopic measurement of anogenital distance; ref. 3, Elger *et al.* (1970), end-point based on microscopic evaluation of sex organs. 5α-DHT = 5α-dihydrotestosterone; 5α-A-3α,17β-diol = 5α-androstane-3α,17β-diol; A-dione = 4-androstene-3,17-dione; 17-MeT = 17α-methyl testosterone; 17-MeDHT = 17α-methyldihydrotestosterone
Quoted from Kincl, 1989.

testosterone. Goldman (1970) found that 100 mg/kg of DHA induced slight clitoral enlargement and increases in the anogenital distance. The sulfate was not active.

5.2.2.1. Influence on Human Babies

A female fetus, and the mother, may become virilized by exposure to an elevated androgen milieu during pregnancy. Increased androgen production can result from abnormal maternal adrenal function (adrenogenital syndrome), arrhenoblastoma, or thecal cell tumor (Murset *et al.*, 1970; Fayez *et al.*, 1974; Verkauf *et al.*, 1977) or if the mother was treated with synthetic progestational agents (see Section 5.3.1 below). Hayles and Nolan (1957; 1958) reported masculinization of a baby girl associated with the use of methyl testosterone during pregnancy.

5.2.3. ANTI-ANDROGENS

Simultaneous administration of anti-androgens blocks the virilizing effects of androgens in the female. Elger *et al.* (1970) injected pregnant rats with methyl testosterone (MT) (1.3 or 10 mg daily) and 30 mg of cyproterone acetate (CA) from days 15 to 21. Microscopic evaluation showed that CA prevented the virilizing consequence of 1 or 3 mg of MT but not of 10 mg. Wolffian ducts regressed in most but not all female fetuses. In some, rudimentary, or even whole, ducts persisted on one side.

5.2.4. ESTROGENS

Exposure of genetic females to estrogens induces teratological changes which persist into adulthood; the vaginal epithelium proliferates abnormally leading to adenosis and ultimately to the development of adenocarcinoma of the vagina and cervix; similar changes may develop in the mammary glands.

5.2.4.1. Estradiol

In mice, the vaginal epithelium is more sensitive to damage than is the reproductive capacity (Kimura, 1975). The reaction is rapid; the mitotic activity recedes within two to three days after exposure. Kimura *et al.* (1980) injected 50 μg of estradiol on day 17 of gestation and found in the offspring irreversible, ovary-independent cornification, or stratification, of the vaginal epithelium. Estradiol had minimal effects on reproductive capacity. When estradiol was injected 2 days earlier (day 15 of gestation) only one of six females had ovaries containing CL at the age of 3–5 months. Injection of the same amount of estradiol after birth (day 3) provoked less severe changes in the vaginal epithelium but blocked the reproductive capacity completely.

The sex cords of rat embryos are sensitive to estrogen exposure in mid-pregnancy. Injection of 0.1 mg of estradiol between days 16 and 19 had no effect on the formation of external genitalia, or the anogenital distance in either sex. Repeated dosing between days 11 and 16 resulted in a shortening of the distance in males and formation of intersexes (Table 3.16).

TABLE 3.16. *Influence of Various Steroids Injected Subcutaneously to Rats from Day 11 of Gestation on the Anogenital Distance of Male and Female Pups Removed by Cesarean Section*

Treatment	Daily dose (mg)	No. of treatment (days)	Anogenital distance (mm $\pm$ SE)					
			Males	(No. of pups)	Females	(No. of pups)	Intersex	(No. of pups)
0	0	0	3.08 ± 0.12	(18)	1.19 ± 0.07	(13)		
Cortisol	5 × 4	4	3.13 ± 0.07	(30)	1.24 ± 0.02	(38)		
	15 × 4	4	2.50 ± 0.09	(21)	1.21 ± 0.04	(34)	1.83 ± 0.01	(3)
Estradiol	0.1 × 5	5	2.42 ± 0.11	(19)	1.06 ± 0.04	(21)	0.0[a]	(1)
	1 × 5	5	2.38 ± 0.16	(8)	1.00 ± 0.0	(9)	1.38 ± 0.11	(16)
Progesterone	5 × 6	6	2.64 ± 0.06	(34)	1.02 ± 0.02	(30)		
	50 × 6	6	2.89 ± 0.06	(41)	1.20 ± 0.05	(28)		

[a]No apparent anogenital openings
Quoted from Kincl, 1989.

5.2.5. NON-STEROIDAL ESTROGENS

Triphenylethylene derivatives which possess estrogen-like (uterotropic activity) are highly teratogenic to the fetus. Diethylstilbestrol (DES) synthesized by Dodds (Dodds *et al.*, 1938) was in extensive use between 1945 and 1971 in pregnant diabetic women, in women with a history of an inability to carry to term, for treatment of post-menopausal syndrome and breast and prostatic cancer, and in beef cattle and poultry to achieve a more pleasing carcass fat distribution.

5.2.5.1. Effects on Experimental Animals

Several groups have demonstrated the development of cervicovaginal adenosis-like lesions in mice as a result of prenatal exposure to DES (Plapinger and Bern, 1979; McLachlan, 1977; McLachlan *et al.*, 1975, 1980; Walker, 1980; Maier *et al.*, 1985; Iguchi *et al.*, 1986a; Iguchi and Takasugi, 1987). Doses needed to develop the lesions in ICR/JCL strain are between $200-2000 \mu g/day$ injected for four days beginning on day 14 of gravidity or $200 \mu g$ if continuously infused (i.v.) also for four days. The regimen induces lesions in the fornical and upper vaginal epithelium in $80-85\%$ of females and stratification of the uterine epithelium in $38-70\%$. The appearance is dose-dependent. The use of lower doses decreases the incidence (Nomura and Kanzaki, 1977; Newbold and McLachlan, 1982). The vaginal epithelium exhibits a mitotic activity at birth and the activity persists in the portion derived from the urogenital sinus in mature females (Tanaka *et al.*, 1984).

In neonatal mice a dose of only $0.1 \mu g$ is often enough to reveal the changes in 36% of animals. In 10-day-old ovariectomized mice a daily injection of $0.001 \mu g$ of estradiol is effective. The observation suggests that ovarian steroids play a role in the induction of the DES syndrome (Iguchi *et al.*, 1986b).

Prenatal DES exposure alters the morphology of the ovaries and their steroidogenic capability. Polyovular follicles (PF), containing two to nine oocytes occur spontaneously in the ICR/JCI strain but the incidence is low. In DES-treated mice the incidence increases $33-112$-fold. PF appear already on day 5 of life in animals exposed to $2000 \mu g/day$. Females injected with $20 \mu g/day$ develop PF when they reach 30 days of age (Iguchi and Takasugi, 1986).

Male mice (ICR/JCL strain), exposed *in utero* between days 9 and 16 to DES, retained both the Müllerian and Wolffian ducts. Some may exhibit sperm abnormalities, nodular lesions with squamous metaplasia of the coagulating glands and ampullae (McLachlan *et al.*, 1975; McLachlan, 1977; Vorherr *et al.*, 1979; Nomura and Masuda, 1980; Rosenfeld and Bronson, 1980; Arai *et al.*, 1983; Newbold *et al.*, 1984). A dose of $100 \mu g/kg$ BW daily (about $3 \mu g$) produced lesions in 75% of adults $9-10$ months old. Pathological findings included hypoplastic, fibrotic intra-abdominal testes, often posterior to the urinary bladder or firmly fixed to the posterior pole of the kidney, nodular enlargement of the seminal vesicles and/or coagulating glands associated with squamous metaplasia. The treatment was toxic; the average number of male offspring born to DES mothers was 2.6 while in controls it was 4.6 (McLachlan *et al.*, 1975). Injections between days 9 through 16 of gestation, or continuous infusion ($10 \mu g/h$) from day 15 to 19 were teratogenic (Takasugi *et al.*, 1983).

5.2.5.2. Effects on Humans

Female babies with masculinized genitalia were born to mothers who took DES during pregnancy (Bongiovanni *et al.*, 1959). Boys may be born with hypospadias (Kaplan, 1959; Yalom *et al.*, 1973).

The most frequent changes include gross structural cervicovaginal abnormalities (vaginal and/or cervical ridges), incomplete cervical collar ('cock's comb') formation, transverse vaginal septa, lack of vaginal pars, and vaginal adenosis, the presence of glandular tissue of Müllerian origin (Sandberg and Hebard, 1977; Singer and Hochman, 1978). The incidence is highest in babies exposed to DES during vaginogenesis (weeks 12–13). Kaufman and Adam (1978) found a T-shaped uterus with bulbous cornual extensions in 23/66 women; in six the uterus was hypoplastic with a cavity of less than 2.5 cm. Early reports indicated a very high incidence of cervicovaginal malformations (almost 90%) in DES babies (Pomerance, 1973). Study of larger groups revealed a lower, yet still unfortunately very high frequency (Table 3.12). Vaginal adenosis is already present at birth. In stillborn babies the incidence (70%) is far above the 4% seen in unexposed babies (Johnson *et al.*, 1979).

In 1973 Henderson *et al.*, predicted there would be an increase of genito-urinary abnormalities and cancer in men born to mothers who took DES during pregnancy. The projection was unfortunately correct. Bibbo *et al.* (1975; 1977) examined 42 DES-exposed men and found epididymal cysts in four, hypoplastic penises and/or testes in two and in one a testicular mass. Gill *et al.* (1976; 1977) examined 159 DES-exposed men (exposed on the average *in utero* to 12 g of DES) and found genital lesions in 25.8% and decreased sperm count, semen volume and sperm motility in 32%. The incidence of overall irregularities was only 7% in a control group of 161 men. Cosgrove *et al.* (1977), Whitehead and Leiter (1981) and Stillman (1982) reached a similar conclusion while Leary *et al.* (1984) did not observe deviations as a result of DES exposure in babies exposed to 1.5 g.

5.3. Induction of Cancer by Estrogens

Cancer was induced by exposure to DES *in utero* in hamsters (Gilloteaux *et al.*, 1982), mice (McLachlan, 1977; Barrett *et al.*, 1981; Lamb *et al.*, 1981; Newbold and McLachlan, 1982; Greenman and Delongchamp, 1986; Greenman *et al.*, 1986, 1987) and rats (Boylan, 1978).

In mice (CD-1 strain) a dose of 5–100 μg/kg BW injected between days 9 and 16 of gestation induced adenosis formation in 10–15% of animals; 2% of exposed offspring developed cancer (Newbold and McLachlan, 1982).

In hamsters, prenatal exposure to 100 μg (injected to mother) between days 8 and 11 increased the sensitivity to a later DES treatment (15 mg pellet of DES at the age of 50 days). Carcinoma developed 150–250 days later. The uteri became hyperplastic with papillae projecting into the lumen. Cystic glandular structures were inside the papillae with no opening into the luminal space. With time the glandular proliferations filled the uterine cavity leading to uterine swelling. In older animals the cystic stroma became hemorrhagic, invaded by inflammatory tissue and fibrous material, and sections of the uterus became hard. While some cysts becme atrophic, others were hyperplastic, incorporating edematous hyperplasia including adenocarcinoma and carcinoma *in situ* (Gilloteaux *et al.*, 1982).

Cancer may develop 20–25 years after transplacental exposure to DES in humans. The tumor is characterized by clear and hobnail cells originating from paramesonephric, rather than mesonephric, epithelium; hence the name clear-cell adenocarcinoma (CCA). Herbst *et al.* (1971; 1972) summarized the history of 91 girls (average age 17 years) with cervical and vaginal carcinomas. Adenosis was detected in 24/26 patients indicating a relationship between the development of CCA and adenosis formation. Sixty-nine mothers were interviewed; 49 had taken DES, dienestrol, hexestrol, or a combination of the drugs. A connection between CCA and the use of triphenylethylenes has been confirmed by others (Folkman, 1971; Hatcher and Conrad, 1971; Yaffee, 1973; Noller and Fish, 1974; Tsukada *et al.*, 1972; Gilson *et al.*, 1973; Henderson *et al.*, 1973; Ulfelder, 1973; 1975; Scully *et al.*, 1974; Herbst et al., 1975, 1986; Horwitz *et al.*, 1988). In older women benign vaginal adenosis may develop into squamous lesions similar to those found in the cervix and become neoplastic (Fetherston, 1975).

5.4. Pregnanes

Greene *et al.* (1939b) found progesterone, a precursor in androgen biosynthesis, androgenic. Later studies did not confirm the results: Revesz and Chappel (1966) injected 100 mg s.c. to gravid rats and found no evidence of virilization. Courrier and Jost (1942) found virilization with pregnenolone. Our own studies (see Table 3.13) confirm these findings.

5.4.1. DERIVATIVES OF PROGESTERONE

Injection of pregnant rats with progestational agent induces masculinization of external genitalia. Virilizing synthetic compounds with progestational activity include acetophenone derivatives obtained from 16α,17-dihydroxy progesterone (Lerner *et al.*, 1962), 17-hydroxy progesterone (Schöler and de Wachter, 1961; Suchowsky and Junkmann, 1961; Whalen *et al.*, 1966) derivatives of 19-nor testosterone (Pincus, 1956; Revesz, *et al.*, 1960; Kincl and Dorfman, 1962; Whalen *et al.*, 1966; Saunders, 1967), and 19-hydroxyiated androgens (Booth, 1976).

5.4.1.1. Influence on Human Embryos

Embryos became exposed to constituents of oral contraceptives (OCs) either during a 'pregnancy test' for threatened miscarriage, while pregnancy was not suspected, or when mothers used OCs during breast-feeding. According to Shiono *et al.* (1979) over 70 000 fetuses were exposed to OCs in the US annually.

The first association between the use of OCs and masculinization was made by Wilkins *et al.* (1958). Other reports soon followed (Bongiovanni *et al.*, 1959; Grumbach *et al.*, 1959; Grumbach and Ducharme, 1960; Jones and Wilkins, 1960; Harlap *et al.*, 1975; Harlap and Eldor, 1980). Before that time there was no recognition that steroid hormones would masculinize girl babies. Physicians prescribed androgens (17α-ethinyl testosterone or methyl testosterone) as anabolic agents during pregnancy. The therapy often continued in the presence of frank masculinizing changes (deepening of the voice, hirsutism, acne and clitoral enlargement) in the mother. Most of the baby girls were born with an enlarged clitoris (often to the point of differentiating as a phallus) with varying degrees of labioscrotal fusion. Virilization often took place without masculinization changes in the mother (see Diamond and Young, 1963). Wilkins (1960) reviewed 70 cases and concluded that OCs induced labioscrotal fusion only during the first trimester. Clitoral hypertrophy was influenced at any time during pregnancy. Jacobson (1961) reported masculinization in 18.5% of girl babies in Norlutin (NET) users. The incidence in unexposed pregnancies was only 1%. Fine *et al.* (1963) confirmed the teratological effect of NET.

Hagler *et al.* (1963) and Burnstein and Wasserman (1964) reported on the virilizing properties of Provera (MAP).

Bongiovanni *et al.* (1959), Neumann *et al.* (1970) and Lanier *et al.* (1973) described masculinization of female infants associated with estrogen therapy alone. Driscoll and Taylor (1980) tested the effect of maternal estrogens upon the male urogenital system.

Prenatal OCs do not influence the sex of offspring (Keserü *et al.*, 1974: Oechsli, 1974; Rothman and Liess, 1976). There is no danger of increased predisposition to cancer to the mother.

5.4.2. ADRENOCORTICAL HORMONES

Elevated concentrations of cortical hormones during pregnancy adversely influence body growth and adrenal function in offspring (Eguchi and Wells, 1965; Hansson and Angervall, 1966; Paul and D'Angelo, 1972), may induce cleft palate (Walker, 1965, 1967, 1971) and produce changes in behavior. The differentiation of the genital apparatus is not influenced. Very high doses of cortisol may produce some virilizing changes in rat offspring (see Table 3.15).

References

ABRAMOVICH, D. R. and ROWE, P. (1973) Foetal plasma testosterone levels at mid-pregnancy and at term: relationship to foetal sex. *J. Endocr.* **56**: 621–622.

ABRAMOVICH, D. R., BAKER, T. G. and NEAL, P. (1974) Effect of human chorionic gonadotrophin on testosterone secretion by the fetal human testis in organ culture. *J. Endocr.* **60**: 179–185.

ACEVEDO, H. F., AXELROD, L. R., ISHIKAWA, E. and TAKAKI, F. (1961) Steroidogenesis in the human fetal testis: The conversion of pregnenolone-7α-^{3}H to dehydroepiendrosterone, testosterone and 4-androstene-3,17-dione. *J. Clin. Endocr. Metab.* **21**: 1611–1613.

ACEVEDO, H. F., AXELROD, L. R., ISHIKAWA, E. and TAKAKI, F. (1963) Studies in fetal metabolism. II. Metabolism of progesterone-4-C^{14} and pregnenolone-7α-H^3 in human fetal testes. *J. Clin. Endocr. Metab.* **23**: 885–890.

ADAM P. A. J., TERAMO, K., RAIHA, N., GITLIN, D. and SCHWARTZ, R. (1969) Human fetal insulin metabolism early in the gestation. Response to acute elevation of the fetal glucose concentration and placental transfer of human insulin ^{131}I. *Diabetes* **18**: 409–416.

ADESANYA, T., GRILLO, I. and SHIMA, K. (1966) Insulin content of enzyme histochemistry of the human foetal pancreatic islet. *J. Endocr.* **36**: 151–158.

AHLUWALIA, B., WILLIAMS, J. and VERMA, P. (1974) *In vitro* testosterone biosynthesis in the human fetal testis. II. Stimulation by cyclic AMP and human chorionic gonadotropin (hCG). *Endocrinology* **95**: 1411–1415.

AKSEL, S. and TYREY, L. (1977) Luteinizing hormone-releasing hormone in the human fetal brain. *Fert. Steril.* **28**: 1067–1071.

ALEXANDER, D. P., BRITTON, H. G., COHEN, N. M., NIXON, D. A. and PARKER, R. A. (1968) Insulin concentrations in the foetal plasma and foetal fluids of the sheep. *J. Endocr.* **40**: 389–390.

ALEXANDER, D. P., BRITTON, H. G., COHEN, N. M. and NIXON, D. A. (1969) Plasma concentrations of insulin, glucose, free-fatty acids and ketone bodies in the foetal and newborn sheep and the response to a glucose load before and after birth. *Biol. Neonatl* **14**: 178–193.

ALEXANDER, D. P., BRITTON, H. G., MASHITER, K., NIXON, D. A. and SMITH, Jr. F. G. (1970) The response of the foetal sheep in utero to intravenous glucose. *Biol. Neonate* **15**: 361–367.

ALEXANDER, D. P., ASSAN, R., BRITTON, H. G. and NIXON, D. A. (1971) Glucagon in the foetal sheep. *J. Endocr.* **51**: 597–598.

ALEXANDER, D. P., FORSLING, M. L., MARTIN, M. J., NIXON, D. A., RATCLIFFE, J. G., REDSTONE, D. and TUNBRIDGE, D. (1972) The effect of maternal hypoxia on fetal pituitary hormone release in the sheep. *Biol. Neonate* **21**: 219–228.

ALEXANDER, D. P., BRITTON, H. G., FORSLING, M., NIXON, D. A. and RATCLIFFE, J. G. (1974) Pituitary and plasma concentrations of adrenocorticotrophin, growth hormone, vasopressin, and ocybocin in fetal and maternal sheep during the latter half of gestation and the response to haemorrhage. *Biol. Neonate* **24**: 206–219.

AMENDOMORI, Y., CHEN, C. L. and MEITES, J. (1970) Serum prolactin levels in rats during different reproductive states. *Endocrinology* **86**: 506–510.

ANDERSEN, C. Y., BYSKOV, A. G. and GRINSTED, J. (1983) Growth pattern of the sex ducts in fetal mouse hermaphrodites. *J. Embryol. Exp. Morphol.* **73**: 59–68.

ANDERSON, A. B. M., PIERREPOINT, O. G., GRIFFITHS, K. and TUNBULL, A. C. (1972) Steroid metabolism in the adrenals of fetal sheep in relation to natural and corticotrophin-induced parturition. *J. Reprod. Fertil.* **16**: 25–37.

ANDERSSON, T. (1956) Intersexuality in pigs. *Kungl. Skogs-osh. Lantg. Tigskr. Arg. Gen.* **21**: 136–153.

ANGLE, M. J. and MEAD, R. A. (1979) The source of progesterone in preimplantation rabbit blastocysts. *Steroids* **33**: 625–637.

ANON. (1988) Origin of chromosome anomalies in human fetuses. *Res. Reprod.* **20**: 1–2.

ARAI, Y., MORI, T., SUZUKI, Y. and BERN, H. A. (1983) Long-term effects of perinatal exposure to sex steroids and diethylistilbestrol on the reproductive system of male mammals. *Int. Rev. Cytol.* **84**: 235–268.

AUBERT, M. L., GRUMBACH, M. M. and KAPLAN, S. L. (1975a) The ontogenesis of human fetal hormones. III. Prolactin. *J. Clin. Invest.* **56**: 155–164.

AUBERT, M. L., GARNIER, P. E., KAPLAN, S. L. and GRUMBACH, M. M. (1975b) Heterogeneity of circulating human prolactin (hPRL); decreased radioreceptor activity of "big" hPRL. *Endocrinology Suppl.* **96**: 80A.

AZUKIZAWA, M., MURATA, Y., IKENOUE, T., MARTIN, C. B. and HERSHMAN, J. M. (1976) Effect of thyrotropin-releasing hormone on secretion of thyrotropin, prolactin, thyroxine, and tri-iodothyronine in pregnant and fetal rhesus monkeys. *J. Clin. Endocr. Metab.* **43**: 1020–1028.

BAILLIE, A. H. (1965) 3β-Hydroxysteroid dehydrogenase activity in the foetal mouse testis. *J. Anat., Lond.* **99**: 507–511.

BAILLIE, A. H., NIEMI, M. and IKONEN, M. (1965) 3β-Hydroxysteroid dehydrogenase activity in the human foetal testis. *Acta Endocr. (Copenh.)* **48**: 429–438.

BAILLIE, A. H., CALMAN, K. C., FERGUSON, M. M. and HART, D. McK. (1966) Histochemical utilization of 3α-, 6β-, 11α-, 12α-, 16α-, 16β-, 17α-, 21- and 24-hydroxysteroids. *J. Endocr.* **34**: 1–12.

BAKER, T. G. (1963) A quantitative and cytological study of germ cells in human ovaries. *Proc. Roy. Soc. (London)* **158**: 417–433.

BAKER, T. G. (1972) Oogenesis and ovarian development. In: *Reproductive Biology*, Balio, H. and Glosse, S. (Eds). Excerpta Med Found., Amsterdam, The Netherlands.

BAKER, B. L. and JAFFE, R. B. (1975) The genesis of cell types in the adenohypophysis of the human fetus as observed with immunocytochemistry. *Am. J. Anat.* **143**: 137–162.

BAKKE, J. L. and LAWRENCE, N. (1966) Persistent thyrotropin insufficiency following neonatal thyroxine administration. *J. Lab. Clin. Med.* **67**: 477–482.

BAKKE J. L., GELLERT, R. J. and LAWRENCE, N. L. (1970) The persistent effects of perinatal hypothyroidism on pituitary, thyroidal and gonadal functions. *J. Lab. Clin. Med.* **76**: 25–33.

BARNES, R. J. (1976) Water and mineral exchange between maternal and fetal fluids. In: *Fetal Physiology and Medicine*, Beard R. W. and Nathanielsz, P. W. (Eds), W. B. Saunders, Philadelphia.

BARRETT, J. C., WONG, A. and McLACHLAN, J. A. (1981) Diethylstilbestrol induces neoplastic transformation without measurable gene mutation at two loci. *Science* **212**: 1402–1404.

BARRY, J. (1976) Systématization et afférences des structures hypothalamique à competénce gonado-trope chez les primates. In: *Systéme Nerveux Activité Sexuelle et Reproduction*, Masson, J. (Ed.), pp. 13–25.

BASSETT, J. M. and MADILL, D. (1974) Influence of prolonged glucose infusions on plasma insulin and growth hormone concentrations of foetal lambs. *J. Endocr.* **62**: 299–309.

BASSETT, J. M. and THORBURN, G. D. (1971) The regulation of insulin secretion by the ovine foetus *in utero*. *J. Endocr.* **50**: 59–74.

BASSETT, J. M. and THORBURN, G. D. (1973) Circulating levels of progesterone and corticosteroids in the pregnant ewe and its fetus. In: *Endocrinology of Pregnancy and Parturition: Experimental Studies in the Sheep*. Pierrepoint C. G. (Ed.), Alpha Omega, Cardiff, pp. 126–140.

BASSETT, J. M., THORBURN, G. D. and WALLACE, A. L. C. (1970) The plasma growth hormone concentration of fetal lamb. *J. Endocr.* **48**: 251–263.

BAST, J. D. and MELAMPY, R. M. (1972) Luteinizing hormone, prolactin and ovarian 20α-hydroxy-steroid dehydrogenase levels during pregnancy and pseudopregnancy in the rat. *Endocrinology* **91**: 1499–1505.

BEACH, F. A. (1975) Bisexual mating behavior in the male rat: effects of castration and hormone administration. *Psychol. Zool.* **18**: 390–402.

BEACH, F. A. and KUEHN, R. E. (1970) Coital behavior in dogs. X. Effects of androgenic stimulation during development of feminine mating response in females and males. *Horm. Behav.* **1**: 347–367.

BEARN, J. G. (1966) The role of the foetal pituitary in the development and growth of the foetal thyroid of rabbit. *J. Endocr.* **36**: 213–214.

BEGEOT, M., DUBOIS, M. P. and DUBOIS, P. M. (1977) Growth hormone and ACTH in the pituitary of normal and anencephalic human fetuses, immunocytochemical evidence for hypothalamic influences during development. *Neuroendocrinology* **24**: 208–220.

BEGEOT, M., DUBOIS, M. P. and DUBOIS, P. M. (1978a) Mise en evidence par immunocytochemie de la β-lipotropine (β-LPH), des α et β endorphines dans l'antehypophysyse de foetus humains normaux et anencephales. *Ann. Endocr.* (*Paris*) **39**: 235–241.

BEGEOT, M., DUBOIS, M. P. and DUBOIS, P. M. (1978b) Immunologic localization of α- and β-endorphins and β-lipotropin in corticotrophic cells of the normal and anencephalic fetal pituitaries. *Cell Tissue Res.* **193**: 413–422.

BEGEOT, M., DUBOIS, M. P. and DUBOIS, P. M. (1979) Influence de l'hypothalamus sur la différenciation des cellules presentant une immunoreactivite de type ACTH, β-LPH (β-lipotropine), α- et β-endorphines dans les ebauches antehypophysaires de foetus de rat en culture organotypique. *J. Physiol.* (*Paris*) **75**: 27–35.

BEGEOT, M., DUPOUY, J. P., DUBOIS, M. P. and DUBOIS, P. M. (1981) Immunocytological determination of gonadotropic and thyrotropic cells in fetal rat anterior pituitary during normal development and under experimental conditions. *Neuroendocrinology* **32**: 285–294.

BERÇU, B. B., MORIKAWA, Y., JACKSON, I. M. D. and DONAHOE, P. K. (1979) Inhibition of Müllerian inhibiting substance secretion by follitropin. *Pediatr. Res.* **13**: 246–249.

BEST, M. M., DUNCAN, E. H. and BEST, M. M. (1969) Accelerated maturation and persistent growth impairment in the rat resulting from thyroxine administration in the neonatal period. *J. Lab. Clin. Med.* **73**: 135–143.

BIBBO, M., Al-NAQEEB, M., BACCARINI, I., GILL, W., NEWTON, M., SLEEPER, K. M., SONEK, M. and WIED, B. L. (1975) Follow-up study of male and female offspring of DES-treated mothers. *J. Reprod. Med.* **15**: 29–32.

BIBBO, M., GILL, W. B., AZIZI, F., BLOUGH, R., FANG, V. S., ROSENFELD, R. L., SCHU-MACHER, G. F. B., SLEEPER, K., SONEK, M. G. and WIED, G. I. (1977) Follow-up study of male and female offspring of DES-exposed mothers. *Obstet Gynecol.* **49**: 1–8.

BIRGE, D. A., PEAKE, G. T., MARIZ, I. K. and DAUGHADAY, W. H. (1967) Radioimmunoassayable growth hormone in the rat pituitary gland: effects of age, sex and hormonal state. *Endocrinology* **81:** 195–204.

BLANCHARD, M. G. and JOSSO, N. (1974) Sources of the anti-Müllerian hormone synthesized by the fetal testis-Müllerian-inhibiting activity of fetal bovine Sertoli cells in tissue culture. *Pediatr. Res* **8:** 968–971.

BLANDAU, R. J., WHITE, B. G. and RUMERY, R. C. (1963) Observations on the movements of the living primordial germ cells in the mouse. *Fertial. Steril.* **14:** 482–489.

BLOCH, E. (1964) Metabolism of 4-^{14}C-progesterone by human fetal testes and ovaries. *Endocrinology* **74:** 833–845.

BLOCH, E. (1966) *In vitro* steroid synthesis by gonads and adrenals during mammalian fetal development. *Excerpta Med. Int. Series* **132:** 675–679.

BLOCH, E. (1967) The conversion of 7-^{3}H-pregnenolone and 4-^{14}C-progesterone to testosterone and androstenedione by mammalian fetal testes *in vitro. Steroids* **9:** 415–430.

BLOCH, E. and BENIRSCHKE, K. (1959) Synthesis *in vitro* of steroids by human fetal adrenal gland slices. *J. Biol. Chem.* **234:** 1085–1089.

BLOCH, E. and BENIRSCHKE K. (1965) *In vitro* steroid synthesis by fetal, newborn and adult armadillo adrenals and by fetal armadillo testes. *Endocrinology* **76:** 43–51.

BLOCH, E., TISSENBAUM, B. and BENIRSCHKE, K. (1962) The conversion of 4-C^{14}-progesterone to 17α-hydroxyprogesterone, testosterone and Δ^4-androstene-3,17-dione by human fetal testes *in vitro. Biochim. Biophys. Acta* **60:** 182–184.

BLOCH, E., LEW, M. and KLEIN, M. (1971) Studies on the inhibition of fetal androgen formation: testosterone synthesis by fetal and newborn mouse testes *in vitro. Endocrinology* **88:** 41–46.

BLOCH, E., GUPTA, C., FELDMAN, S. and van DAMME, O. (1974) Testosterone production by testes of fetal rats and mice. *INSERM (Paris)* **32:** 177–190.

BLOM, A. K., HOVE, K. and NEDKVITNE, J. J. (1976) Plasma insulin and growth hormone concentrations in pregnant sheep II: Post-absorptive levels in mid-and late pregnancy. *Acta Endocr. (Copenh.)* **82:** 553–560.

BONGIOVANNI, M., DiGEORGE, M. and GRUMBACH, M. M. (1959) Masculinization of the female infant associated with estrogenic therapy alone during gestation: four cases. *J. Clin. Endocr.* **189:** 1004–1011.

BOOTH, J. E. (1976) Effects of 19-hydroxylated androgens on sexual differentiation in the neonatal female rat. *J. Endocr.* **70:** 319–320.

BOTTIGLIONI, F., COLLINS, W. P., FLAMIGNI, C., NEUMANN, F. and SOMMERVILLE, I. F. (1971) Studies on androgen metabolism in experimentally feminized rats. *Endocrinology* **89:** 553–559.

BOWERS, S., FRIESEN, H. and HWANG, P. (1971) Prolactin and thyrotropin release in man by synthetic pyroglutamyl-histidyl-prolinamide. *Biochem. Biophys. Res. Commun.* **45:** 1033–1041.

BOYLAN, E. S. (1978) morphological and functional consequences of prenatal exposure to diethylstilbestrol in the rat. *Biol. Reprod.* **19:** 854–863.

BRASSEL, J. A. and BOYD, D. B. (1975) Influence of thyroid hormone on fetal brain growth and development. In: *Perinatal Thyroid Physiology and Disease.* Fisher, D. A. and Burrow, G. N. (Eds), Raven Press, New York, pp. 59–71.

BRINKMANN, A. D. (1977) *In vitro* synthesis and secretion of testosterone by foetal testes of rats and guinea-pigs under the influence of luteinizing hormone. *J. Endocr.* **72:** 19P.

BRINKMANN, A. D. and van STRAALEN, R. J. C. (1979) Development of the LH-response in fetal guinea pig testes. *Biol. Reprod.* **21:** 991–997.

BROUGHTON, P. F., LUMBERS, E. R. and MOTT, J. C. (1974) Factors influencing plasma renin and anglotensin II in the conscious pregnant ewe and its fetus. *J. Physiol.* **243:** 619–636.

BROWN, R. S., SANDER, E. and ARGOS, P. (1985) The primary structure of transcription factor TFIIIA 12 consecutive repeats. *FEBS Lett.* **186:** 271–274.

BROWN-GRANT, K. and SHERWOOD, M. R. (1971) The early androgen syndrome in the guinea-pig. *J. Endocrinol.* **49**: 277–291.

BRUBAKER, P. L., BAIRD, A. C., BENNETT, H. P. J., BROWNE C. A. and SOLOMON, S. (1982) Corticotropic peptides in the human fetal pituitary. *Endocrinology* **111**: 1150–1155.

BRUHN, T., PARVIZI, N. and ELLENDORFF, F. (1983) Ontogeny of hypothalamus-pituitary function in the fetal pig: gonadotropin release in response to electrical and electrochemical stimulation of the hypothalamus. *Endocrinology* **112**: 639–644.

BRUNET, N., GOURDJI, D., MOREAU, M., GROUSELLE, D., BOURNAUD, F. and TIXIER-VIDAL, A. (1977) Effect of 17-β-estradiol on prolactin secretion and thyroliberin responsiveness in two rat prolactin continuous cell lines. Definition of an experimental model. *Ann. Biol. Anim. Biochim. Biophys.* **17**: 413–419.

BRUNNER, J. A. and WITSCHI, E. (1946) Testosterone-induced modifications of sex development in female hamsters. *Am. J. Anat.* **79**: 293–320.

BUDDINGH, F., PARKER, H. R., ISHIZAKI, G. and TYLER, W. S. (1971) Long term studies of the functional development of the fetal kidney in sheep. *Am. J. Vet. Res.* **32**: 1993–1998.

BUDZIK, G. D., HUTSON, J. M., IKAWA, H. and DONAHOE, P. K. (1982) The role of zinc in Müllerian duct regression. *Endocrinology* **110**: 1521–1525.

BUGNON, C., BLOCH, B. and FELLMANN, D. (1977) Cyto-immunological study of the ontogenesis of the gonadotropic hypothalamo-pituitary axis in the human fetus. *J. Steroid. Biochem.* **8**: 565–575.

BUHL, A. E., PASZTOR, L. M. and RESKO, J. A. (1979) Sex steroids in guinea pig fetuses after sexual differentiation of the gonads. *Biol. Reprod.* **21**: 903–908.

BURSTEIN, R. and WASSERMAN, H. C. (1964) The effect of provera on the fetus. *Obstet. Gynecol.* **23**: 931–934.

BYSKOV, A. G. and GRINSTED, J. (1981) Feminizing effect of mesonephros on cultured differentiating mouse gonads and ducts. *Nature (Lond.)* **212**: 817–818.

CAGNONI, M., FAMTINI, F. and MORACE, G. (1964) Studi sulla caratterizzazione sessuale delle strutture nervose deputate alla regolazione della funzione gonadica. Nota I. Gli effetti della somministrazione di testosterone in ratte proveniente da madri trattate nell'ultimo periodo della gravidanza. *Ras. Neurol. Veget.* **XVIII**: 275–284.

CARR, B. R., OHASHI, M. and SIMPSON, E. R. (1982) Low density lipoprotein binding and *de novo* synthesis of cholesterol in the neocortex and fetal zones of the human fetal adrenal gland. *Endocrinology* **110**: 1994–1998.

CATT, K. J., DUFAU, M. L., NEAVES, W. B., WALSH, P. C. and WILSON, J. D. (1975) LH-hCG receptors and testosterone content during differentiation of the testis in the rabbit embryo. *Endocrinology* **97**: 1157–1165.

CHALLIS, J. R. G. and THORBURN, G. D. (1976) The fetal pituitary-adrenal axis and its functional interactions with the neurohypophysis. In: *Fetal Physiology and Medicine*, Beard, R. and Nathaniels, P. W. (Eds), Saunders, London,

CHALLIS J. R. G., KIM, C. K., NAFTOLIN, F., JUDD, H. L. and YEN, S. S. C., BENIRSCHKE K. (1974) The concentration of androgens, oestrogens, progesterone and luteinizing hormone in the seurm of foetal calves throughout the course of gestation. *J. Endocr.* **60**: 107–115.

CHALLIS, J. R. G., KENDALL, J. Z., ROBINSON, J. S. and THORBURN, G. D. (1977a) The regulation of corticosteroids during late pregnancy and their role in parturition. *Biol. Reprod.* **16**: 57–69.

CHALLIS, J. R. G., JONES, C. T., ROBINSON, J. S. and THORBURN, G. D. (1977b) Development of fetal pituitary-adrenal function. *J. Steroid. Biochem.* **8**: 471–478.

CHALLIS, J. R. G., HUHTANEN, D., SPRAGUE, C., MITCHELL, B. F. and LYE, S. J. (1985) Modulation by cortisol of adrenocorticotropin-induced activation of adrenal function in fetal sheep. *Endocrinology* **116**: 2267–2272.

CHAPLIN, S. and SMITH, J. M. (1987) Drugs and the fetus. *IPPF Med. Bull.* **21**(4): 1–2.

CHARD, T. (1972) The posterior pituitary in human and animal parturition. *J. Reprod. Fertil. (Suppl.)* **16:** 121–138.

CHARRIER, J. (1973) Evolution fetale et postnatale du contenu en hormone de croissance de l'hypophyse ovine. *Ann. Biol. Anim. Biochim. Biophys.* **13:** 155–163.

CHATELAIN, A., DUBOIS, M. P. and DUPOUY, J.-P. (1976) Hypothalamus and cytodifferentiation of the foetal pituitary gland study *in vivo. Cell. Tiss. Res.* **169:** 335–344.

CHATELAIN, A., DUBOIS, M. P. and DUPOUY, J.-P. (1977) Les cellules à prolactine chez la ratte gestante, le foetus, le noiuveau-né et le jeune. *Ann. Biol. Anim. Bioch. Biophys.* **17:** 403–412.

CHATELAIN, A., DUPOUY, J.-P. and DUBOIS, M. P. (1979) Ontogenesis of cells producing polypeptide hormones (ACTH, MSH, LPH, GH, PRL) in the fetal hypophysis of the rat: influence of the hypothalamus. *Cell Tissue Res.* **196:** 409–427.

CHEZ, R. A., HUTCHINSON, D. L., SALAZAR, H. and MINTZ, D. H. (1970a) Some effects of fetal and maternal hypophysectomy in pregnancy. *Am. J. Obstet. Gynecol.* **108:** 643–650.

CHEZ, R., MINTZ, D. H., HORGER, III, E. O. and HUTCHINSON, D. L. (1970b) Factors affecting the response to insulin in the normal subhuman pregnant primate. *J. Clin. Invest.* **49:** 1517–1527.

CHIAPPA, S. A. and FINK, G. (1977) Releasing factor and hormonal changes in the hypothalamic pituitary-gonadotropin and adrenocorticotrophin systems before and after birth and puberty in male, female and androgenized female rats. *J. Endocr.* **72:** 211–224.

CHOWDHURY, M. and STEINBERGER, E. (1975) Biosynthesis of gonadotrophins by rat pituitaries *in vitro. J. Endocr.* **66:** 369–374.

CLARK, S. O., EILIN, N., STYNE, D. M., GLUCKMAN, P. D., KAPLAN, S. L. and GRUMBACH, M. M. (1984) Hormone ontogeny in the ovine fetus. XVII. Demonstration of pulsatile luteinizing hormone secretion by the fetal pituitary gland. *Endocrinology* **115:** 1774–1779.

CLARKE, I. J., SCARAMUZZI, R. J. and HORT, R. V. (1976) Effects of testosterone implants in pregnant ewes on their female offspring. *J. Embryol. Exp. Morph.* **36:** 87–99.

CLARKE, I. T., SCARAMUZZI, R. J. and SHORT, R. V. (1977) Ovulation in prenatally androgenized ewes. *J. Endocr.* **73:** 385–389.

CLEMENTS, J. A., REYES, F. I., WINTER, J. S. and FAIMAN, C. (1976) Studies on human sexual development. III. fetal pituitary and serum, and amniotic fluid concentrations of LH, CG, and FSH. *J. Clin. Endocr. Metab.* **42:** 9–19.

CLEMENTS, J. A., REYES, F. I., WINTER, J. S. D. and FAIMAN, C. (1980) Ontogenesis of gonadotropin-releasing hormone in the human fetal hypothalamus. *Proc. Soc. Exp. Biol. Med.* **163:** 437–444.

COHEN, A. (1963) Corrélation entre l'hypophyse et le cortex surrénal chez le foetus de rat. Le cortex surrénal du nouveau-né. *Arch. Anat. Micr. Morph. Exp.* **52:** 277–285.

COHEN, A., DUPOUY, J.-P. and JOST, A. (1971) Influence de l'hypothalamus sur l'activité corticostimulante de l'hypophyse faetale du rat au cours de la gestation. *C. R. Acad. Sci. (Paris)* **273:** 883–886.

COLENBRANDER, B., CRUIP, T. A. M., DIELEMAN, S. S. and WENSING, C. J. G. (1977) Changes in serum LH concentrations during normal and abnormal sexual development in the pig. *Biol. Reprod.* **17:** 506–513.

COLENBRANDER, B., van de WIEL, D. F. M., van ROSSUM-KOK, C. M. J. E. and WENSING, C. J. G. (1982) Changes in serum FSH concentrations in the pig during development. *Biol. Reprod.* **26:** 105–109.

COMLINE, R. S. and SILVER, M. (1961) The release of adrenaline and noradrenaline from the adrenal glands of the foetal sheep. *J. Physiol.* **156:** 424–444.

COMLINE, R. S. and SILVER, M. (1972) The composition of foetal and maternal blood during parturition in the ewe. *J. Physiol.* **222:** 233–256.

CONKLIN, P. M., SCHINDLER, W. J. and HULL, S. F. (1973) Hypothalamic thyrotrophin releasing factor: activity and pituitary responsiveness during development in the rat. *Neuroendocrinology* **11:** 197–211.

COSGROVE, M. D., BENTON, B. and HENDERSON, B. E. (1977) Male genitourinary abnormalities and maternal diethylstilbestrol. *J. Urol.* **117:** 220–222.

COURRIER, R. and JOST, A. (1942) Intersexualité foetale provoqué par la pregnenolone au cours de la grossesse. *Soc. Biol. (Paris)* **136:** 395–396.

CUNHA, G. R. (1975) Age-dependent loss of sensitivity of female urogenital sinus to androgenic conditions as a function of the epithelial–stromal interaction in mice. *Endocrinology* **97:** 665–673.

CUTTLER, L., EGLI, C. A., STYNE, D. M., KAPLAN, S. L. and GRUMBACH, M. L. (1985) Hormone ontogeny in the ovine fetus. XVIII. The effect of an opioid antagonist on luteinizing hormone secretion. *Endocrinology* **116:** 1997–2002.

DAIKOKU, S., KAWANO, H. and ABE, K. (1980). Studies on the development of hypothalamic regulation of the hypophysial gonadotropic activity in rats. *Arch. d'Anat. Microsc. Morph. Exp.* **69:** 89–97.

D'ANGELO, S. A. and WALL, N. R. (1971) Simultaneous effects of thyroid and adrenal inhibitors on maternal-fetal endocrine interrelations in the rat. *Endocrinology* **89:** 591–597.

D'ANGELO, S. A. and WALL, N. R. (1972) Maternal-fetal endocrine interrelations: thyroid system of the rat. *Neuroendocrinology* **9:** 197–206.

D'ANGELO, S. A., PAUL, D. H. and WALL, N. R. (1973) Maternal-fetal endocrine interrelations— influence of maternal adrenocorticosteroids on fetal ACTH secretion. *Am. J. Physiol.* **224:** 543–547.

DANTCHAKOFF, V. (1936) L'hormone male adulte dans l'histogènese sexuelle du mammifere. *C. R. Soc. Biol.* **123:** 873–876.

DANTCHAKOFF, V. (1937a) Sur l'obtention experimentale des freemartins chez le cobaye et sur la nature du facteur conditionnant leur histogènese sexuelle. *C. R. Acad. Sci. (Paris)* **204:** 195–196.

DANTCHAKOFF, V. (1937b) Sur l'édification des glandes annexes du tractus génital dans les "free-martins" et sur les facteurs formatifs dans l'histogènese sexuelle male. *C. R. Soc. Biol.* **124:** 407–411.

DANTCHAKOFF, V. (1938a) Sur les effets de l'hormone male dans un jeune cobaye male traité depuis un stade embryonnaire (production d'hypermales). *C. R. Soc. Biol.* **127:** 1259–1262.

DANTCHAKOFF, V. (1938b) Sur les effets de l'hormone male dans une jeune cobaye femelle traité dupuis un stade embryonnaire (inversions sexuelles). *C. R. Soc. Biol.* **127:** 1255–1258.

DANTCHAKOFF, V. (1938c), Sur le mecanisme des déviations sexuelles dans une femelle génétique à la suite: a. de testosterinisation; b. du free-martinisme; c. des tumeurs de la surrenale (virilism). *C. R. Acad Sci. (Paris)* **206:** 1411–1413.

DANTCHAKOFF, V. (1938d) Effet du traitement hormonal de l'embryon de cobaye par la testosterone sur ses facultés procréatrices et sur sa progeniture. *C. R. Soc. Biol.* **128:** 891–893.

DANTCHAKOFF, V. (1939) Les bases biologiques du "free-martinisme" et de "l'intersexualité hormonale": sont-elles les mêmes? *C. R. Soc. Biol.* **130:** 1473–1474.

DAVIES, I. J. and RYAN, K. J. (1973) Glucocorticoid synthesis from pregnenolone by sheep fetal adrenals *in vitro*. *J. Endocr.* **58:** 485–491.

DEANESLY, R. (1939) Uterus masculinus of the rabbit and its reactions to androgens and estrogens. *J. Endocr.* **1:** 300–306.

DIAMOND, M. and YOUNG, W. C. (1963) Differential responsiveness of pregnant and nonpregnant guinea pigs to the masculinizing action of testosterone propionate. *Endocrinology* **72:** 429–438.

DICKMANN, Z. and DEY, S. K. (1974a) Steroidogenesis in the preimplantation rat embryo and its possible influence on morula-blastocyst transformation and implantation. *J. Reprod. Fertil.* **37:** 91–93.

DICKMANN, Z. and DEY, S. K. (1974b) Evidence that Δ^5-3β-hydroxysteroid dehydrogenase activity in rat blastocysts is autonomous. *J. Endocr.* **61:** 513–514.

DICKMANN, Z., DEY, S. K. and GUPTA, J. S. (1976) A new concept: control of early pregnancy by steroid hormones originating in the preimplantation embryo. *Vit. Horm.* **34:** 215–242.

DODDS, E. C., GOLDBERG, L., LAWSON, W. and ROBINSON, R. (1938) Estrogenic activity of certain synthetic compounds. *Nature* **141:** 247–248.

DONAHOE, P. K., ITO, Y., MARFATIA, S. and HENDREN, W. H. III (1976) The production of Müellerian inhibiting substance by the fetal, neonatal and adult rat. *Biol. Reprod.* **15:** 329–334.

DONAHOE, P. K., ITO, Y., PRICE, J. M. and HENDREN, W. H. III (1977) Müllerian inhibiting substance in human testes after birth. *J. Pediatr. Surg.* **12:** 323–330.

DONAHOE, P. K., BUDAIK, G. P., TREISTAD, R., MUDGETT-HUNTER, M., FULLER, A. Jr., HUTSON, J. M., IKAWA, H., HAYASHI, A. and MacLAUGHLIN, D. (1982) Müllerian-inhibiting substance: an update. *Rec. Prog. Horm. Res.* **38:** 279–330.

DONAHOE, P. K., CATE, R. L., McLAUGHLIN, D. T., EPSTEIN, J., FULLER, A. F., TAKE-HASHI, M., COUGHLIN, J. P., NIMFA, E. and TAYLOR, L. A. (1987) Müllerian inhibiting substance: gene structure and mechanism of action of fetal regressor. *Rec. Prog. Horm. Res.* **43:** 431–467.

DREW, J. S., LONDON, W. T., LUSTBADER, E. D., HESSER, J. E. and BLUMBER, B. S. (1978) Hepatitis B virus and sex ration of offspring. *Science* **201:** 687–692.

DRISCOLL, S. G. and TAYLOR, S. F. (1980) Effects of prenatal maternal estrogen on the male urogenital system. *Obstet. Gynec.* **56:** 537–542.

DROST, M. and HOLM, L. W. (1968) Prolonged gestation in ewes after foetal adrenalectomy. *J. Endocr.* **40:** 293–296.

DUBOIS, P. M. and DUBOIS, M. P. (1974) Mise en evidence par immunofluorescence de l'activité gonadotropes dans l'antehypophyse foetale humaine. *INSERM (Paris)* **32:** 37–62.

DUBOIS, P. M., PAULIN, C., ASSAN, R. and DUBOIS, M. P. (1975) Evidence for immunoreactive somatostatin in the endocrine cells of human foetal pancreas. *Nature* **256:** 731–732.

DUFAU, M. L., WARREN, D. W., KNOX, G. F., LOUMAYE, E., CASTELLON, M. L., LUNA, S. and CATT, K. J. (1984) Receptors and inhibitory actions of gonadotropin-releasing hormone in the fetal Leydig cell. *J. Biol. Chem.* **259:** 2896–2899.

DUPOUY, J.-P. (1971) Inhibition directe, par le cortisol, de la libération d'ACTH par l'hypophyse foetal du Rat soumise à un extrait hypothalamique. *C. R. Acad. Sci. (Paris)* **272:** 1886–1889.

DUPOUY, J.-P. (1974) Sites of the negative feedback action of corticosteroids on the hypothalamo-hypophysial system of the rat fetus. *Neuroendocrinology* **16:** 148–155.

DUPOUY, J.-P. (1975) CRF activity in fetal rat hypothalamus, in late pregnancy. *Neuroendocrinology* **19:** 303–313.

DUPOUY, J.-P. (1976) Evolution de la teneur de l'hypophyse foetale en ACTH. Etude chez le rat, enfin de gestation. *C. R. Acad. Sci. (Paris)* **282:** 211–214.

DUPOUY, J.-P. and COHEN, A. (1975) Comparison de l'activité corticosurrénalienne foetale et maternelle au cours du nyctyhémère et durant la gestation. *C. R. Acad. Sci. (Paris)* **280:** 463–466.

DUPOUY, J.-P. and DUBOIS, M. P. (1975) Ontogenesis of the α-MSH, β-MSH and ACTH cells in the foetal hypophysis of the rat. Correlation with the growth of the adrenals and adrenocortical activity. *Cell Tissue Res.* **161:** 373–384.

DUPOUY, J.-P. and MAGRE, S. (1973) Ultrastructure des cellules granulées de l'hypophyse foetale du rat. Indentification des cellules corticotropes et thyréotropes. *Arch. d'Anat. Micr. Morph. Exp.* **62:** 185–205.

DURAND, P., CATHIARD, A. M., LOCATELLI, A. and SAEZ, J. M. (1982) Modifications of the steroidogenic pathway during spontaneous and adrenocorticotropin-induced maturation of ovine fetal adrenal. *Endocrinology* **110:** 500–505.

DÜRENBERGER, H. and KRATOCHWILL, K. (1980) Specificity of tissue interaction and origin of mesenchymal cells in the androgen response of the embryonic mammary gland. *Cell* **19:** 465–471.

EGUCHI, Y. and WELLS, L. J. (1965) Response of the hypothalamic-hypophyseal adrenal axis to stress-observations in fetal and caesarean newborn rats. *Proc. Soc. Exp. Biol. Med.* **120:** 675–679.

EGUCHI, Y., SAKAMOTO, Y., ARISHIMA, K., MORIKAWA, Y. and HASHIMOTO, Y. (1975) Hypothalamic control of the pituitary testicular relation in fetal rats: measurement of collective volume of Leydig cells. *Endocrinology* **96:** 504–507.

EICHWALD, E. J. and SILMER, C. R. (1955) Untitled communication. *Transplant Bull.* **2:** 148–149.

ELGER, W., STEINBECK, H., CUPCEANCU, B. and NEUMANN, F. (1970) Influence of methyltestosterone and cyproterone acetate on Wolffian duct differentiation in female rat foetuses. *J. Endocr.* **47:** 417–422.

ELLINWOOD, W. E. and RESKO, J. A. (1980) Sex differences in biologically active and immunoreactive gonadotropins in the fetal circulation of rhesus monkeys. *Endocrinology* **107**: 902–907.

ELLINWOOD, W. E., BAUGHMAN, W. L. and RESKO, J. A. (1982) The effects of gonadectomy and testosterone treatment on luteinizing hormone secretion in fetal rhesus monkeys. *Endocrinology* **110**: 183–189.

ELSAESSER, F., ELLENDORFF, F., POMERANTZ, D. K., PARVIZI, N. and SMIDT, D. (1976) Plasma levels of luteinizing hormone, progesterone, testosterone and 5α-dihydrotestosterone in male and female pigs during sexual maturation. *J. Endocr.* **68**: 347–348.

ELSAESSER, F., PARVIZI, N. and ELLENDORFF, F. (1978) Effects of prenatal testosterone on the stimulatory estrogen feedback on LH release in the pig. In: *Hormones and Brain Development*, Dorner, G. and Kawashima, M. (Eds), Elsevier/North Holland Biomedical Press, Amsterdam, pp. 61–67.

ENGLER, D., SCANLON, M. F. and JACKSON, I. M. D. (1981) Thyrotropin-releasing hormone in the systematic circulation of the neonatal rat is derived from the pancreas and other extraneural tissues. *J. Clin. Invest.* **67**: 800–808.

ENGSTRÖM, N. H. and ENGSTRÖM, W. W. (1959) Effects of estrogen and testosterone on circulating thyroid hormone. *J. Clin. Endocr. Metab.* **19**: 783–796.

EPSTEIN, M. F., CHEZ, R. A., OAKEO, G. K. and VAITUKAITIS, J. L. (1976) Hypothalamic-pituitary control of perinatal prolactin secretion in *Macaca mulatta*. *Endocrinology* **99**: 743–751.

ERENBERG, A., OMORI, K., MENKES, J. H., OH, W. and FISHER, D. A. (1974) Growth and development of the thyroidectomized ovine fetus. *Pediat. Res.* **8**: 783–789.

ERICKSON, R. P. and VERGA, V. (1989) Minireview: Is zinc-finger Y the sex-determining gene? *Am. J. Hum. Genet.* **45**: 671–674.

EUKER, J. S., MEITES, J. and RIEGLE, G. D. (1975) Effects of acute stress on serum LH and prolactin in intact, castrate and dexamethasone-treated male rats. *Endocrinology* **96**: 85–92.

EVANS, C. A. and KENNEDY, T. G. (1980) Blastocyst implantation in ovariectomized, adrenalectomized hamsters treated with inhibitors of steroidogenesis during the pre-implantation period. *Steroids* **36**: 41–52.

EVANS, H. J., BUCKTON, K. E., SPOWART, G. and CAROTHERS, A. D. (1979) Heteromorphic S chromosomes in 46, XX males: evidence for the involvement of X–Y interchange. *Hum. Genet.* **49**: 11–31.

EVANS, T. C., KRETZCHMAR, R. M., HODGES, R. D. and SONG, C. W. (1967) Radioiodine uptake studies of the human fetal thyroid. *J. Nucl. Med.* **8**: 157–165.

FALCONI, G. and ROSSI, G. L. (1965) Some effects of oestradiol 3-benzoete on the rat foetus. *Proc. Eur. Soc. Study Drug Tox.* **6**: 150–156.

FAYEZ, J. A., BRUNCH, T. R. and MILLER, G. L. (1974) Virilization in pregnancy associated with polycystic ovary disease. *Obstet. Gynec.* **44**: 511–521.

FELDMAN, S. C. and BLOCH E. (1978) Developmental pattern of testosterone synthesis by fetal rat testes in response to luteinizing hormone. *Endocrinology* **102**: 999–1007.

FETHERSTON, W. C. (1975) Squamous neoplasia of vagina related to DES syndrome. *Am. J. Obstet. Gynecol.* **122**: 176–181.

FINE, E. H., LEVIN, M. and McCONNELL, E. L. (1963) Masculinization of female infants associated with norethindrome acetate. *Obstet. Gynecol.* **22**: 210–213.

FISER, Jr., R. H., ERENBERG, A., SPERLING, M. A., OH, W. and FISHER, D. A. (1974) Insulin-glucagon substrate interrelations in the fetal sheep. *Pediat. Res.* **8**: 951–955.

FISHELL, S. B., EDWARDS, R. G. and EVANS, C. J. (1984) Human chorionic gonadotropin secreted by preimplantation embryos cultured *in vitro*. *Science* **223**: 816–818.

FISHER, D. A. (1974) Fetal thyroid metabolism. *Contemp. Obst. Gynec.* **3**: 47–54.

FISHER, D. A. and DUSSAULT, J. H. (1979) Development of the mammalian thyroid gland. In: *Handbook of Physiology, Endocrinology III*, Physiological Society, Washington, pp. 321–338.

FISHER, D. A., HOBEL, C. J., GARZA, R. and PIERCE, C. (1970) Thyroid function in the pre-term fetus. *Pediatrics* **46**: 208–216.

FLICKINGER, C. J. (1974) Fine structural aspects of cytodifferentiation. In: *Male Accessory Sex Organs*, Brandes, D. (Ed.), Academic Press, New York, pp. 115–131.

FLORSHEIM, W. H., FAIRCLOTH, M. A., CORCORRAN, V. L. and RUDKO, P. (1966) Perinatal thyroid function in the rat. *Acta Endocr. (Copenh.)* **52**: 375–382.

FOLKMAN, J. (1971) Transplacental carcinogenesis by stilbestrol. *N. Engl. J. Med.* **285**: 404–405.

FOSTER, D. L., CRUZ, T. A. C., JACKSON, G. L., COOK, B. and NALBANDOV, A. V. (1972a) Regulation of luteinizing hormone in the fetal and neonatal lamb. III. Release of LH by the pituitary *in vivo* in response to crude ovine hypothalamic extract or purified porcine gonadotrophin releasing factor. *Endocrinology* **90**: 673–683.

FOSTER, D. L., JACKSON, G. L., COOK, B. and NALBANDOV, A. V. (1972b) Regulation of luteinizing hormone (LH) in the fetal and neonatal lamb. IV. Levels of LH releasing activity in the hypothalamus. *Endocrinology* **90**: 684–691.

FRANCHIMONT, P. and PASTEELS, J. L. (1972) Sécrétion indépendante des hormones gonodotropes et de leurs sous-unités. *C. R. Acad. Sci. (Paris)* **275**: 1799–1802.

FRIEND, J. P. (1977) Persistence of maternally derived [+]3[+]H-estradiol in fetal and neonatal rats. *Experientia* **33**: 1235–1236.

FUKUCHI, M., INOUE, T., ABE, H. and KUMAHARA, Y. (1970) Thyrotropin in human fetal pituitaries. *J. Clin. Endocr. Metab.* **31**: 565–569.

GARDNER, R. L. (1977) Developmental potency of normal and neoplastic cells of the early mouse embryo. In: *Birth Defects*, Littlefield, M. and de Grouch L. (Eds), Excerpta Med. Int. Congr. Ser. **432**: 154–166.

GELOSO, J. P. (1961) Date de l'entrée en fonction de la thyroide chez le foetus de rat. *C. R. Soc. Biol.* **155**: 1239–1244.

GELOSO, J. P., HEMON, P., LEGRAND, J., LEGRAND, C. and JOST, A. (1968) Some aspects of thyroid physiology during the perinatal period. *Gen. Comp. Endocr.* **10**: 191–197.

GENAZZANI, A. R., FRAIOLI, F., FIORETTI, P. and FELBER, J. P. (1975) Placental impermeability to maternal ACTH in the rabbit. *Experientia* **31**: 245–247.

GEORGE, F. W. and OJEDA, S. R. (1982) Changes in aromatase activity in the rat brain during embryonic, neonatal, and infantile development. *Endocrinology* **111**: 522–529.

GEORGE, F. W., MILEWICH, L. and WILSON, J. D. (1978a) Oestrogen content of the embryonic rabbit ovary. *Nature (Lond)* **274**: 172–173.

GEORGE, F. W., CATT, K. J., NEAVES, W. B. and WILSON, J. D. (1978b) Studies on the regulation of testosterone synthesis in the fetal rabbit testis. *Endocrinology* **102**: 665–673.

GEORGE, F. W., SIMPSON, E. R., MILEWICH, L. and WILSON, J. D. (1979) Studies on the regulation of the onset of steroid hormone biosynthesis in fetal rabbit gonads. *Endocrinology* **105**: 1100–1106.

GILL, W. B., SCHUMACHER, G. F. B. and BIBBO, M. (1976) Structural and functional abnormalities in the sex organs of mail offspring of DES (diethylstilbestrol) treated mothers. *J. Reprod. Med.* **16**: 147–153.

GILL, W. B., SCHUMACHER, G. F. B. and BIBBO, M. (1977) Pathological semen and anatomical abnormalities of the genital tract in human male subjects exposed to diethylstilbestrol in utero. *J. Urol.* **117**: 477–480.

GILLOTEAUX, J. PAUL, R. J. and STEGGLES, A. W. (1982) Upper genital tract abnormalities in the syrian hamster as a result of *in utero* exposure to diethylstilbestrol. I. Uterine cystadenomatous papilloma and hypoplasia. *Virchows Arch. Pathol. Anat.* **398**: 163–183.

GILSON, M. D., DIBONA, D. D. and KNAB, D. R. (1973) Clear-cell adenocarcinoma in young females. *Obstet. Gynec.* **41**: 494–500.

GITLIN, D. and BIASUCCI, A. (1969a) Ontogenesis of immunoreactive thyroglobulin in the human conceptus. *J. Clin. Endocr. Metab.* **29**: 849–853.

GITLIN, D. and BIASUCCI, A. (1969b) Ontogenesis of immuno-reactive growth hormone, folliculo-stimulating hormone, thyroid-stimulating hormone, luteinizing hormone, chorionic prolactin and chorionic gonadotropin in the human conceptus. *J. Clin. Endocr. Metab.* **29**: 926–935.

GLUCKMAN, P. D., MARTI-HENNEBERG, C., KAPLAN, S. L. and GRUMACH, M. M. (1979a) Hormone ontogeny in the ovine fetus: XIV. The effect of 17β-estradiol infusion on fetal plasma gonadotropins and prolactin and the maturation of sex steroid-dependent negative feedback. *Endocrinology* **105**: 1173–1177.

GLUCKMAN, P. D., MUELLER, P. L., KAPLAN, S. L., RUDOLPH, A. M. and GRUMBACH, M. M. (1979b) Hormone ontogeny in the ovine fetus. I. circulating growth hormone in mid-and late gestation. *Endocrinology* **104**: 162–167.

GLUCKMAN, P. D., MARTI-HENNEBERG, C., KAPLAN, S. L., LI, C. H. and GRUMBACH, M. M. (1980a) Hormone ontogeny in the ovine fetus. X. The effects of beta endorphin and naloxone on circulating growth hormone, prolactin and chorionic somatomammotropin. *Endocrinology* **107**: 76–80.

GLUCKMAN, P. D., MARTI-HENNEBERG, C., LEISTI, S., KAPLAN, S. L. and GRUMBACH, M. M. (1980b) Alpha-melanocyte stimulating hormone inhibits prolactin secretion in fetal and infant lambs. *Life Sci.* **27**: 1429–1433.

GLUCKMAN, P. D., GRUMBACH, M. M. and KAPLAN, S. L. (1981) The neuroendocrine regulation and function of growth hormone and prolactin in the mammalian fetus. *Endocr. Rev.* **2**: 363–395.

GLUCKMAN, P. D., MARTI-HENNEBERG, C., KAPLAN, S. L. and GRUMBACH, M. M. (1983) Hormone ontogeny in the ovine fetus: XIV. The effect of 17β-estradiol infusion on fetal plasma gonadotropins and prolactin and the maturation of sex steroid-dependent negative feedback. *Endocrinology* **112**: 1618–1623.

GLYDON, R. S. (1957) The development of the blood supply of the pituitary in the albino rat with special reference to the portal vessels. *J. Anat. London.* **91**: 237–244.

GOLDMAN, A. S. (1970) Virilization of the external genitalia of the female rat fetus by dehydroepiandrosterone. *Endocrinology* **87**: 432–435.

GOLDMAN, A. S. and BAKER, M. K. (1971) Androgenicity in the rat fetus of metabolites of testosterone and antagonism by cyproterone acetate. *Endocrinology* **89**: 276–280.

GOLDMAN, A. S., BAKER, M. K., CHEN, J. C. and WIELAND, R. G. (1972) Blockade of masculine differentiation in male rat fetuses by maternal injection of antibodies to testosterone-3-bovine serum albumin. *Endocrinology* **90**: 716–721.

GOLDMAN, A. S., SHAPIRO, B. H. and NEUMANN, F. (1976) Role of testosterone and its metabolites in the differentiation of the mammary gland in rats. *Endocrinology* **99**: 1490–1495.

GOODFELLOW, P., BANTING, G., SHEER, D., ROPERS, H. H., CAINE, A., FERGUSON-SMITH, M. A., POVEY, S. and VOSS, R. (1983) Genetic evidence that a Y-linked gene in man is homologous to a gene on the X chromosome. *Nature* **302**: 346–349.

GOODYER, C. G., HALL, C. St. G., GUYDA, H., ROBERT, F. and GIROUD, C. J.-P. (1977) Human fetal pituitary in culture: hormone secretion and response to somatostatin, luteinizing hormone releasing factor, thyrotropin releasing factor and dibutyryl cyclic AMP. *J. Clin. Endocr. Metab.* **45**: 73–85.

GOWEN, J. W. (1961) Genetic and cytologic foundations for sex. In: *Sex and Internal Secretion*, Vol. I., Young, W. C. (Ed.), Williams & Wilkins Co., Baltimore, MD, pp. 3–75.

GOY, R. W. and PHOENIX, C. H. (1971) The effects of testosterone propionate administered before birth on the development of behavior in genetic female rhesus monkeys. In: *Steroid Hormones and Brain Functions*, Sawyer, C. and Gorski, R. (Eds), University of California Press, Berkeley, California, pp. 193–202.

GOY, R., BRIDSON, W. and YOUNG, W. (1964) Period of maximal susceptibility of the prenatal guinea pig to masculinizing actions of testosterone propionate. *J. Comp. Physiol. Psychol.* **57**: 166–174.

GREENBERG, A. H., CZERNICHOW, P., REBA, R. C., TYSON, J. and BLIZZARD, R. M. (1970) Observations on the maturation of thyroid function in early fetal life. *J. Clin. Invest.* **49**: 1790–1803.

GREENE, R. R., BURRILL, M. W. and IVY, A. C. (1939a) Experimental intersexuality: the effects of antenatal androgens on sexual development of female rats. *Am. J. Anat.* **65**: 415–469.

GREENE, R. R., BURRILL, M. W. and IVY, A. C. (1939b) Progesterone is androgenic. *Endocrinology* **24**: 351–357.

GREENE, R. R., BURRILL, M. W. and IVY, A. C. (1939c) Experimental intersexuality: modification of sexual development of the white rat with a synthetic estrogen. *Proc. Soc. Exp. Biol. Med.* **41:** 169–170.

GREENE, R. R., BURRILL, M. W. and IVY, A. C. (1939d) Experimental intersexuality. The paradoxical effects of estrogens on the sexual development of the female rat. *Anat. Rec.* **74:** 429–438.

GREENE, R. R., BURRILL, M. W. and IVY, A. C. (1940) Experimental intersexuality: the effects of estrogens on the antenatal sexual development of the rat. *Am. J. Anat.* **67:** 305–345.

GREENE, R. R., BURRILL, M. W. and IVY, A. C. (1941) Experimental intersexuality: the effects of combined estrogens and androgens on the embryonic sexual development of the rat. *J. Exp. Zool.* **87:** 211–232.

GREENGARD, O. (1975) Cortisol treatment of neonatal rats: effects on enzymes in kidney, liver and heart. *Biol. Neonate* **27:** 352–360.

GREENMAN, D. L. and DELONGCHAMP, R. R. (1986) Interactive responses to diethylstilboestrol in C3H mice. *Food Chem. Toxicol.* **24:** 931–934.

GREENMAN, D. L., HIGHMAN, R. and CHEN, J. J., SCHIEFERSTEIN, G. J., NORVELL, M. J. (1986) Influence of age on induction of mammary tumors by diethylstilbestrol in C3H/HeN mice with low murine mammary tumor virus titer. *J. Nat. Cancer Inst.* **77:** 891–898.

GREENMAN, D. L., KODELL, R. L., HIGHMAN, B., SCHIEFERSTEIN, G. J. and NORVELL, M. J. (1987) Mammary tumorigenesis in C3H/HeN-MTV mice treated with diethylstilboestrol for varying periods. *Food Chem. Toxicol.* **25:** 229–232.

GRINSTED, J. (1982) Influence of mesonephros on foetal and neonatal rabbit gonads. II. Sex-steroid release by the ovary *in vitro. Acta Endocr. (Copenh.)* **99:** 281–287.

GRINSTED, J., BYSKOV, A. G., CHRISTENSEN, I. J. and JENSENIUS, J. C. (1982) Influence of mesonephros on foetal and neonatal rabbit gonads. I. Sex-steroid release by the testis *in vitro. Acta Endocr. (Copenh.)* **99:** 272–280.

GROOM, G. V. and BOYNS, A. R. (1973) Effect of hypothalamic releasing factors and steroids on release of gonadotrophins by organ cultures of human foetal pituitaries. *J. Endocr.* **59:** 511–522.

GROOM, G. V., GROOM, M. A., COOKE, I. D. and BOYNS, A. R. (1971) The secretion of immuno-reactive luteinizing hormone and follicle stimulating hormone by the human foetal putuitary in organ culture. *J. Endocr.* **49:** 335–344.

GRUMBACH, M. M. and DUCHARME, R. (1960) The effects of androgens on fetal sexual development: androgen-induced female pseudohermaphroditism. *Fertil. Steril.* **11:** 157–180.

GRUMBACH, M. M. and KAPLAN, S. L. (1973) Ontogenesis of growth hormone, insulin, prolactin and gonadotropin secretion in the human fetus. In: *Foetal and Neonatal Physiology*, Comline, R. S., Cross, K. W., Dawes, G. D. and Nathanielsz, P. W. (Eds), Cambridge University Press, Cambridge, pp. 462–487.

GRUMBACH, M. M., DUCHARME, R. and MOLOSHOK, R. E. (1959) On the fetal masculinization action of certain oral progestins. *J. Clin. Endocr. Metab.* **19:** 1369–1380.

GULYAS B. J., TULLNER, W. W. and HODGEN, G. D. (1977) Fetal or maternal hypophysectomy in rhesus monkeys (*Macaca mulatta*): effects on the development of testes and ohter endocrine organs. *Biol. Reprod.* **17:** 650–660.

HADZISELIMOVIC, F. and GUGGENHEIM, R. (1980) Transmission and scanning electron microscopy of epididymis in male mice receiving estrogen during gestation. *Acta Biol. Acad. Sci. Hung.* **31:** 133–140.

HAGEN, C. and McNEILLY, A. S. (1975) Identification of human luteinizing hormone, follide-stimulating hormone, luteinizing hormone β-subunit and gonadotrophin α-subunit in foetal and adult pituitary gland. *J. Endocr.* **67:** 49–57.

HAGEN, C. and McNEILLY, A. S. (1977) The gonadotrophins and their subunits in foetal pituitary glands and circulation. *J. Steroid. Biochem.* **8:** 537–544.

HAGLER, S. A., SCHULTZ, A., HANKIN, H. and KUNSTADTER, R. H. (1964) Fetal effects of steroid therapy during pregnancy. *Am. J. Dis. Child.* **106:** 586–590.

HANSSON, C. G. and ANGERVALL, L. (1966) The parathyroids in corticosteroid-treated pregnant rats and their offspring. II. Effect of deoxycorticosterone acetate (DOCA). *Acta Endocr. (Copenh.)* **53:** 553–560.

HAOUR, F. and SAXENA, B. B. (1974) Detection of a gonadotropin in rabbit blastocyst before implantation. *Science* **185:** 444–445.

HARLAP, S. and ELDOR, J. (1980) Births following oral contraceptive failures. *Obstet. Glynec.* **55:** 447–452.

HARLAP, S., PRYWES, R. and DAVIES, A. M. (1975) Birth defects and oestrogens and progesterones in pregnancy. *Lancet* **1:** 682–683.

HATCHER, R. A. and CONRAD, C. C. (1971) Adenocarcinoma of the vagina and stilbestrol as a "morning-after" pill. *N. Engl. J. Med.* **285:** 1264–1265.

HAUSER, H. and GANDELMAN, R. (1983) Contiguity to males in utero affects avoidance responding in adult female mice. *Science* **220:** 437–438.

HAYASHI, M., SHIMA, H., HAYASHI, K., TRELSTAD, R. L. and DONAHOE, P. K. (1984) Immunocytochemical localization of Müellerian inhibiting substance in the rough endoplasmic recticulum and Golgi apparatus in Sertoli cells of the neonatal calf testis using a monoclonal antibody. *J. Histochem. Cytochem.* **32:** 649–654.

HAYLES, A. B. and NOLAN, R. B. (1957) Female pseudohermaphroditism: Report of case in an infant born of a mother receiving methyltestosterone during pregnancy. *Proc. Staff. Mayo Clin.* **32:** 41–44.

HAYLES, A. B. and NOLAN, R. B. (1958) Masculinization of female fetus, possibly related to administration of progesterone during pregnancy. *Proc. Staff. Mayo Clin.* **33:** 200–203.

HENDERSON, B. E., BENTON, B. D. A., WEAVER, P. T., LINDEN, G. and WOLAN, J. F. (1973) Stilbestrol and urogenital-tract cancer in adolsescents and young adults. *New. Eng. J. Med.* **288:** 354–356.

HERBST, A. L., ULFELDER, H. and POSKANZER, D. C. (1971) Adenocarcinoma of the vagina. Association of maternal stilbestrol therapy with tumor appearance in young women. *N. Engl. J. Med.* **284:** 878–881.

HERBST, A. L., KURMAN, R. J. and SCULLY, R. E. (1972) Vaginal and cervical abnormalities after exposure to stilbestrol in utero. *Obstet. Gynecol.* **40:** 287–298.

HERBST, A. L., POSKANZER, D. C., ROBBOY, S. J., FRIEDLANDER, L. and SCULLY, P. E. (1975) Prenatal exposure to stilbestrol: A prospective comparison of exposed female offspring with unexposed controls. *N. Engl. J. Med.* **292:** 334–339.

HERBST, A. L., ANDERSON, S., HUBBY, M. M, HAENSZEL, W. M., KAUFMAN, R. H. and NOLLER, K. L. (1986) Risk factors for the development of diethylstilbestrol associated clear cell adenocarcinoma: a case-control study. *Am. J. Obstet. Gynecol.* **154:** 814–822.

HERTIG, A. T., ROCK, J. and ADAMS, J. C. (1956) A description of 34 human ova within the first 17 days of development. *Am. J. Anat.* **98:** 435–493.

HILL, D. E. (1976) Insulin and fetal growth. In: *Diabetes and Other Endocrin Disorders During Pregnancy and in the Newborn*, Alan, R. Liss, New York, NY, pp. 127–139.

HIROSE, T. (1977) Cortisol and corticosterone productions of isolated adrenal cells in neonatal rabbits. *Acta Endocr. (Copenh.)* **84:** 349–356.

HITZEMAN, Str., J. W. (1962) Development of enzyme activity in the Leydig cells of the mouse. *Anat. Rec.* **143:** 351–362.

HOBSON, B. and WIDE, L. (1975) Relationship of the sex of the foetus to the amount of human chorionic gonadotrophin in placentae; single and dizygotic twin placentae compared. *J. Endocr.* **64:** 117–123.

HORWITZ, R. I., VISCOLI, C. M., MARINO, M., BRENNAN, Ta., FLANNERY, J. T. and ROBBOY, S. J. (1988) Clear cell adenocarcinoma of the vagina and cerfix: incidence, undetected disease, and diethylstilbestrol. *J. Clin. Epidemiol.* **41:** 593–597.

HUFF, R. L. and EIK-NESS, K. B. (1966) Metabolism *in vitro* of acetate and certain steroids by six-day-old rabbit blastocysts. *J. Reprod. Fertil.* **11:** 57–63.

HUGHES, W. (1929) The free martin condition in swine. *Anat. Rec.* **41**: 213–245.

HUHTANIEMI, I. (1977) Studies on steroidogenesis and its regulation in human fetal adrenal and testis. *J. Steroid Biochem.* **8**: 491–497.

HUHTANIEMI, I., IKONEN, M. and VIHKO, R. (1970) Presence of testosterone and other neutral steroid in human fetal testes. *Biochem. Biophys. Res. Commun.* **38**: 715–720.

HUHTANIEMI, I. T., KORENBROT, C. C. and JAFFE, R. B. (1977) HCG binding and stimulation of testosterone biosynthesis in the human fetal testis. *J. Clin. Endocr. Metab.* **44**: 963–967.

HUHTANIEMI, I. T., KORITNIK, D. R., KORENBROT, C. C., MENNIN, S., FOSTER, D. B. and JAFFE, R. B. (1979) Stimulation of pituitary-testicular function with gonadotropin-releasing hormone in fetal and infant monkeys. *Endocrinology* **105**: 109–114.

HUNTER, R. H. F., BAKER, T. G. and COOK, B. (1982) Morphology, histology and steroid hormones of the gonads in intersex pigs. *J. Reprod. Fertil.* **64**: 217–222.

HURLEY, T. W., D'ERCOLE, A. J., HANDWERGER, S., UNDERWOOD, L. E., FURLANETTO, R. W. and FELLOWS, R. E. (1977) Ovine placental lactogen induces somatomedin: a possible role in fetal growth. *Endocrinology* **101**: 1635–1638.

HUTSON, J. M. and DONAHOE, P. K. (1983) Is Müllerian inhibiting substance a circulating hormone in the chick quail *Coturnix coturnix japonica* a chimera? *Endocrinology* **113**: 1470–1475.

HUTSON, J., IKAWA, H. and DONAHOE, P. K. (1981) The ontogeny of Müllerian inhibiting substance in the gonads of the chicken. *J. Pediatr. Surg.* **16**: 822–827.

HYYPPA, M. (1972) Hypothalamic monoamines in human fetuses. *Neuroendocrinology* **9**: 257–266.

IGUCHI, T. and TAKASUGI, N. (1986) Polyovular follicles in the ovary of immature mice exposed prenatally to diethylstilbestrol. *Anat. Embryol.* **175**: 53–55.

IGUCHI, T. and TAKASUGI, N. (1987) Postnatal development of uterine abnormalities in mice exposed to DES in utero. *Biol. Neonate* **52**: 97–103.

IGUCHI, T., TAKASE, M. and TAKASUGI, N. (1986a) Development of vaginal adenosis-like lesions and uterine epithelial stratification in mice exposed perinatally to diethylstilbestrol. *Proc. Soc. Exp. Biol. Med.* **181**: 59–65.

IGUCHI, T., TAKEI, T., TAKASE, M. and TAKASUGI, N. (1986b) Estrogen participation in induction of cervicovaginal adenosis-like lesions in immature mice exposed prenatally to diethylstilbestrol. *Acta Anat.* **127**: 110–114.

IKONEN, M. and NIEMI, M. (1966) Metabolism of progesterone and 17α-hydroxypregnenolone by the foetal human testis "in vitro". *Nature* **212**: 716–717.

ISHIKAWA, H., SHIINO, M. and RENNELS, E. G. (1977) Effects of fetal brain extract on the growth and differentiation of rat pituitary anlage cells. *Proc. Soc. Exp. Biol. Med.* **155**: 511–515.

JACOBS, P. A. and STRONG, J. A. (1959) A case of human intersexuality having a possible XXY sex-determining mechanism. *Nature* **183**: 302–303.

JACOBSON, D. B. (1961) Abortion: its prediction and managment: clinical experience with norlutin. *Fertil. Steril.* **12**: 474–485.

JAFFE, R., YUEN, B., KEYE, W. and MIDGLEY, A. R. (1973) Physiology and pathologic profiles of circulating human prolactin. *Am. J. Obstet. Gynec.* **117**: 757–773.

JAFFE, R. B., SERÓN-FERRÉ, M., CRICKARD, K., KORITNIK, D., MITCHELL, B. F. and HUHTANIEMI, I. P. (1981) Regulation and function of the primate fetal adrenal gland and gonad *Rec. Prog. Horm. Res.* **37**: 41–103.

JANERICH, D. T., PIPER, J. M. and GLEBATIS, D. M. (1974) Oral contraceptives and congenital limb-reduction defects. *N. Engl. J. Med.* **291**: 697–700.

JEAN, C. (1971a) Analyse des malformations mammaires du nouveau né provoquées par l'injection d'oestrogenes à la mère gravide chez le rat et la souris. *Arch. Anat. Micr. Morphol. Exper.* **60**: 147–168.

JEAN, C. (1971b) Developpement mammaire post-natal de la souris issue de mère traitée par l'oestradiol pendant la gestation. *Arch. Sci. Physiol.* **25**: 145–185.

JEAN, C. and DELOST, P. (1964) Atrophie de la glande mammaire des descendants adultes issus de mères traitées par les oestrogenos au cours de la gestation chez la souris. *J. Physiol. (Paris)* **56**: 377–384.

JENKINS, J. S. and HALL, C. J. (1977) Metabolism of (14C) testosterone by human foetal and adult brain tissue. *J. Endocr.* **74:** 425–429.

JIRÁSEK, J. E. (1962) Die verteilung der Urgeschlechtszellen in den Keimdrusen menschlicher Fetus. Eine histomezymologische Studie. *Acta Histochem (Jena)* **13:** 220–225.

JIRÁSEK, J. E. (1967) The relationship between the structure of the testis and differentiation of the external genitalia and phenotype in man. *Ciba Found Colloq. Endocr.* **16:** 3–27.

JIRÁSEK, J. E. (1971) Development of the genital system and male pseudohermaphroditism. Cohen, M. (Eds), The Johns Hopkins Press, Baltimore, MD.

JIRÁSEK, J. E. (1977) Morphogenesis of the genital system in the human. In: *Morphogenesis and Malformations of the Genital System*, Blandau, R. S. and Bergsma, D. (Eds), The National Foundation March of Dimes. Birth Defects: Original Article Series, Vol. XIII, Alan, R. Liss, New York.

JIRÁSEK, J. E. (1983) *Atlas of Human Prenatal Morphogenesis*, M. Nijhoff Publishers, Boston.

JIRÁSEK, J. E. (1985) Prenatal development: growth and differentiation. In: *Gynecology and Obstetrics*, Sciarra, J. W. (Ed.), Harper and Row, Philadelphia, Vol. 2, Ch. 14, pp. 1–12.

JIRÁSEK, J. E. (1988) *Human Sex Differentiation: Gonadal Histogenesis*. The 1987 Distinghished Visiting Professorship Lectures, University of Tennessee, Memphis, pp. 69–79.

JOHNSON, L. D., DRISCOLL, S. G., HERTIG, A. T., COLE, P. T. and NICKERSON, R. J. (1979) Vaginal adenosis in stillborns and neonates exposed to diethylstilbestrol and steroidal estrogens and progestins. *Obstet. Gynecol.* **53:** 671–679.

JONES, H. W. and WILKINS, L. (1960) The genital anomaly associated with prenatal exposure to progestogens. *Fertil. Steril.* **11:** 148–156.

JOSIMOVICH, J. B. (1974) Passage of hormones through the placenta. In: *Handbook of Physiology, Endocrinology II*, Part 2, The Physiological Society, Washington DC, pp. 277–284.

JOSSO, N. (1970) Action of testosterone in the Wolffian duct of the rat fetus in organ culture. *Arch. Anat. Microsc. Morphol. Exp.* **59:** 37–50.

JOSSO, N. (1971) Interspecific character of the Müllerian-inhibiting substance action of the human fetal testis, ovary and adrenal on the fetal rat Müllerian ducts in organ culture. *J. Clin. Endocr. Metab.* **32:** 404–409.

JOSSO, N. (1972) Permeability of membranes to the Müllerian-inhibiting substance synthesized by the human fetal testis *in vitro*. A clue to its biochemical nature. *J. Clin. Endocr. Metab.* **34:** 265–270.

JOSSO, N. (1973) *In vitro* synthesis of Müllerian-inhibiting hormone by seminiferous tubules isolated from the calf fetal testis. *Endocrinology* **93:** 829–834.

JOSSO, N. (1974) Müllerian-inhibiting activity of human fetal testicular tissue deprived of germ cells by *in vitro* irradiation. *Pediat. Res.* **8:** 755–758.

JOSSO, N., PICARD, J. Y. and TRAN, D. (1977) The anti-Müllerian hormone. In: *Morphogenesis and Malformations of the Genital System*. Blandau, R. J. and Bergsma, D. (Eds), The National Foundation March of Dimes. Birth Defects: Original Article Series, Vol. XIII, Alan R. Liss, New York.

JOSSO, N., VIGIER, B., TRAN, D. and PICARD, J. Y. (1985) Initiation of production of anti-Müllerian hormone by the fetal gonad. *Arch. d'Anat. Micr. Morph. Exper.* **74:** 96–100.

JOST, A. (1947) Recherches sur la différentiation sexuelle de l'embryon de Lapin. III. Rôle des gonades foetales dans la differenciation somatique. *Arch. Anat. Micr. Morphol. Exper.* **36:** 271–316.

JOST, A. (1953) Problems of fetal endocrinology: the gonadal and hypophyseal hormones. *Rec. Prog. Horm. Res.* **8:** 379–418.

JOST, A. (1966) Problems of fetal endocrinology: the adrenal glands. *Rec. Prog. Horm Res.* **22:** 541–574.

JOST, A. (1972a) Use of androgen antagonists and antiandrogens in studies on sex differentiation. *Gynec. Invest.* **2:** 180–201.

JOST, A. (1972b) Données préliminaires sur les stades initiaux de la differentiation du testicule chez le rat. *Arch. Anat. Micr. Morphol. Exper.* **61:** 415–438.

JOST, A., VIGIER, B., PRÉPIN, J. and PERCHELLET, J. P. (1973) Studies on sex differentiation in mammals. *Rec. Prog. Horm. Res.* **29:** 1–41.

KADONAGA, J. T., CARNER, K. R., MASIAR, F. R. and TJIAN, R. (1987) Isolation of cDNA encoding transcription factor Sp1 and functional analysis of the DNA binding domain. *Cell* **51:** 1079–1090.

KAJIHARA, A., KOJIMA, A., ONAYA, T., TAKEMURA, Y. and YAMADA, T. (1972) Placental transport of thyrotropin releasing factor in the rat. *Endocrinology* **90:** 592–594.

KAPLAN, N. M. (1959) Male pseudohermaphroditism: report of a case with observation of pathogenesis. *N. Engl. J. Med.* **261:** 641–644.

KAPLAN, S. L., GRUMBACH, M. M. and AUBERT, M. L. (1976a) The ontogenesis of pituitary hormones and hypothalamic factors in the human fetus: maturation of central nervous system regulation of anterior pituitary function. *Rec. Prog. Horm. Res.* **32:** 161–243.

KAPLAN, S. L., GRUMBACH, M. M. and AUBERT, M. L. (1976b) α- and β-glycoprotein hormone subunits (hLH, hFSH, hCG) in the serum and pituitary of the human fetus. *J. Clin. Endocr. Metab.* **42:** 995–998.

KAUFMAN, R. H. and ADAM, E. (1978) Genital tract anomalies associated with in utero exposure to diethylstilbestrol. *Isr. J. Med. Sci.* **14:** 353–362.

KELLER, K. and TANDLER, J. (1916) Uber das Verhalten der Eihaute bei der Zwillingstrachtigkeit des Rindes. *Mschr. Ver. Tierarztl. Ost.* **3:** 513–519.

KELLY, S. J. (1977) Studies of the developmental potentional of 4- and 8-cell mouse blastomers. *J. Exp. Zool.* **200:** 365–376.

KERVRAN, A. and GIRARD, J. R. (1974) Glucose-induced increase of plasma insulin in the rat foetus in utero. *Endocrinology* **62:** 545–551.

KESERU, T. L., MARAZ, A. and SZABO, J. (1974) Oral contraception and sex ratio at birth. *Lancet* **1:** 369.

KHODR, G. S. and SILER-KHODR, T. M. (1980) Placental luteinizing hormone-releasing factor and its synthesis. *Science* **207:** 315–317.

KHORRAM, O., DEPALATIS, L. R. and McCANN, S. M. (1984) Hypothalamic control of prolactin secretion during the perinatal period in the rat. *Endocrinology* **115:** 1698–1704.

KIM, C. K., YEN, S. S. C. and BENIRSCHKE, K. (1972) Serum testosterone in fetal cattle. *Gen. Comp. Endocr.* **18:** 404–407.

KIMURA, T. (1975) Persistent vaginal cornification in mice treated with estrogen prenatally. *Endocr. Japon* **22:** 497–502.

KIMURA, T., KAWASHIMA, S. and NISHIZUKA, Y. (1980) Effects of prenatal treatment with estrogen on mitotic activity of vaginal anlage cells in mice. *Endocr. Japon* **27:** 739–745.

KINCL, F. A. (1989) Hormone toxicity in the newborn. In: *Monographs on Endocrinology*, Vol. 31, Gross, F., Grumbach, M. M., Labhart, A., Mann, T. and Zander J. (Eds), Springer-Verlag, Berlin, Heidelberg, New York.

KINCL, F. A. and DORFMAN, R. I. (1962) Influence of progestational agents on the genetic female foetus of orally treated pregnant rats. *Acta Endocr (Copenh)* **41:** 274–279.

KING, K. C., BUTT, J., RAIVIC, K., RAIHA, N., ROUX, J., TERAMO, K., YAMAGUCHI, K. and SCHWARTZ, R. (1971) Human maternal and fetal insulin response to arginine. *N. Engl. J. Med.* **285:** 607–612.

KISER, T. E., CONVEY, E. M., LIN, Y. C. and OXENDER, W. D. (1975) Luteinizing hormone and androgens in the bovine fetus after gonadotropin-releasing hormone. *Proc. Soc. Exp. Biol. Med.* **149:** 785–789.

KOIKE, S. and JOST, A. (1982) Precocious production of Müllerian inhibitor by the rabbit fetal testis. *C. R. Seances Acad. Sci. Ser. III Sci.* **295:** 701–706.

LAMB, J. C. IV, NEWBOLD, N. N. and McLACHLAN, J. A. (1981) Visualization by light and scanning electron microscopy of reproductive tract lesions in female mice treated transplacentally with diethylstilbestrol. *Cancer Res.* **41:** 4057–4062.

LANIER, A. P., NOLLER, K. L., DECKER, D. G., ELVEBACK, L. R. and KURLAND, L. T. (1973) Cancer and stilbestrol: A follow-up of 1,719 persons exposed to estrogens *in utero* and born 1943–1959. *Mayo Clin. Proc.* **48:** 793–799.

LEARY, F. J., RESSEGUIE, L. J., KURLAND, L. T., O'BRIEN, P. C., EMSLANDER, R. F. and NOLLER K. L. (1984) Males exposed in utero to diethylstilbestrol. *J. Am. Med. Assoc.* **252:** 2984–2989.

LEE, J. B. (1974) Prostaglandins and the renal antihypertensive and natriuretic endocrine function. *Rec. Prog. Horm. Res.* **30:** 481–532.

LEISTI, L., MILLER, W. L. and JOHNSON, L. K. (1982) Synthesis of growth hormone prolactin and proopiomelanocortin by ovine fetal anterior and neurointermediate lobes. *Endocrinology* **111:** 1368–1375.

LEONTIC, E. A., SCHRUEFER, J. J., ANDREASSEN, B., PINTO, H. and TYSON, J. E. (1979) Further evidence for the role of prolactin on human fetoplacental osmoregulation. *Am. J. Obstet. Gynec.* **133:** 435–438.

LERNER, L. T., PHILIPPO, M., YIACS, E., BRENNAN, D. and BORMAN, A. (1962) Comparison of the acetophenone derivatives of 16-17-dihydroxyprogesterone with other progestational steroids for masculinization of the rat fetus. *Endocrinology* **71:** 448–451.

LEVINA, S. E. (1968) Endocrine features in development of human hypothalamus, hypophysis and placenta. *Gen. Comp. Endocr.* **11:** 151–159.

LEVINA, S. E. (1972) Times of appearance of LH and FSH activities in human fetal circulation. *Gen. Comp. Endocr.* **19:** 242–246.

LILLIE, F. R. (1916) The theory of the free-martin. *Science, NY* **43:** 611–613.

LILLIE, F. R. (1917) The free-martin, a study of action of the sex hormones in the foetal life of cattle. *J. Exp. Zool.* **23:** 371–451.

LIMONTA, P., DONDI, D., MAGGI, R., MARTINI, L. and PIVA, F. (1989) Neonatal organization of the brain opioid systems controlling prolactin and luteinizing hormone secretion. *Endocrinology* **124:** 681–686.

LINKIE, D. M. and NISWENDER, G. D. (1972) Serum levels of prolactin luteinizing hormone, and follicle stimulating hormone during pregnancy in the rat. *Endocrinology* **90:** 632–637.

LIPSETT, M. C. and TULLNER, W. W. (1965) Testosterone synthesis by the fetal rabbit gonad. *Endocrinology* **77:** 273–277.

LLANOS, A. J., RAMACHANDRAN, J., CREASY, R. K., RUDOLPH, A. M. and SÉRON-FERRÉ, M. (1979) α-Melanocyte-stimulating hormone and adrenocorticotropin in the regulation of glucocorticoid secretion during the perinatal period in sheep. *Endocrinology* **105:** 613–617.

LOWREY, G. H., ASTER, R. H., CARR, E. A., ROMAN, G., BEIERWALTES, W. H. and SPAFFORD, N. R. (1958) Early diagnostic criteria of congenital hypothyroidism: a comprehensive study of forty-nine cretins. *Am. J. Dis. Child.* **96:** 131–143.

LYON, M. F. (1972) X-chromosome inactivation and developmental patterns in mammals. *Biol. Rev.* **47:** 1–35.

MACHO, L. (1979) Development of thyroid and adrenal functions during ontogenesis. *Treatises on Medicine* **XVI/I,** VEDA, Slovak Academy of Sciences, Bratislava, Czechoslovakia, pp. 1–145.

MADILL, D., BASSETT, J. M. (1973) Corticosteroid release by adrenal tissue from foetal and newborn lambs in response to corticotrophin stimulation in a perifusion system *in vitro. J. Endocr.* **58:** 75–87.

MAGRE, S. and DUPOUY, J.-P. (1973) Étude cytochimique de l'adénohypophyse foetale du rat. *Arch. d'Anat. Micr. Morph. Exp.* **62:** 217–232.

MAIER, D. B., NEWBOLD, R. R. and McLACHLAN, J. A. (1985) Prenatal diethylstilbestrol exposure alters murine uterine responses to prepubertal estrogen stimulation. *Endocrinology* **116:** 1878–1886.

MATSUMOTO, A. and ARAI, Y. (1981) Effect of androgen on sexual differentiation of synaptic organization in the hypothalamic arcuate nucleus: An ontogenetic study. *Neuroendocrinology* **33**: 166–169.

MATSUZAKI, F., IRIE, M. and SHIZUME, K. (1971) Growth hormone in human fetal pituitary glands and cord blood. *J. Clin. Endocr.* **33**: 908–911.

McCLUNG, C. E. (1902) The accessory chromosome-sex determinant? *Biol. Bull.* **3**: 43–84.

McEVOY, R. C. and MADSON, K. L. (1980) Pancreatic insulin-, glucagon- and somatostatin-positive islet cell populations during the perinatal development of the rat. I. Morphometric quantitation. *Biol. Neonate* **38**: 248–254.

McEWEN, B. S., LIEBERBURG, I., CHAPTAL, C. and KREY, L. C. (1977) Aromatization: important for sexual differentiation of the neonatal rat brain. *Horm. Behav.* **9**: 249–263.

McGREGOR, W. G., KUHN, R. W. and JAFFE, R. B. (1983) Biologically active chorionic gonadotropin: synthesis by the human fetus. *Science* **220**: 306–308.

McLACHLAN, J. A. (1977) Prenatal exposure to diethylstilbestrol in mice: toxicological studies. *J. Toxicol. Env. Health.* **2**: 527–537.

McLACHLAN, J. A., NEWBOLD, R. R. and BULLOCK, B. (1975) Reproductive tract lesions in male mice exposed prenatally to diethylstilbestrol. *Science* **190**: 991–992.

McLACHLAN, J. A., NEWBOLD, R. R. and BULLOCK, B. C. (1980) Long-term effects on the female mouse genital tract associated with prenatal exposure to diethylsilbestrol. *Cancer Res.* **40**: 3988–3999.

McNEILLY, A. S., GILMORE, D., DOBBIE, G. and CHARD, T. (1977) Prolactin releasing activity in the early human foetal hypothalamus. *J. Endocr.* **73**: 533–534.

MELMED, S., HARADA, A., MURATA, Y., SOCOL, M., REED, A., CARLSON, H. E., AZUK-IZAWA, M., MARTIN, C., JORGENSEN, E. and HERSHMAN, J. M. (1979) Fetal response to thyrotropin-releasing hormone after thyroid hormone administration to the rhesus monkey: lack of pituitary suppression. *Endocrinology* **105**: 334–341.

MILEWICH, L., GEORGE, F. W. and WILSON, J. D. (1977) Estrogen formation by the ovary of the rabbit embryo. *Endocrinology* **100**: 187–196.

MILLER, J., McLACHIAN, A. D. and KLUG, A. (1985) Repetitive zinc-binding domains in the protein transcription factor IIIA from *Xenopus oocytes*. *EMBO J.* **41**: 1609–1614.

MILNER, R. D. G. and HALES, C. N. (1965) Effect of intravenous glucose on concentration of insulin in arterial and umbilical-cord plasma. *Br Med. J.* **i**: 284–286.

MILNER, R. D. G., ASHWORTH, M. A. and BARSON, A. J. (1972) Insulin release from human fetal pancreas in response to glucose, leucine, and arqinine. *J. Endocr.* **52**: 497–505.

MINTZ, D. H., CHEZ, R. A. and HORGER, E. O. (1969) Fetal insulin and growth hormone metabolism in the sub-human primate. *J. Clin. Invest.* **48**: 176–186.

MOORE, C. R. (1939) Modification of sex development in the opposum by sex hormones. *Proc. Soc. Exp. Biol. Med.* **40**: 544–546.

MORGAN, T. H. (1910) Sex-limited inheritance in *Drosophila*. *Science* **32**: 120–122.

MOTT, J. C. (1975) The place of the renin-angiotensin system before and after birth. *Br. Med. Bull.* **31**: 44–50.

MUELLER, P. L., GLUCKMAN, P. D., KAPLAN, S. L., GRUMBACH, A. M. and GRUMBACH, M. M. (1979) Hormone ontogeny in the ovine fetus. V. Circulating prolactin in mid- and late gestation and the newborn. *Endocrinology* **105**: 129–134.

MUELLER, P. L., SKLAR, C. A., GLUCKMAN, P. D., KAPLAN, S. L. and GRUMBACH, M. M. (1981) Hormone ontogeny in the ovine fetus. IX. Luteinizing hormone and follicle-stimulating hormone response to luteinizing hormone-releasing factor in mid- and late gestation and in the neonate. *Endocrinology* **108**: 881–886.

MULCAHEY, J. J., DiBLASIO, A. M., MARTIN, M. C., BLUMENFELD, Z. and JAFFE, R. B. (1987) Hormone production and peptide regulation of the human fetal pituitary gland. *Endocr. Rev.* **8**: 406–425.

MÜLLER, U., ASCHMONEIT, I., ZENZES, M. T. AND WOLF, U. (1978) Binding studies of H-Y antigen in rat tissues: indication for a gonad specific receptor. *Human Genet.* **43**: 151–157.

MURSET, G., ZACHMANN, M., PRADER, A., FISCHER, J. and LABHART, A. (1970) male external genitalia of a girl caused by a virilizing adrenal tumour in the mother. *Acta Endocr. (Copenh.)* **65**: 627–638.

NAFTOLIN, F., RYAN, K. J. and PETRO, Z. (1972) Aromatization of androstenedione by the anterior hypothalamus of adult male and female rats. *Endocrinology* **90**: 295–298.

NATAF, B. M. (1968) Fetal rat thyroid gland in organ culture. *Gen. Comp. Endocr.* **10**: 159–173.

NATHANIELSZ, P. W., ABEL, M. H., BASS, F. G., KRANE, E. J., THOMAS, A. C. and LIGGINS, G. C. (1978) Pituitary stalk-section and some of its effects on endocrine function in the fetal lamb. *Q. J. Exp. Physiol.* **63**: 211–219.

NECKLAWS, E. C., LaQUAGLIA, M. P., MacLAUGHLIN, D., HUDSON, P., MUDGETT-HUNTER, M. and DONAHOE, P. K. (1986) Detection of Müllerian inhibiting substance in biological samples by a solid phase sandwich radioimmunoassay. *Endocrinology* **118**: 791–796.

NEUMANN, F. and STEINBECK, H. (1974) Antiandrogens. In: *Handbook of Experimental Pharmacology*, Vol XXV/Z, Eichler, O., Farah, A., Herken, H. and Welch, A. D. (Eds), Springer Verlag, Heidelberg, pp. 1–484.

NEUMANN, F., ELGER, W. and STEINBECK, H. (1970) Effects of oral contraceptives on the fetus. *Lancet* **2**: 1258–1259.

NEWBOLD, R. R. and McLACHLAN, J. A. (1982) Vaginal adenosis and adenocarcinoma in mice exposed prenatally or neonatally to diethylstilbestrol. *Cancer Res.* **42**: 2003–2011.

NEWBOLD, R. R., SUZUKI, Y. and McLACHLAN, J. A. (1984) Müllerian duct maintenance in heterotypic organ culture after *in vivo* exposure to diethylstilbestrol. *Endocrinology* **115**: 1863–1868.

NIEMI, I. and IKONEN, M. (1962) Cytochemistry of oxidative enzyme systems in the Leydig cells of the rat testis and their functional significance. *Endocrinology* **70**: 167–174.

NOLLER, K. L. and FISH, C. R. (1974) Diethylstilbestrol usage: its interesting past, important present and questionable future. *Med. Clin. N. Am.* **58**: 793–810.

NOMURA, T. and KANZAKI, T. (1977) Induction of urogenital anomalies and some tumors in the progeny of mice receiving diethylstilbestrol during pregnancy. *Cancer Res.* **37**: 1099–1104.

NOMURA, T. and MASUDA, M. (1980) Carcinogenic and teratogenic activities of diethylstilbestrol in mice. *Life Sci.* **26**: 1955–1962.

NOMURA, T., WEISZ, J., LLOYD, C. W. (1966) *In vitro* conversion of 7-^{3}H-progesterone to androgen by the rat testis during the second half of fetal life. *Endocrinology* **78**: 245–253.

NORMAN, R. L. and SPIES, H. G. (1979) Effect of luteinizin hormone-releasing hormone on the pituitary-gonadal axis in fetal and infant rhesus monkeys. *Endocrinology* **105**: 655–659.

OBENSHAIN, S. S., ADAM, P. A. J., KING, K. C., TERAMO, K., RAIVIO, K. O., RÄIHÄ, N. and SCHWARTZ, R. (1969) Human fetal insulin response to sustained maternal hyperglycemia. *N. Engl. J. Med.* **285**: 566–569.

OECHSLI, F. W. (1974) Oral contraception and sex ratio at birth. *Lancet* **1**: 1004–1005.

OHNO, S. (1976) Major regulatory genes for mammalian sexual development. *Cell* **7**: 315–321.

ORTH, J. M. (1984) The role of follicle-stimulating hormone in controlling Sertoli cell proliferation in testes of fetal rats. *Endocrinology* **115**: 1248–1255.

ORTH, J. M., GUNSALUS, G. L. and LAMPERTI, A. A. (1988) Evidence from Sertoli cell-depleted rats indicates that spermatid number in adults depends on numbers of Sertoli cells produced during perinatal development. *Endocrinology* **122**: 787–794.

OSAMURA, R. Y. (1977) Functional prenatal development of anencephalic and normal anterior pituitary glands. *Acta Pathol. Japon* **27**: 495–502.

PAGE, D. C. (1988) Is ZFY the sex-determining gene on the human Y chromosome? *Phil. Trans. Roy. Soc. London B* **322**: 155–157.

PAGE, D. C., MOSHER, R., SIMPSON, E. M., FISHER, E. M. C., MARDON, G., POLLACK, J.,

McGILLIVRAY, B., DE LA CHAPELLE, A. and BROWN, L. G. (1987) The sex-determining region of the human Y chromosome encodes a finger protein. *Cell* **51**: 1091–1104.

PAINTER, T. (1923) Studies in mammalian spermatogenesis. II. The spermatogenesis of man. *J. Exp. Zool.* **37**: 291–335.

PARSONS, B., McEWEN, B. S. and PFAFF, D. W. (1982) A discontinuous schedule of estradiol treatment is sufficient to activate progesterone-facilitated feminine sexual behavior and to increase cytosol receptors for progestins in the hypothalamus of the rat. *Endocrinology* **110**: 613–619.

PARVIZI, N. (1986) Differential effects of catecholoestradiol-17β and oestradiol-17 on concentrations of plasma LH in the fetal pig. *J. Endocr.* **111**: 297–300.

PASQUALINI, J. R. and OJASOO, T. (1991) Hormone responses of the offspring after administration of hormones and anti-hormones during gestation, in humans and in different animal species. In: *Hormones and Fetal Pathophysiology*, Pasqualini, J. R. and Scholler, R. (Eds), Marcel Dekker Inc., New York, in press.

PASTEELS, J. L., BRAUMAN, H. and BRAUMAN, J. (1963) Etude compareé de la secrétion d'hormone somatotrope par l'hypophyse humaine *in vitro*, et de son activité lactogenique. *C. R. Acad. Sci. (Paris)* **256**: 2031–2039.

PASTEELS, J. L., GAUSSET, P., DANGUY, A. and ECTORS, F. (1974) Gonadotropin secretion by human foetal and infant pituitaries. In: *Endocrinologie Sexuelle de la Periode Perinatale. INSERM (Paris)*, **32**: 13–32.

PASTEELS, J. L., SHERIDAN, R., GASPAR, S. and FRANCHIMONT, P. (1977) Synthesis and release of gonadotropins and their subunits by long-term organ cultures of human fetal hypophyses. *Mol. Cell Endocr.* **9**: 1–19.

PAUL, D. H. and D'ANGELO, S. A. (1972) Dexamethasone and corticosterone administration to pregnant rats—effects on pituitary-adrenocortical function in the newborn. *Proc. Soc. Exp. Biol. Med.* **140**: 1360–1364.

PAVLOVA, F. G., PRONINA, T. S. and SKOBELSKAYA, Y. B. (1968) Histo-structure of adenohypophysis of human fetuses and contents of somatotropic and adrenocroticotropic hormones. *Gen. Comp. Endocr.* **10**: 269–276.

PAYNE, D. W. and KATZENELLENBOGEN, J. A. (1979) Binding specificity of rat α-fetoprotein for series of estrogen derivatives: studies using equilibrium and nonequilibrium binding techniques. *Endocrinology* **105**: 743–753.

PAZ, G. F., THILIVERIS, J. A., WINTER, J. S. D., REYES, F. I. and FAIMAN, C. (1980) Hormonal control of testosterone secretion by the fetal rat testis in organ culture. *Biol. Reprod.* **23**: 1087–1095.

PEARSE, A. G. E. and TAKOR, T. (1976) Neuroendocrine embryology and the APUD concept. *Clin. Endocrinol. Suppl.* **5**: 2295–2445.

PERLARDY, G. and DELOST, P. (1978) Secretion of the androgens in the male guinea-pig during the perinatal period. *Acta Endocr. (Copenh.)* **89**: 770–779.

PHOENIX, C. H., GOY, R. W., GERALL, A. A. and YOUNG, W. C. (1959) Organizing action of prenatally administered testosterone propionate on the tissues mediating mating behavior in the female guinea pig. *Endocrinology* **65**: 369–382.

PICARD, J.-Y. and JOSSO, N. (1980) Hormone anti-Müllérienne et lectines: nouvelles perspectives. *Ann. Endocr. (Paris)* **41**: 538–544.

PICARD, J. Y., TRAN, D. and JOSSO, N. (1978) Biosynthesis of labelled anti-Müllerian hormone by fetal testes: evidence for the glycoprotein nature of the hormone and for its disulfide-bonded structure. *Mol. Cell Endocr.* **12**: 17–30.

PICKERING, D. E. (1968) Thyroid physiology in the developing monkey fetus. *J. Gen. Comp. Endocr.* **10**: 182–190.

PICON, R. (1969) Action au testicule foetal sur de development *in vitro* des canaux de Müller chez le rat. *Arch. Anat. Micr. Morph. Exp.* **58**: 1–9.

PICON, R. (1976) Testosteone secretion by foetal rat testes *in vitro*. *J. Endocr.* **71**: 231–238.

PICON, R. and HABERT, R. (1981) A sensitive bioassay for luteinizing hormone-like activity applied to systemic plasma of foetal rats. *Acta Endocr. (Copenh.)* **97**: 176–180.

PIERSON, M., MALAPRADE, D., GRIGNON, G., HARTEMANN, P., BELLEVILLE, F., LEMOINE, D. and NABET, P. (1973) Etude de la sécrétion hyophysaire du foetus humain, corrélations entre morphologie et activité secretoire. *Ann. Endocr. (Paris)* **34**: 418–427.

PINCUS, G. (1956) Some effects of progesterone and related components upon reproduction and early development in mammals. *Acta Endocr. (Copenh.) Suppl.* **28**: 18–36.

PLAPINGER, L. and BERN, H. A. (1979) Adenosis-like lesions and other cervicovaginal abnormalities in mice treated perinatally with estrogen. *J. Natl. Cancer Inst.* **63**: 507–518.

POINTIS, G. and MAHOUDEAU, J. A. (1975) Influence des hormones gonadotropes de l'hypophyse foetale sur la production de testostérone par le testicule foetale de souris de 18 jours en culture organotypique. *C. R. Acad. Sci. (Paris)* **280**: 2361–2364.

POINTIS, G. and MAHOUDEAU, J. A. (1976) Demonstration of pituitary gonadotrophin hormone activity in the male foetal mouse. *Acta Endocr. (Copenh.)* **83**: 158–165.

POINTIS, G. and MAHOUDEAU, J. A. (1977) Responsiveness of foetal mouse testis to gonadotrophins at various times during sexual differentiation. *J. Endocr.* **74**: 149–150.

POINTIS, G., LATREILLE, M.-T. and CEDARD, L. (1980) Gonado-pituitary relationships in the fetal mouse at various times during sexual differentiation. *J. Endocr.* **86**: 483–488.

POLÁCKOVÁ M. and VOJTÍSKOVÁ, M. (1968) Inhibitory effect of early orchidectomy on the expression of the male antigen in mice. *Folia Biol. (Praha)* **14**: 93–100.

POLANI, P. E. (1979) Role of sex chromosomes in the determination and differentiation of sex in mammals. *Dev. Med. Child Neurol.* **21**: 249–263.

POLITZER, G. (1933) Die Keimbahn des Menschen. *Z. Anat. Entwicklungsgesch.* **100**: 331–361.

POLITZER, G. (1953) Die Entwicklung des Wolffischen Ganges beim Menschen. *Acta Anat.* **18**: 343–360.

POMERANCE, W. (1973) Post-stilbestrol secondary syndrome. *Obstet. Gynecol.* **42**: 12–17.

POMERANTZ, D. K. and NALBANDOV, K. (1975) Androgen levels in the sheep fetus during gestation. *Proc. Soc. Exp. Biol. Med.* **149**: 413–416.

PRICE, D., ORTIZ, E. and DEANE, H. W. (1964) The presence of Δ^5-3β-hydroxysteroid dehydrogenase in fetal guinea pig testes and adrenal glands. *Am. Zool.* **4**: 327.

PRICE, J. M., DONAHOE, P. K. and ITO, Y. (1979) Involution of the female Müllerian duct of the fetal rat in the organ culture assay for the detection of Müllerian inhibiting substance. *Am. J. Anat.* **156**: 265–283.

RAESIDE, J. I. and MIDDLETON, A. T. (1979) Development of testosterone secretion in the fetal pig testis. *Biol. Reprod.* **21**: 985–989.

RALL, L. B., PICTET, R. L. and RUTTER, W. J. (1979) Synthesis and accumulation of proinsulin and insulin during development of the embryonic rat pancreas. *Endocrinology* **105**: 835–841.

RAYNAUD, A. (1939a) Effect of estradiol dipropionate injected into mice during gestation. *C. R. Soc. Biol.* **130**: 872–875.

RAYNAUD, A. (1939b) Structure of the genital apparatus (gonads and ducts of Wolff and Müller) of male intersex mice obtained by the injection of estradiol dipropionate into the mother during gestation. *C. R. Soc. Biol.* **130**: 1012–1015.

RAYNAUD, A. (1942) Modification experimental de la différentiation sexuelle des embryons de souris, par action des hormones androgènes et oestrogènes. *Actual Scient. Indus.* Nos. 925, 926, Hermann Cie, Paris pp. 66–134.

RAYNAUD, A. (1947) Effect des injections d'hormones sexuelles à la souris gravide, sur le dévélopment des ébauches de la glande mammaire des embryones. L'action des substances androgènes. *Ann. Endocr. (Paris)* **8**: 248–253.

RAYNAUD, A. (1949) Nouvelles observations sur l'appareil mammaire des souris provenant de mères ayant reçu des injections de testostérone pendant la gestation. *Ann. d'Endocr. (Paris)* **10**: 54–62.

RAYNAUD, A. (1957) Sur le dévélopment et la différentiation sexuelle de l'appareil gubernaculaire du foetus de souris. *C. R. Acad. Sci.* **245**: 2100–2103.

RAYNAUD, A. (1958) Effects, sur l'appareil gubernaculaire des foetus, des hormones oestrogènes injectées à la souris gravide. *C. R. Soc. Biol.* **152:** 1461–1464.

REDDY, V. V. R., NAFTOLIN, F. and RYAN, K. J. (1974) Conversion of androstenedione to estrone by neural tissues from fetal and neonatal rats. *Endocrinology* **94:** 117–121.

REICHLIN, S. (1974) Regulation of somatotrophic hormone secretion. In: *Handbook of Physiology, Endocrinology*, Vol. 7, American Physiol Soc., Washington DC, pp. 405–447.

RESKO, J. A. (1970) Androgen secretion by the fetal and neonatal rhesus monkey. *Endocrinology* **87:** 680–687.

RESKO, J. A., MALLEY, A., BEGLEY, D. and HESS, D. L. (1973) Radioimmunoassay of testosterone during fetal development of the Rhesus monkey. *Endocrinology* **93:** 156–161.

REUSENS, B., KUHN, E. R. and MOET, J. J. (1979) Fetal plasma plactin levels and fetal growth in relation to maternal CB-154 treatment in the rat. *Gen. Comp. Endocr.* **39:** 118–120.

REVESZ, C. and CHAPPEL, C. I. (1966) Biological activity of medrogestone: a new orally active progestin. *J. Reprod. Fert.* **12:** 473–487.

REVESZ, C., CHAPPEL, C. I. and GAUDRY, R. (1960) Masculinization of female fetuses in the rat by progestational compounds. *Endocrinology* **66:** 140–144.

REYES, F. I., BORODITSKY, R. S., WINTER, J. S. O. and FAIMAN, C. (1974) Studies on human sexual development. II. Fetal and maternal serum gonadotropin and sex steroid concentrations. *J. Clin. Endocr. Metab.* **38:** 612–617.

RIEUTORT, M. (1974) Pituitary content and plasma levels of growth hormone in foetal and weanling rats. *J. Endocr.* **60:** 261–268.

RIGAUDIERE, N. (1981) Quantification of endogenous testosterone and dihydrotestosterone in fetal tissues from male guinea-pig. *Steroids* **38:** 185–194.

RODESCH, F., CAMUS, M., ERMANS, A. M., DODION, J. and DELANGE, F. (1976) Adverse effect of amniofetography on fetal thyroid function. *Am. J. Obstet. Gynec.* **126:** 723–726.

ROSENBERG, U. B., SCHRÖDER, C., PREISS, A., LIENLIN, A., CÔTE, S., RIEDE, E. and JÄCKLE, H. (1986) Structural homology of the product of the *Drosophila Krüppel* gene with *Xenopus* transcription factor IIIA. *Nature* **319:** 336–339.

ROSENFELD, D. I. and BRONSON, R. A. (1980) Reproductive problems in the DES-exposed female. *Obstet. Gynecol.* **55:** 453–456.

ROTHMAN, K. J. and LIESS, J. (1976) Gender of offspring after oral contraceptive use. *N. Engl. J. Med.* **295:** 859–861.

SAITOH, H., HIRATO, K., YANAIHARA, T. and NAKAYAMA, T. (1982) A study of 5α-reductase in human fetal brain. *Endocr. Japon* **29:** 461–467.

SALAZAR, H., MacAULAY, M. A., CHARLES, D. and PARDO, M. (1969) The human hypophysis in anencephaly. I. Ultrasturcture of the pars distalis. *Arch Pathol.* **87:** 201–211.

SANDBERG, E. C. and HEBARD, J. C. (1977) Examination of young women exposed to stilbestrol in utero. *Am. J. Obstet. Gynec.* **128:** 364–370.

SANYAL, M. K. and VILLEE, C. A. (1977) Stimulation of androgen biosynthesis in rat fetal testes *in vitro* by gonadotropins. *Biol. Reprod.* **16:** 174–181.

SARA, V. R., KING, T. L., STUART, M. C. and LAZARUS, L. (1976) Hormonal regulation of fetal brain cell proliferation: presence in serum of a trophin responsive to pituitary growth hormone stimulation. *Endocrinology* **99:** 1512–1518.

SATAW, Y., OKAMOTO, N., IDEDA, T., UENO, TY. and MIYABURA, S. (1972) Electron microscopic studies of anterior pituitaries and adrenal cortices of normal and anencephalic human fetuses. *J. Electron Microsc. (Tokyo)* **21:** 29–39.

SAUNDERS, F. J. (1967) Effects of norethynodrel combined with mestranol on the offspring when administered during pregnancy and lactation in rats. *Endocrinology* **80:** 447–452.

SCHNEIDER, G. and MULROW, P. S. (1973) Regulation of aldosterone production during pregnancy in the rat. *Endocrinology* **92:** 1208–1215.

SCHÖLER, H. F. and de WACHTER, A. M. (1961) Evaluation of androgenic properties of progestational compounds in the rat by the female foetal masculinization test. *Acta Endocr. (Copenh.)* **38:** 128–136.

SCHULTZ, F. M. and WILSON, J. D. (1974) Virilization of the Wolffian duct in the rat fetus. *Endocrinology* **94:** 979–986.

SCHWANZEL-FUKUDA, M., ROBINSON, J. A. and SILVERMAN, A. J. (1981) The fetal development of the luteinizing hormone-releasing hormone (LHRH) neuronal systems of the guinea pig brain. *Brain Res. Bull.* **7:** 293–315.

SCULLY, R. E., ROBBOY, S. J. and HEREST, A. L. (1974) Vaginal and cervical abnormalities including clear-cell adenocarcinoma related to prenatal exposure to stilbestrol. *Ann. Clin. Lab. Sci.* **4:** 222–233.

SÉTALÓ, G. and NAKANE, P. K. (1976) Functional differentiation of the fetal anterior pituitary cells in the rat. *Endocr. Exptl.* **10:** 155–166.

SHAHA, C., LIOTTA, A. S., KRIEGER, D. T. and BARDIN, C. W. (1984) The ontogeny of immunoreactive β-endorphin in fetal, neonatal, and pubertal testes from mouse and hamster. *Endocrinology* **114:** 1584–1591.

SHAPIRO, B. H., LEVINE, D. C. and ADLER, N. T. (1980) The testicular feminized rat: a naturally occurring model of androgen independent brain masculinization. *Science* **209:** 418–420.

SHEMESH, M., AILENBERG, M., MILAGUR, F., AYALON, N. and HANSEL, W. (1978) Hormone secretion by cultured bovine pre- and post-implantation gonads. *Biol. Reprod.* **19:** 761–767.

SHEPARD, T. H., ANDERSEN, H. J. and ANDERSEN, H. (1964) The human fetal thyroid. 1. its weight in relation to body weight, crown-rump length, food length and estimated gestation age. *Anat. Record* **148:** 123–128.

SHIONO, P. H., HARLAP, S., RAMCHARAN, S., BERENDES, H., GUPTA, S. and PELLEGRIN, F. (1979) Use of contraceptives prior to and after conception and exposure to other fetal hazards. *Contraception* **20:** 105–120.

SHORE, L. and SHEMESH, M. (1981) Altered steroidogenesis by the fetal bovine freemartin ovary. *J. Reprod. Fertil.* **63:** 309–314.

SIEGLER, A. M., WANG, C. F. and FRIBERG, J. (1979) Fertility of the diethylstilbestrol-exposed offspring. *Fert. Ster.* **31:** 601–607.

SIITERII, P. K. and WILSON, J. D. (1974) Testosterone formation and metabolism during male sexual differentiation in the human embryo. *J. Clin. Endocr. Metab.* **38:** 113–125.

SILER, T. M., MORGENSTERN, L. L. and GREENWOOD, F. C. (1972) The release of prolactin and other peptide hormones from human anterior pituitary tissue cultures. *Ciba Found. Symp. Lactogenic Hormones*, Wolstenholme, G. E. W. and Knight, J. (Eds), Churchill, London, pp. 206–222.

SILER-KHODR, T. M. and KHODR, G. S. (1980) Studies in human fetal endocrinology. II. LH and FSH content and concentration in the pituitary. *Obstet. Gynecol.* **56:** 176–181.

SILER-KHODR, T. M., MORGENSTERN, L. L. and GREENWOOD, F. C. (1974) Hormone synthesis and release from human fetal adenohypophyses *in vitro. J. Clin. Endocr. Metab.* **39:** 891–905.

SILER-KHODR, T. M., MORGANSTERN, L. L. and GREENWOOD, F. C. (1979) Hormone synthesis and release from human fetal adenohypophyses *in vitro. J. Clin. Endocr. Metab.* **39:** 891–899.

SILMAN, R. E., CHARD, T., LOWRY, P. J., MULLEN, P. E., SMITH, I. and YOUNG, I. M. (1977) Human fetal corticotrophin and related pituitary peptides. *J. Steroid Biochem* **8:** 553–557.

SILMAN, R. E., HOLLAND, D., CHARD, T., LOWRY, P. J., HOPE, J., REES, L. H., THOMAS, A. and NATHANIELSZ, P. (1979) Adrenocorticotrophin-related peptides in adult and foetal sheep pituitary glands. *J. Endocr.* **81:** 19–34.

SINGER, M. S. and HOCHMAN, M. (1978) Incompetent cervix in a hormone-exposed offspring. *Obstet. Gynecol.* **51:** 625–626.

SKLAR, C. A., MUELLER, P. L., GLUCKMAN, P. D., KAPLAN, S. L., RUDOLPH, A. M. and GRUMBACH, M. M. (1981) Hormone ontogeny in the ovine fetus. VII. Circulating luteinizing hormone and follicle-stimulating hormone in mid and late gestation. *Endocrinology* **108:** 874–880.

SLEBODZINSKI, A. and SREBRO, Z. (1968) The thyroid gland and the neurosecretory activity of the hypothalamus in the newborn rabbit. *J. Endocr* **42**: 193–203.

SLOB, A. K., GOY, R. W. and VAN DER WERFF TEN BOSCH, J. J. (1973) Sex differences in growth of guinea-pigs and their modification by neonatal gonadectomy and prenatally administered androgen. *J. Endocrinol* **58**: 11–19.

SLOB, A. K., OOMS, M. P. and VREEBURG, J. T. M. (1980) Prenatal and early postnatal sex differences in plasma and gonadal testosterone and plasma luteinizing hormone in female and male rats. *J. Endocr.* **87**: 81–87.

STEVENS, N. M. (1905) Studies in spermatogenesis with especial reference to the accessory chromosome. *Carnegie Inst. Report* No. 36 Washington, DC.

STILLMAN, R. J. (1982) *In utero* exposure to diethylstilbestrol: adverse effects on the reproductive tract and reproductive performance in male and female offspring. *Am. J. Obstet. Gynecol* **142**: 905–921.

STINNAKRE, M. G. (1972) Etude de l'action "paradoxale" des estrogènes sur les canaux de Wolff des foetus femelles de Rat, l'aide d'un anti-androgène l'acetate de "cyprotérone". *C. R. Hebd. Seance Acad. Sci (Paris) D* **275**: 101–103.

STINNAKRE, M. G. (1975) Period of sensitivity of rat fetal Wolffian duct to androgens. *Arch. Anat. Microsc. Morphol.* **64**: 45–59.

STOKES, H. and BODA, J. M. (1968) Immunofluorescent localization of growth hormone and prolactin in the adenohypophysis of fetal sheep. *Endocrinology* **83**: 1362–1366.

STREETER, G. L. (1951) Development horizons in human embryos. Age XI to XXIII. *Contrib. Embryol.* Carnegie Inst., Washington, DC.

STRICKLAND, D. M., SAEED, S. A., CASEY, M. L. and MITCHELL, M. D. (1983) Stimulation of prostaglandin biosynthesis by urine of the human fetus may serve as a trigger for parturition. *Science* **220**: 521–522.

SUCHOWSKY, G. R. and JUNKMANN, K. (1961) A study of the virilizing effect of progestogens on the female rat fetus. *Endocrinology* **68**: 341–349.

SULLMAN, F. G. (1956) Experiments on the mechanism of the push and pull principle. *J. Endocr. (Proc.)* **14**: XXVII–XXVIII.

SUZUKI, Y., ISHII, H. and ARAI, Y. (1983) Prenatal exposure of male mice to androgen increases neuron number in the hypogastric ganglion. *Dev. Brain Res.* **10**: 151–154.

SWAAB, D. F., VAN LEEUWEN, F. W., DOGTEROM, J. and HONNFBIER, W. J. (1977) The fetal hypothalamus and pituitary during growth and differentiation. *J. Steroid Biochem.* **8**: 545–551.

SWANSON, H. E. and VAN DER WERFF TEN BOSCH, J. J. (1964) The "early-androgen" syndrome; differences in response to prenatal and postnatal administration of various doses of testosterone propionate in female and male rats. *Acta Endocr. (Copenh.)* **47**: 37–50.

SWANSON, H. E. and VAN DER WERFF TEN BOSCH, J. J. (1965) The "early-androgen" syndrome; effects of prenatal testosterone propionate. *Acta Endocr. (Copenh.)* **50**: 379–390.

TAGUCHI, O., NISHIZUKA, Y. and TAKASUGI, N. (1977) Irreversible lesions in female reproductive tracts of mice after prenatal exposure to testosterone propionate. *Endocr. Japon* **24**: 385–391.

TAKASUGI, N., TANAKA, M. and KATO, C. (1983) Effects of continuous intravenous infusion of diethylstilbestrol into pregnant mice on fetus: testicular morphology at fetal and postnatal period. *Endocr. Japon* **30**: 35–42.

TAKETO, T. and KOIDE, S. S. (1981) *In vitro* development of testis and ovary from indifferent fetal mouse gonads. *Dev. Biol.* **84**: 61–66.

TAMURA, T., MINAGUCHI, H. and SAKAMOTO, S. (1973) Responsiveness of human fetal pituitary to hypothalamic hormones *in vitro*. *Endocr. Japon* **20**: 545–553.

TANAKA, M., IGUCHI, T. and TAKASUGI, N. (1984) Early changes in the vaginal epithelium of mice exposed prenatally to diethylstilbestrol. *IRCS Med. Sci.* **12**: 814–815.

TANOOKA, N. and GREER, M. A. (1978) Evidence that control of fetal thyrotropin secretion is independent of both fetal and maternal hypothalamus. *Endocrinology* **102**: 852–858.

TAUTZ, D., LEHMANN, R., SCHNÜRCH, H., SCHUH, R., SEIFERT, E., KIENLIN, A., JONES, K. and JÄCKLE, H. (1987) Finger protein of novel structure encoded by *hunchback*, a second member of the gap class of *Drosophila* segmentation genes. *Nature* **327**: 383–389.

THIVERIS, J. A. and CURRIE, R. W. (1980) Observations on the hypothalamohypophyseal portal vasculature in the developing human fetus. *Am. J. Anat.* **157**: 441–444.

THOMAS, A. L., JACK, P. M. B., MANNS, J. G. and NATHANIELSZ, P. W. (1975) Effect of synthetic thyrotrophin releasing hormone on thyrotrophin and prolactin concentrations in the peripheral plasma of the pregnant ewe, lamb fetus and neonatal lamb. *Biol. Neonate* **26**: 109–116.

THOMAS, K., de GASPARO, M. and HOET, J. J. (1967) Insulin levels in the umbilical vein and in the umbilical artery of newborns of normal and gestational diabetic mothers. *Diabetologia* **3**: 299–304.

THOMSETT, M. J., MARTI-HENNEBERG, C., GLUCKMAN, P. D., KAPLAN, S. L., RUDOLPH, A. M. and GRUMBACH, M. M. (1980) Hormone ontogeny in the ovine fetus. VIII. The effect of thyrotropin-releasing factor on prolactin and growth hormone release in the fetus and neonate. *Endocrinology* **106**: 1074–1078.

THORBURN, G. D. and HOPKINS, D. S. (1973) Thyroid function in the foetal lamb. In: *Foetal and Neonatal Physiology.* Comline, R. S., Cross, K. W., Dawes, G. S. and Nathanielsz, P. W. (Eds) Cambridge University Press, Cambridge, pp. 488–507.

THORELL, J. I. (1970) Plasma insulin levels in normal human foetuses. *Acta Endocr. (Copenh.)* **63**: 134–140.

THORELL, J. I., PERSSON, B. (1970) Transient stimulation of insulin release by fructose in newborn pigs. *Endocrinology* **86**: 897–898.

TRAN, D. and JOSSO, N. (1982) Localization of anti-Müllerian hormone in the rough endoplasmic reticulum of the developing bovine Sertoli cell using immunocytochemistry with a monoclonal antibody. *Endocrinology* **111**: 1562–1567.

TSENG, M. T. (1977) Effects of luteinizing hormone releasing hormone on the ultrastructure of gonadotrophs in the foetus of the rhesus monkey near term. *J. Endocr.* **74**: 369–373.

TSUKADA, Y., HEWETT, W. J., BARLOW, J. J. and PICKREN, J. W. (1972) Clear-cell adenocarcinoma ("mesonephroma") of the vagina. 3 Cases associated with maternal synthetic nonsteroid estrogen therapy. *Cancer* **29**: 1208–1214.

TYSON, J. E. and PINTO, H. (1978) Identification of the possible significance of prolactin in human reproduction. *Clin. Obstet. Gynaecol.* **5**: 411–420.

TYSON, J. E., FRIESEN, H. G. and ANDERSON, M. S. (1972) Human lactational and ovarian response to endogenous prolactin release. *Science* **117**: 897–899.

UCHIBORI, M. and KAWASHIMA, S. (1985) Stimulation of removal process growth by estradiol-17β in dissociated cells from fetal rat hypothalamus-preoptic area. *Zool. Sci.* **2**: 381–388.

UENO, S., TAKAHASHI, M., MANGANARO, T. F., RAGIN, R. C. and DONAHOE, P. K. (1989) Cellular localization of Müllerian inhibiting substance in the developing rat ovary. *Endocrinology* **124**: 1000–1006.

ULFELDER, H. (1973) Stilbestrol adenosis and adenocarcinoma. *Amer. Obstet. Gynec.* **117**: 794–800.

ULFELDER, H. (1975) Das Stilbostrol-adenosis-karzinom-syndrom. *Geburt. Frauenheil.* **35**: 329–333.

VAN DER WERFF TEN BOSCH, J. J. and GOLDFOOT, D. A. (1975) Effects of various androgens administered to pregnant guinea-pigs on their female offspring. *J. Endocr.* **64**: 35P.

VAN VLIET, G., STYNE, D. M., KAPLAN, S. L. and GRUMBACH, M. M. (1983) Hormone ontogeny in the ovine fetus. XVI. Plasma immunoreactive somatomedin C/insulin-like growth factor I in the fetal and neonatal lamb and in the pregnant ewe. *Endocrinology* **113**: 1716–1720.

VANNIER, R. and RYANAUD, J. P. (1975) Effect of estrogen plasma binding on sexual differentiation of the rat fetus. *Mol. Cell Endocr.* **3**, 323–337.

VANNIER, B. and RAYNAUD, J. P. (1980) Long-term effects of prenetal oestrogen treatment on genital morphology and reproductive function in the rat. *J. Reprod. Fertil.* **59**: 43–49.

VARMA, S. K., MURRAY, R. and STANBURY, J. B. (1978) Effect of maternal hypothyroidism and triiodothyronine on the fetus and newborn in rats. *Endocrinology* **102**: 23–30.

VAUGHAN, M. K., VAUGHAN, G. M. and O'STEEN, W. K. (1971) Pituitary adrenal pineal and renal weights in offspring of rats treated with testosterone and/or melatonin during pregnancy. *J. Endocr.* **51:** 211–212.

VERKAUF, B. S., REITER, E. D., HERNANDEZ, L. and BURNS, S. A. (1977) Virilization of mother and fetus associated with lutema of pregnancy: a case report with endocrinologic studies. *Am. J. Obstet. Gynec.* **129:** 274–280.

VEYSSIÈRE, G., JEAN, C. H. and JEAN, C. L. (1974) Evaluation quantitative de la croissance des ébauches mammaires des foetus de souris apres injection de testostèrone de dihydrotestostérone et d'acetate de cyproterone à la mère gravide. *Arch. Anat. Micr. Morph. Exp.* **63:** 63–78.

VEYSSIÈRE, G., BERGER, M., JEAN-FAUCHER, C. H., DeTURCKHEIM, M. and JEAN, C. L. (1975) Dosage radioimmunologique de la testostèrone dans le plasma, les gonades et les surrénales de foetus en fin de gestation et de nouveau-nés, chez le lapin. *Arch. Int. Physiol. Biochim.* **83:** 667–672.

VEYSSIÈRE, G., BERGER, M., JEAN-FAUCHER, C. H., DeTURCKHEIM, M. and JEAN, C. L. (1976) Levels of testosterone in the plasma, gonads, and adrenals during fetal development of the rabbit. *Endocrinology* **99:** 1263–1268.

VEYSSIÈRE, G., BERGER, M., CORRE, M., JEAN-FAUCHER, C. H., DeTURCKHEIM, M. and JEAN, C. (1979) Percentage binding of testosterone and dihydrotestosterone and unbound testosterone and dihydrotestosterone in rabbit maternal and fetal plasma during sexual organogenesis. *Steroids* **34:** 308–317.

VEYSSIÈRE, G., BERGER, M., JEAN-FAUCHER, C. H. DeTURCKHEIM, M. and JEAN, C. L. (1980a) Ontogeny of pituitary gonadotrophin hormone activity and of testicular responsiveness to gonadotrophins in foetal rabbit. *Acta Endocr. (Copenh.)* **94:** 412–418.

VEYSSIÈRE, G., CORRE, M., BERGER, M., JEAN-FAUCHER, C. W., DeTURCKHEIM, M. and JEAN C. L. (1980b) Sexual organogenesis and circulating androgens in the rabbit fetus; study after active immunization of mothers against testosterone. *Arch. Anat. Micr. Morphol. Exp.* **69:** 17–28.

VEYSSIÈRE, G., BERGER, M., JEAN-FAUCHER, C. H., DeTURCKHEIM, M. and JEAN, C. L. (1982a) Testosterone and dihydrotestosterone in sexual ducts and genital tubercle of rabbit fetuses during sexual organogenesis: effects of fetal decapitation. *J. Steroid Biochem.* **17:** 149–154.

VEYSSIÈRE, G., BERGER, M., JEAN-FAUCHER, C. H., DeTURCKHEIM, M. and JEAN, C. L. (1982b) Pituitary and plasma levels of luteinizing hormone and follicle-stimulating hormone in male and female rabbit fetuses. *J. Endocr.* **92:** 381–387.

VIGIER, B., LEGEAI, L., PICARD, J.-Y. and JOSSO, N. (1982) A sensitive radioimmunoassay for bovine anti-Müllerian hormone, allowing its detection in male and freemartin fetal serum. *Endocrinology* **111:** 1409–1411.

VILLEE, D. B. (1974) The control of androgen synthesis in human fetal testicular cells in culture. *INSERM (Paris)* **32:** 247–472.

VILLEE, D. B., ENGEL, L. L. and VILLEE, C. A. (1959) Steroidhydroxylation in human fetal adrenals. *Endocrinology* **65:** 465–472.

VILLEE, D. B., ENGEL, L. L. and VILLEE, C. A. (1959) Steroid hydroxylation in human fetal adrenals. *Endocrinology* **65:** 465–472.

VOJTÍŠKOVÁ, M. and POLÁČKOVÁ, M. (1966) An experimental model of the epigenetic mechanism of autotolerance using the H-Y antigen in mice. *Folia Biol. (Praha)* **12:** 137–140.

VOJTÍŠKOVÁ, M. and POLÁČKOVÁ, M. (1971) Association of the expression of male-specific antigen and androgenic activity. *Folia Biol. (Praha)* **17:** 273–278.

VOJTÍŠKOVÁ, M. and POLÁČKOVÁ, M. (1972) Testosterone-abolished female responsiveness to syngeneic male-skin grafts. *Folia Biol. (Praha)* **23:** 209–212.

VOM SAAL, P. S. and BRONSON, F. H. (1980) Sexual characteristics of adult female mice are correlated with their blood testosterone levels during prenatal development. *Nature* **208:** 597–599.

VOM SAAL, F. S., GRANT, W. M., McMULLEN, O. W. and LAVES, K. S. (1983) High fetal estrogen concentrations: correlation with increased adult sexual activity and decreased aggression in male mice. *Science* **220:** 1306–1309.

VORHEES, C. V., BRUNNER, R. L., McDANIEL, C. R. and BUTCHER, R. E. (1978) The relationship of gestational age to vitamin A induced postnatal dysfunction. *Teratology* **17**: 271–275.

VORHERR, H. (1973) Contraception after abortion and post partum. *Am. J. Obstet. Gynecol.* **117**: 1002–1025.

VORHERR, H., MESSER, R. H., VORHERR, U. F., JORDAN, S. W. and KORNFELD, M. (1979) Teratogenesis and carcinogenesis in rat offspring after transplacental and transmammary exposure to diethylstilbestrol. *Biochem Pharmacol* **28**: 1865–1877.

WACHTEL, S. S. (1983) *H-Y Antigen and the Biology of Sex Determination*. Grume Stratton, New York, pp. 1–302.

WALKER, B. E. (1965) Cleft palate produced in mice by human equivalent dosage with triamcinolone. *Science* **149**: 862–863.

WALKER, B. E. (1967) Induction of cleft palate in rabbits by several glucocorticoids. *Proc. Soc. Exp. Biol. Med.* **125**: 1281–1284.

WALKER, B. E. (1971) Induction of cleft palate in rats with anti inflammatory drugs. *Teratology* **4**: 39–42.

WALKER, B. E. (1980) Reproductive tract anomalies in mice after prenatal exposure to DES. *Teratology* **21**: 313–321.

WALLACE, A. L. C., NANCARROW, O. D., EVISON, B. M. and RADFORD, H. M. (1979) The effect of thyrotropin releasing hormone on pituitary and thyroid function in pre- and post-natal lambs. *Acta Endocr. (Copenh.)* **92**: 119–129.

WALSH, S. W., NORMA., R. L. and NOVY, M. J. (1979) *In utero* regulation of rhesus monkey fetal adrenals: effects of dexamethasone, adrenocorticotropin, thyrotropin-releasing hormone, prolactin, human chorionic gonadotropin, and α-melanocyte-stimulating hormone on fetal and maternal plasma steroids. *Endocrinology* **104**: 1805–1813.

WARREN, D. W., HALTMEYER, G. C. and EIK-NES, K. B. (1973) Testosterone in the fetal rat testis. *Biol. Reprod.* **8**: 560–565.

WARREN, D. W., HALTMEYER, G. C. and EIK-NES, K. B. (1975) The effect of gonadotropins on the fetal and neonatal rat testis. *Endocrinology* **96**: 1226–1229.

WARTENBERG, H. (1978) Human testicular development and the role of the mesonephros in the origin of a dual Sertoli cell system. *Andrologia* **10**: 1–21.

WARTENBERG, H. (1985) Origin of gonadal blastemal cells in mammalian gonadogenesis. *Arch. d'Anat. Micr. Morph. Expt.* **74**: 60–63.

WATANABE, Y. G. and DAIKOKU, S. (1979) An immunohistochemical study on the cytogenesis of adenohypophysial cells in fetal rats. *Dev. Biol.* **68**: 557–567.

WEISZ, J. and WARD, I. L. (1980) Plasma testosterone and progesterone titers of pregnant rats, their male and female fetuses, and neonatal offspring. *Endocrinology* **106**: 306–316.

WELSHONS, W. J. and RUSSELL, L. B. (1959) The Y-chromosome as the bearer of male determining factors in the mouse. *Proc. Natl. Acad. Sci. (USA)* **45**: 560–566.

WENIGER, J. P. and ZEIS, A. (1974) Sur la sensibilité de testicule embryonnaire de souris à l'hormone lutéinisante, LH. *C. R. Acad. Sci. (Paris)* **279**: 1629–1631.

WENIGER, J. P. and ZEIS, A. (1975) Effet des gonadotropines sur la synthèse d'androgenes par les testicules embryonnaires de souris et de rat. *Arch. Anat. Micr. Morph. Exp.* **64**: 61–66.

WEZEMAN, F. H. and REYNOLDS, W. A. (1971) Stability of fetal calcium levels and bone metabolism after maternal administration of thyrocalcitonin. *Endocrinology* **89**: 445–452.

WHALEN, R. E., PECK, C. K. and LOPICCOLO, J. (1966) Virilization of female rats by prenatally administered progestin. *Endocrinology* **78**: 965–970.

WHITEHEAD, E. D. and LEITER, E. (1981) Genital abnormalities and abnormal somen analyses in male patients exposed to diethylstilbestrol *in utero*. *J. Urol.* **125**: 47–50.

WIDE, L. and HOBSON, B. (1974) Relationship between the sex of the foetus and the amount of human chorionic gonadotrophin in placentae from the 10th to the 20th week of pregnancy. *J. Endocr.* **61**: 75–81.

WILKINS, I. (1960) Masculinization of female fetus due to use of orally given progestins. *J. Am. Med. Assoc.* **172:** 1028–1032.

WILKINS, L., JONES, W., HOLMAN, G. and STEMPFEL, S. (1958) Masculinization of the female fetus associated with administration of oral and intramuscular progestins during gestation: Non-adrenal female pseudohermaphroditism. *J. Clin. Endocr. Metab.* **18:** 559–585.

WILLES, R. F., BODA, J. M. and MANNS, J. G. (1969a) Insulin secretion by the ovine fetus in utero. *Endocrinology* **84:** 520–527.

WILLES, R. F., BODA, J. M. and STOKES, H. (1969b) Cytological localization of insulin and insulin concentration in the fetal ovine pancreas. *Endocrinology* **84:** 671–675.

WILSON, J. D. (1973) Testosterone uptake by the urogenital tract of the rabbit embryo. *Endocrinology* **92:** 1192–1199.

WILSON, J. D. (1978) Sexual differentiation. *Ann. Rev. Physiol.* **40:** 279–306.

WILSON, J. D. and LASNITZKI, I. (1971) Dihydrotestosterone formation in fetal tissues of the rabbit and rat. *Endocrinology* **89:** 659–668.

WILSON, J. D., GRIFFIN, J. E., GEORGE, F. W. and LESHIN, M. (1981) The role of gonadal steroids in sexual differentiation. *Recent Prog. Horm. Res.* **37:** 1–39.

WINTER, J. S. (1982) Hypothalamic-pituitary function in the fetus and infant. *J. Clin. Endocr. Metab.* **11:** 41–48.

WINTERS, A. J., ESKAY, R. L. and PORTER, J. C. (1974a) Concentration and distribution of TRH and LH–RH in the human fetal brain. *J. Clin. Endocr. Metab.* **39:** 960–963.

WINTERS, A. J., OLIVER, G., COLSTON, C., MacDONALD, P. C. and PORTER, J. C. (1974b) Plasma ACTH levels in the human fetus and neonate as related to age and parturition. *J. Clin. Endocr. Metab.* **39:** 269–273.

WINTOUR, E. M., BROWN, E. H., DENTON, D. A., HARDY, K. J., McDOUGALL, J. G., ODDIE C. J. and WHIPP, G. T. (1975) The ontogeny and regulation of corticosteroid secretion by the ovine foetal adrenal. *In vitro* and *in vivo* studies. *Acta Endocr. (Copenh.)* **79:** 301–316.

WITSCHI, E. (1948) Migrations of the germ cells of human embryos from the yolk-sac to the primitive gonadal folds. *Contr. Embryol.* Carnegie Inst., Washington, **32:** 67–80.

WOODBURY, D. M. and VORNADAKIS, A. (1966) Effects of steroids on the central nervous system. In: *Methods in Hormone Research*, Dorfman, R. I. (Ed.), Academic Press, New York, Vol. V, pp. 1–57.

YAFFEE, S. (1973) Stilbestrol and adenocarcinoma of the vagina. *Pediat.* **51:** 297–298.

YASUDA, Y., KIHARA, T. and NISHIMURA, H. (1977) Effect of prenatal treatment with ethinyl estradiol on the mouse uterus and ovary. *Am. J. Obstet. Gynecol.* **127:** 832–836.

YASUDA, Y., KIHARA, T., TANIMURA, T. and NISHIMURA, H. (1985) Gonadal dysgenesis induced by prenatal exposure to ethynyl estradiol in mice. *Teratology* **32:** 219–228.

YALOM, I. D., GREEN, R. and FISK, N. (1973) Prenatal exposure to female hormones: effect on psychosexual development in boys. *Arch. Gen. Psychiat.* **28:** 554–561.

YOUNG, W. C., GOY, R. W. and PHOENIX, C. H. (1964) Hormones and sexual behavior. *Science* **143:** 212–218.

ZAAIJER, J. J. P., deGOEIJ, A. F. P. M. and ORTIZ, E. (1985) Müllerian duct regression in the fetal male guinea pig linked to early pituitary FSH production. *Current Trends in Comparative Endocrinology*, Lofts, B. and Holmes, W. N. (Eds), Hong Kong Univ Press, pp. 605–609.

ZENZES, M. T., MULLER, U., ASCHMONEIT, I. and WOLF, U. (1978) Studies on H-Y antigen in different cell fractions of the testis during pubescence. Immature germ cells are H-Y antigen negative. *Human Genet.* **45:** 297–303.

Index